Islands of Love,
Islands of Risk

Islands of Love, Islands of Risk

CULTURE AND HIV IN THE TROBRIANDS

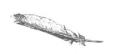

KATHERINE LEPANI

VANDERBILT UNIVERSITY PRESS

Nashville

© 2012 by Vanderbilt University Press
Nashville, Tennessee 37235
All rights reserved
First printing 2012

This book is the recipient of the Norman L. and Roselea J. Goldberg Prize
from Vanderbilt University Press for the best project in the area of medicine.

This book is printed on acid-free paper.
Manufactured in the United States of America

Library of Congress Cataloging-in-Publication Data on file

LC control number 2012028971

ISBN 978-0-8265-1874-3 (cloth)
ISBN 978-0-8265-1875-0 (paperback)
ISBN 978-0-8265-1876-7 (e-book)

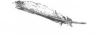

DEDICATED TO THE MEMORY OF

YAWAGU SARAH WATSON

1929–2010

<hr />

Contents

Acknowledgments

My heartfelt gratitude goes to the people of the Trobriand Islands, whose contribution to this research is beyond measure. I hold deep appreciation and respect for all the men, women, and young people who were willing to sit down with me and talk openly about their culture and their lives in a spirit of trust and collective concern. *Agutoki saina kwaiveka*. Sincere appreciation is extended to the Trobriand Paramount Chief, Guyau Pulayasi Daniel, for his endorsement of the project. I am indebted to my research collaborators, Diana Siyotama Lepani, Florence Mokolava, and Ethel Jacob, for their commitment to the project, their invaluable advice and untiring support, and their lasting friendship. Our teamwork was strengthened by the memory of Asi Toyola, whose dedicated career as a nurse touched the lives of many people in Papua New Guinea (PNG). I also acknowledge Lisepa Tony and Nelson Toposona for helping to facilitate discussions, and the women's fellowship groups, church deacons, and ward councillors who received me with the greatest hospitality when I visited their villages. The residents of Orabesi village and the women of OKO Women's Fellowship always made me feel right at home, and I greatly value their kindness and generosity.

I wish to acknowledge the government authorities in the Trobriands for their logistical help and support, including Thomas Pilai, district administrator; Haydon Abraham, area manager; and Sergeant George Bayagau, Royal PNG Police Constabulary. I am appreciative of the help provided by Tirah Elliot, district health manager, and the staff of Losuia District Health Center, who graciously accommodated my frequent visits and requests for information. The principal and staff at Kiriwina High School were also very helpful, and I appreciate their support and interest in the project. I am particularly indebted to the kindness of Sarah and Rodney Clark and the staff at Konki, who provided ongoing practical support for my communication and transportation requirements as well as many friendly conversations. I also thank the late Sir Dennis Young and the staff at Digogwa and Kiriwina Lodge for providing practical assistance and transportation, often on short notice.

It has been a privilege to be associated with the many dedicated individuals and organizations involved in the national response to HIV in Papua New Guinea, and I appreciate the support and encouragement of them all. I hold immense respect for the late Carol Jenkins, whose extensive knowledge of PNG and HIV provided critical vision from the beginning of the national response and whose indomitable spirit will always be a source of inspiration. I also pay tribute to the late Sue Crockett, who will be remembered by many friends and colleagues for her vital contribution in paving the foundation for the national response. Sincere thanks are extended to the founding director of the National AIDS Council Secretariat, Dr. Clement Malau, and subsequent directors, secretariat staff, and team members of the National HIV/AIDS Support Project. I am grateful to the PNG National AIDS Council Research Advisory Committee for a grant to support my fieldwork in 2003. At the provincial level, I wish to acknowledge the members of the Milne Bay Provincial Government Research Committee; Dr. Festus Pawa, provincial health manager; Dr. Noel Yaubihi, chair of the Milne Bay Provincial AIDS Committee; Stephen Nesai, manager of the Provincial Management Information System; Lois Elaine Bate, statistician; and Lester Bisibisera, provincial disease control officer.

Special thanks to my wonderful group of women friends in Port Moresby, who manage to hold things together with remarkable resilience, dignity, and finesse. In particular, I am grateful to Lady Roslyn Morauta for her ongoing support and friendship throughout this long process, and I wish to acknowledge her important leadership in PNG's national response to HIV.

I appreciate the institutional support of the Australian National University (ANU) and feel fortunate to have my academic home in such an excellent collegial environment. I am thankful for the ANU International Postgraduate Research Scholarship and financial assistance for fieldwork from the former Research School of Pacific and Asian Studies. I thank my program advisers, Christine Helliwell and Mark Mosko, and ANU colleagues, past and present, for their critical intellectual support and friendship, in particular Sue Andrews, Greg Dvorak, Richard Eves, Vicki Luker, Doreen Montag, Christine Phillips, Elizabeth Reid, Bill Standish, Frances Steel, Christine Stewart, Jack Taylor, and Katerina Teaiwa. I am especially grateful to John Ballard for his resolute encouragement at every stage and his meticulous reading of my work. I also wish to thank Reverend Ralph Lawton for his generous counsel on Kiriwina language.

My deepest respect and gratitude are reserved for Professor Margaret Jolly, who has been a stellar mentor and supervisor. Her consummate knowledge, academic integrity, and empathic understanding have closely guided me from the beginning, and she will always be a beacon of inspiration. I am grateful for her ongoing support toward the fruition of this project and the exceptional opportunity to enhance my research on gender, sexuality, and personhood as a member of her Australian Research Council Laureate Fellowship Project.

I would also like to acknowledge other academic mentors and colleagues whose guidance and friendship have been immensely important along the way, including Peter Aggleton, Warwick Anderson, Holly Buchanan, Leslie Butt, Linus Digim'Rina, Lawrence Hammar, Gilbert Herdt, Shirley Lindenbaum, Martha Macintyre, Kirin Narayan, Will Parks, and Jane Thomason. Special thanks to Ann Herring and Alan Swedlund for the opportunity to participate in the Wenner-Gren Foundation Symposium on Plagues in 2007.

I am grateful to my editor, Michael Ames, for his enthusiastic interest and astute guidance in producing the final manuscript. I take this opportunity to also acknowledge my anonymous reviewers for their critical acumen and comprehensive responses. Special thanks to Holly Wardlow, Robert Foster, and Lynn Morgan for their timely and candid advice on publishing and for pointing me in the direction of Vanderbilt University Press.

This book reflects the love and support of all my family, far-flung and close, in the United States, Australia, and Papua New Guinea. I express enduring gratitude to my parents, Joyce and Wallace Kennedy, for sustaining me with oceans of love and their engaged interest in my work. Their shared passion for reading and their gifts as writers have long nurtured me. My siblings, Ellen Michel and John Kennedy, and their spouses and children have been a source of great support from afar. Special thanks to my sister and her family for lovingly caring for my daughter, Veitania, for six months during my fieldwork.

I am forever grateful to Charles, my husband, for his steadfast faith in my endeavor. He is my sharpest critic, offering invaluable insights and knowledge with humor and goodwill. This book is a reciprocal gift of love. I thank our children, Andrew, Nathaniel, and Veitania, for giving me purpose and supporting me in untold ways. Andrew and my dear daughter-in-law, Susanna, and their children, Thierry, Thealani, and Tyemani, keep us connected to our home in PNG, and my beloved grandchildren give me more joy than ever I could have imagined. Andrew's own participation in the national response to HIV in Papua New Guinea fills me with great pride. Nathaniel lightened my endeavor by helping me to stay focused and providing support when I needed it most. Veitania has been my anchor from the beginning. She grew up during the process but possessed maturity and confidence beyond her years when she embarked on her own journey, traveling overseas by herself to live with her aunt, uncle, and cousins in Indiana after living for three months with her Bubu Sarah and me in the Trobriands.

Finally, I wish to express special appreciation to all my *vevai* in the Trobriands, including those who have sadly departed, for giving me the gift of belonging. My ultimate respect and gratitude is saved for the loving memory of my mother-in-law, the late Sarah Watson, and her immeasurable generosity, graciousness, and dignity of spirit.

Author's Notes

Terminology

The language of HIV comprises a contested and inconsistent terminology, which changes as the collective experience with the global pandemic evolves. The use of the terms "HIV" and "AIDS" has undergone several revisions since the virus and syndrome were first defined in the early 1980s, and still there is no consensus on the most appropriate terminology to describe the global phenomena. In 2006, UNAIDS issued Editors' Notes about the use of the terms, with preference given to "HIV" to name the epidemic and references to "AIDS" limited to describing the effects of the virus on the human immune system in diagnosed cases. UNAIDS reissued these terminology guidelines in March 2007 (see UNAIDS 2007). The changing terminology has been apparent at different times and in different ways in the various contexts where I have worked—academia, development agencies, the Papua New Guinea (PNG) national policy and program response, and community awareness activities in the Trobriands. When I first became involved in the national response in PNG in the mid-1990s, "HIV/AIDS" was consistently used to refer to the epidemic. The UNAIDS guidelines now discourage the use of the slash, as well as reference to "HIV and AIDS," because of concern that it suggests two distinct epidemics. In the book, I use "HIV" primarily in reference to the viral infection, and I limit the use of "AIDS" to how the phenomenon has been constructed and represented in discourse. Occasionally, I use both words together with the conjunction "and" to reflect their discursive representation and to acknowledge them as relational terms. When I use the slash, it reflects the context of usage that I am describing.

Research Participants' Names and Statements

Throughout the book, I use pseudonyms for individual speakers, both to protect the identity of research participants and because at times I was unable to record the names of all participants in large group discussions. Exceptions to this rule are when I introduce people by both their first names and surnames, including my research collaborators and individuals interviewed in their professional or leadership roles. I present quoted statements from interviews and group discussions in English. If the statements were spoken in Kiriwina, I indicate in the reference that they were translated into English.

Prologue

Wosituma

Inade
kwaumego m'bigo biga Tuma
nakapo duwayago
Inagwe
kwaumego m'bigo biga Tuma
nakapo duwayago

Song for Tuma

My mother [my ancestral maternal source]
Bring me your word, your wisdom, from Tuma
For me to quench my parched throat, my yearning voice
My mother [*beseechingly*]
Bring me your word, your wisdom, from Tuma
For me to quench my parched throat, my yearning voice
(*Repeated three times before break in movement*)

On the Losuia Primary School oval, the children solemnly make their entrance, one behind the other in close succession, from tallest to shortest, oldest to youngest—twenty young bodies resplendent in traditional finery. They position themselves in an open-ended circle that spirals outward, surrounding a cluster of adult men and women—teachers, fathers, mothers, aunts and uncles—who are the singers, drummers, and sponsors, or *kepou*, for the performance event. Men holding the small *katuneniya* drums beat a rolling crescendo with their fingertips to signal the commencement of the dance, hushing the throng of admiring spectators. The sharp taut beat of the larger *kaisosau* drums breaks through with a steady rhythm as the high-pitched melodic chant of *Wosituma* rises from the center. Pandanus streamers fluttering in uplifted hands, the young dancers begin an undulating orbit around the *kepou*. Metered steps lift up, swing forward, and alight firmly on the ground, shifting slightly to the left, to the right. The movement resonates with the clink and chime of shell armbands and necklaces and the swish of banana-fiber skirts. The pungent perfume of *vinavana* and *kwebila* leaves, tucked in the dancers' armbands, wafts into the crowd with each step. The dancers' entreating eyes follow the line of their outstretched arms and beyond the *bisila* streamers in their hands, searching toward the horizon and Tuma, the island of the spirits.

The date is 9 December 2003. The Oiabia Elementary School children, aged five to seven years, are dancing *wosimwaya* to honor their older siblings and friends on the occasion of the Losuia Primary School end-of-year closing ceremony and grade 8 graduation. Earlier in the morning, there was a bustle of excitement and pride as the children's *tabusia*, or fathers' sisters, prepared them for the dance. The women dressed the boys and girls in *doba*, brightly colored banana- and pandanus-fiber skirts tied around the hips; *doridori*, belts woven from gold and black orchid fiber tied at the waist; and *kapikapi*, headbands with crests made from bits of colored paper cut into ornate diamond and circle shapes. The women rubbed them with coconut oil, sprinkled their chests with the fine golden confetti leaves of the *liga* tree, and whispered beauty magic into their necks. They painted intricate black, white, and red designs on the young faces, and black bands and white dots on their legs. They adorned the boys with halos of white cockatoo plumage, and both girls and boys with sweet-smelling floral garlands, the spicy *vinavana* and *kwebila* leaves, and strings of betel nut crisscrossing their shoulders. Finally, the children's *tabusia* bestowed on them the carriage of shell valuables, or *veguwa*, the armbands and necklaces symbolizing the rank and renown of their fathers' matrilineages.

Wosimwaya is a genre of traditional Trobriand dance, or *kaiwosi*, performed to mark occasions of communal ceremony and celebration—the annual yam harvests, school graduations, dedications of new church buildings, interisland visitations, and cultural festivals.[1] Referred to in English as "circle dance" to describe the rotation of bodies around the central *kepou*, the choreography moves in a spiral, not a closed circle. The spiral is a quintessential Trobriand aesthetic form—used abundantly in carvings, etchings, and facial decorations as well as choreographed movement—which evokes notions of social process and the passage of time. After three rounds of the stanza, there is a suspended pause when the dancers assume a holding pattern, moving only their right foot up and down the side of their left leg, until the *kepou* resumes the drumming and chanting for another three rounds. The vibrancy of *midimidi*, the fluttering motion of the *bisila* streamers, is the distinctive feature of the dance, demonstrating impetus and vitality. Not an exuberant performance event, the dance embodies a transcendent serenity that channels youthful energy into an expression of ancestral wisdom. *Wosimwaya* illustrates how the "crafting of moving bodies into a dance reflects a theoretical stance toward identity in all its register" (Foster, ed. 1996:xiii). A reverential celebration of matrilineal identity, the cyclical movement of the dance conveys the potential for regeneration, charting future pathways by reconnecting with the past.

On this community occasion, the solemnity of the dance offsets the festive atmosphere that fills the school grounds, teeming with activity since early morning when hundreds of people began arriving for the event. Family groups have settled on mats under the rain trees that line the oval, the women tending cooking fires and preparing food for the students. Others sit under the shade of umbrellas and sell packets of chips, lollipops, balloons, baked scones, and betel nut. Tarpaulins bedecked with hibiscus and frangipani flowers, pandanus streamers, and balloons provide shade from the glaring afternoon sun for the students and teachers. The official guests and head teachers sit on plastic chairs on the timber dais, erected close to the flagpole in front of the classrooms and framed by coconut fronds, flowers, and huge bunches of betel nut. I have been invited to take a seat in the shade along with the teachers and school committee members, next to the table that holds the graduation certificates and awards.

The formal program commences with the fifty grade 8 graduates marching impassively in alphabetical order to take their seats on rows of benches adjacent to the dais. Uniformly clad in black and white clothes prepared especially for the occasion, the students appear stifled amid the swarming color and activity of the crowd. The assorted black trousers and skirts, white shirts and blouses, and occasional pair of heavy black dress shoes have been borrowed from older siblings, bought at the secondhand clothes shop, or sent by relatives residing in urban centers. Some students' fathers or uncles have made the two-day boat trip to Alotau to purchase the items new from the large trade stores in the provincial capital.

The monochrome appearance of the young graduates sharply contrasts with the festive attire they wore for the sports carnival several months earlier. Then the grade 8 students arrived at school in their Trobriand finery, their bodies shimmering with coconut oil and *liga* leaves, shell necklaces and armbands chiming, and bright red skirts swishing with each step. To the applause of an appreciative crowd, they paraded around the oval in their four sports "houses," each the namesake of a founding Methodist missionary, before changing into shorts and T-shirts for the athletic events. The black and white clothing of the graduation ceremony contrasts as well with that worn for the weeklong grade 8 exams during the previous month, when the students dressed in brightly colored clothes sewn by grandmothers and other female relatives, a brand-new dress or shirt for each day. Then, too, relatives arrived from distant villages laden with garden produce to cook for the students throughout the week. The provision of new clothes and cooked food and the embodied presence of family and relatives were significant features of the occasion, sustaining the students throughout the exams. In a manner similar to preparing young bodies for *wosimwaya*, the dedicated investments in the students' scholarly performance registered collective identity and belonging. One father explained, "We do it this way to show our children they are part of us and we are part of them."

The cultural ethos of identity and belonging has deep resonance in the Trobriand Islands, a group of low-lying coral atolls in the Solomon Sea off the east coast of mainland Papua New Guinea (PNG) with a population of approximately thirty thousand people (see Map 1). Trobriand social organization combines a matrilineal kinship system, a hereditary chieftainship that passes from a male chief to his sister's son, and a complex system of reciprocal exchange underpinned by a subsistence economy of yam gardening and fishing. Every Trobriand person belongs to one of four *kumila*, or ranked exogamous matrilineal clans, known as Malasi, Lukuba, Lukwasisiga, and Lukulabuta. *Kumila* consist of numerous subclans or lineages, called *dala*, which are the main units of social identity and economic exchange (Malinowski 1929:417; Weiner 1976:51). Together, *kumila* and *dala* identity constitute the primary substance of personhood, which transcends corporeal

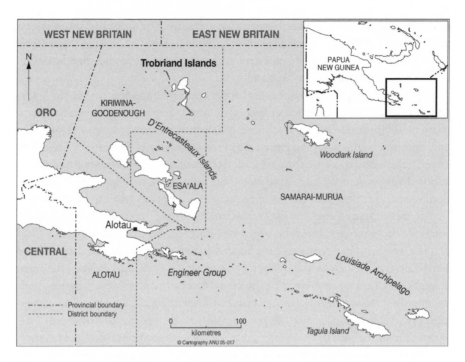

MAP 1. • Trobriand Islands, Kiriwina-Goodenough District, Milne Bay Province, Papua New Guinea. Courtesy of Cartographic-GIS Services, The Australian National University.

life at death and regenerates at conception through matrilineal ancestral spirits, or *baloma*, who reside on the far northwest island of Tuma.

The Trobriand group of islands are part of Kiriwina-Goodenough District in Milne Bay Province, one of nineteen provinces in the independent Pacific Island country of Papua New Guinea. The district is represented in PNG's national parliament by an elected member, and it also has an elected local government council. There are thirty-three administrative wards in the Trobriands and ninety-two *valu*, or villages, comprising small hamlets or residential clusters based on subclan groupings. Village populations range in size from 150 to 1,000, with four villages having approximately 1,000 inhabitants each.[2] The majority of Trobrianders live on the main island of Kiriwina, where the district headquarters of Losuia is located. The population of Losuia is about 600 people, mainly government employees and their families, many of whom are from the Trobriands. The township comprises two main roads that meet at an intersection at the district government offices down by the public market and wharf on the southern lagoon side of Kiriwina. Also located in Losuia are the district health center, the village birth attendants center, Kiriwina High School, and the islands' three trade stores that sell imported food products and manufactured goods.

For more than 150 years, Trobriand society has mediated and absorbed the Western influences of colonization, Christianity, and the cash economy with remarkable resilience. The cultivation of yams for exchange continues to provide the foundation of the Trobriand economy, with yams being "the symbol *par excellence* of the reproductiveness of social relations" (Weiner 1979:333). The distribution of yams through extensive exchange networks reinforces intergenerational and interclan relations between fathers and sons, fathers and daughters, and brothers and their sisters' spouses (Weiner 1976, 1979). Yam exchanges underpin the large-scale mortuary exchange feasts, called *sagali*, which take place immediately after a death and then again to lift the mourning period, which formally lasts between six and twelve months. Constituting the basis for the reproduction of social relations and the regeneration of matrilineal identity, the work of *sagali* compels people to invest *dala* resources in social and economic relationships with non-kin (Weiner 1976, 1980b).

The key role performed by Trobriand women in *sagali* exemplifies their strong social and economic position. Women manufacture *doba*, small bundles of dried banana leaves that are accumulated by the thousands to use as the currency for *sagali* distributions. *Doba* also refers to the banana- and pandanus-fiber skirts worn by girls and women and by male dancers; the skirts are used as well for *sagali* distributions. Cotton fabric, called *karekwa* after the English "calico," has been incorporated into *sagali* over the last several decades and is now regarded as an essential exchange valuable. Purchased by the bolt or acquired through exchange, the fabric is cut into two-meter lengths to augment *doba* transactions. Through *sagali* distributions of *doba*, clan members of the deceased acknowledge and compensate people of different clans who have maintained important social relations with the deceased throughout their lifetime. Also acknowledged and compensated are the people who have taken an active part in mourning—those who carried the dead body, cried over it, and buried it; those who observed various taboos during the extended mourning period; and those who brought food for the mourners.[3]

Internal networks of exchange in the Trobriands link to wider spheres of interaction in the island region known ethnographically as the Massim. Most notable is the renowned Kula trade ring that has connected the widely dispersed Massim island groups for over two thousand years through the circulation of shell necklaces and armbands between exchange partners (see Campbell 2002; Kuehling 2005; Leach and Leach, eds. 1983; Malinowski 1922). Maritime travel by motorized dinghies, small boats, and outrigger canoes is frequent between the Trobriands and other Milne Bay islands, for engaging in Kula transactions, trading betel nut, pigs, and clay pots, and participating in regional church, sports, and educational activities. Dinghies and canoes are important modes of transport for linking coastal villages and the outer islands in the Trobriand group and are used extensively for fishing. Small commercial vessels and barges carrying trade-store goods arrive at Losuia wharf on a regular basis and provide passenger services for travel to other islands throughout the province and to the mainland, where the provincial capital is located. Cruise liners bring groups of tourists to the Trobriands for short visits several times a year, and the occasional yacht anchors off Kaibola on the north shore or at Boli Point, west of the lagoon.

The two airstrips on Kiriwina were built during World War II. One ceased use a long time ago, but the overgrown site is a favorite gathering place for young people. The other airstrip is used by a commercial air service, which in 2003 operated flights twice a week between Kiriwina, Alotau, and Port Moresby, the national capital of Papua New Guinea. The considerable movement of people and goods between the Trobriands and urban centers is indicative of the highly mobile social landscape in contemporary PNG, as people pursue livelihood strategies and new opportunities and maintain extensive social relations and exchange networks. Cargo arriving with passengers at Losuia airport typically includes purchased goods not readily available on the island, including bolts of fabric for *sagali*. Cargo leaving the island comprises garden produce as well as *sagali* exchange items—fiber skirts, clay pots, and *kuvi*, long ceremonial yams—destined for relatives living in urban centers.

With limited wage employment opportunities in the Trobriands, remittances sent by relatives who work elsewhere in PNG or overseas are a primary source of cash income for villagers. Many families collect *bêche de mer*, or sea cucumber, which they boil and smoke to sell by the kilo to local agents. The average gross annual income from *beche de mer* sales, during the six months of the year when harvesting is permitted, is estimated to be close to one million kina.[4] Trobriand artisans are well known for their intricately carved wooden bowls and other carvings, which they produce for sale to provide an important source of cash income. Many women earn small incomes from selling woven baskets and mats. Betel nut consumption in the Trobriands is robust, and roadside sellers conduct a brisk trade to keep up with demand. Garden produce and fish are also sold at the public market at Losuia wharf. Cash income is primarily used to purchase basic household items and food products from the local trade stores. School fees are the single largest annual expense for families to meet. In 2003, fees were K40 per year for elementary school, K100 for primary school, and K800 for high-school boarding students.

The church has a central presence in Trobriand villages and provides an important organizational framework for numerous community endeavors. The majority of Trobriand villages are member congregations of the United Methodist Church. Several villages are solely or predominantly Catholic, while two villages are Seventh-Day Adventist. Over the last two decades, Pentecostalism has been introduced in some villages by Trobrianders returning home from urban centers, but the initial popularity of evangelical forms of worship has not had a lasting appeal for most people. Christianity has syncretized with Trobriand cosmology, including beliefs about the supernatural powers of witchcraft and sorcery. While the church holds a moral authority in the lives of the people, Christian doctrine has not suppressed customary practices or supplanted cultural ideals of sexuality, nor has it generated a repressive attitude to sexuality (Ketobwau 1994:16).

Losuia Primary School is located on the old Methodist mission station at Oiabia, a ten-minute walk from Losuia. Established in 1956 by resident Australian missionaries, Losuia Primary became a government community school in 1981, six years after PNG gained independence from Australia. With an enrolment of over 300 students in grades 3 to 8, and almost equal numbers of boys and girls, it is the largest primary school in the Trobriands, serving Losuia government station and six surrounding villages. It was the first school in the Trobriands to undertake the national education reforms and become a "top-up" primary school, transferring lower primary education to the newly established elementary schools in each village community and adding grades 7 and 8. The school feeds into Kiriwina High School, the government boarding and day school for grades 9 and 10, which draws its enrolment of approximately 150 students, who qualify through examinations, from the primary schools throughout the district.

When the grade 8 graduates were assembled on the benches, the master of ceremonies stepped up to the microphone, powered by a portable diesel generator, and welcomed the gathering of friends and relatives. He called on the pastor of the Oiabia United Church to lead the opening prayer and say a few words about the joyous occasion, and then he invited the principal of Kiriwina High School to deliver the keynote address. The theme of the principal's speech was human resources development and the need to strike a balance between traditional and modern ways of living. The principal began by reflecting on the value of yams in Trobriand society and how the knowledge of yam gardening continues to sustain each new generation. He added that Trobriand women are very important because "they produce the cash crop—our children." He then warned of the consequences of population pressure on the small islands and stressed the importance of formal education to secure the future of the Trobriands. Noting that Trobriand students consistently score poorly on English exams, he exclaimed emphatically, with a hint of reproof, "We love our Kiriwina language too much!" His concluding message was that the strength of culture provides the basis for learning new knowledge to go forward into the future.

The immediate future of the grade 8 students is already sealed. Fast-forward two weeks and large expectant crowds gather around official notices posted on the exterior walls of the trade stores and at the district administration office to scrutinize the names of students selected for next year's enrollment at Kiriwina High School. Typed out in triplicate on the school's manual typewriter, the list of names represents less than a third of the grade 8 graduates from Losuia Primary School, with selection based on examination results and a quota for all feeder schools in the district. Already resigned to the likelihood of not seeing their names on the list, some students have plans to apply for further training at various vocational centers throughout the province. Other students will travel by sea or air to live with relatives in urban centers in expectation of possible skills training or job opportunities. A few girls already have received plane tickets sent by working relatives in distant Port Moresby and will be traveling to the city to serve as live-in caregivers for newborn babies and small children in the host families. The majority of students who do not continue their formal education will settle back into village life, putting their productive energy into gardening and fishing, and enjoying the ease and freedom that are the privilege of unmarried youth.

Expectations about the unfolding future influence the way young Trobrianders carry themselves in the social landscape. A broad distinction is made between those enrolled at school and those who are fully engaged in village life. An unsettling tension exists between the disciplined demands of formal education and the freedom granted to village youth. The tension is felt particularly by parents and community leaders when balancing the complex and at times competing concerns of Trobriand ideology, Christianity, and modernity. Expectations and inevitable tensions are also borne and buffered by young people themselves. Along with clan and lineage affiliation and identity, the Trobriand social category of *tubwa*, or age group of mixed gender, provides a vital social orientation that guides members through life stages, nurturing and shaping bodies, personalities, and potential. *Tubwa* affiliation provides the framework for young people's expanding social relations, and it influences the commencement of sexual activity and the formation of sexual networks for both males and females. The Trobriand construct does not represent a group formally constituted through ritualized initiation or rites of passage, as found in many Melanesian societies (see, for example, Herdt, ed. 1992; Tuzin 1980). By contrast, *tubwa* assumes its form and vitality through the agency and activity of the cohorts themselves, largely independent of adult orchestration, except within the institutional frameworks of church and school.

Not all the grade 8 *tubwa* affiliates are sitting on the benches today in black and white graduation clothing. Several of them have not completed their primary education for various personal reasons—an illness, a death in the family, relocation to another village, or the inability to settle outstanding school fees before examinations. Two students are not with their cohort today because they were expelled by the school management committee earlier in the final term. A male student was expelled after several reprimands for smoking at school during recess. A female student was expelled for going to Losuia wharf at night when a coastal cargo vessel arrived with the monthly shipment of trade-store goods from Alotau. Because she defied warnings after a previous incident, her repeated action was viewed with serious concern by teachers and community leaders and was discussed at the weekly community meeting in her village. Without mentioning the particular student concerned, the ward councillor spoke generally about the problem of schoolgirls visiting the boats and making friends with the crew—young and older men mostly from other islands and provinces in Papua New Guinea. The possible consequences of such action were not stated outright, but the inference was clear in the proscription: "Young girls must take care to look after themselves properly. Parents must look after their girls and tell them to limit themselves to friendships in the village. Schoolgirls must put their minds on their education first and forget about friendships until their schooling is finished."

At least there were no pregnancies this year at Losuia Primary School, several teachers and health workers confided to me with relief, although there were four pregnancies at Kiriwina High School, but that was a considerable drop from 2001, when there were thirteen. The girls wear tight clothes under loose T-shirts to hide their pregnancies and stay in school as long as they can before maternity transforms their embodied social identity and they settle into the sedentary life of early motherhood in the village. If paternity is acknowledged and the relationship between the two young parents is steady, the new father's social identity is transformed as well, bringing new responsibility for cultivating yam gardens and entering into a complex web of interclan exchange relations as a young adult.

The beseeching cry to the ancestral mother tapers off and the drumbeats abruptly cease. The *kepou* members relax between rounds as the young dancers hold their positions, methodically moving their feet up and down, up and down. Several people in the crowd toss betel nut and pepper fruit to the huddle of men and women, who catch them appreciatively and bite into the hard, juicy husks while passing around small plastic containers of lime powder, which is mixed with the betel and pepper. Some of the men have their own carved lime sticks and gourds, elaborately decorated with shells and pandanus streamers. With a swift motion, they wet the sticks between their lips, rattle them majestically inside the gourds to coat them with lime, and lick them clean. The betel-nut paste turns bright red as they chew with zestful pleasure. Women step forward to adjust the skirts on some of the young dancers or rearrange skewed feathers. The spectators converse and mill about, crossing nonchalantly through the performance space.

Another round of the melodic chant starts up and the dancers resume their steady rotation. The spatial boundary between the encircling audience and the performers becomes distinct once again as the spectators move back. Suddenly a woman breaks through the crowd, sashays over to one of the taller dancers at the front of the moving line, and places a string of betel nut around his neck. The dancers continue their curvilinear movement without a break. A few more beats into the round and a second woman struts forward and removes the betel nut from the unfazed dancer. The crowd revels in delight as she scurries back, proudly clutching her prize. From another position in the audience, a third woman glides into the performance space, removes a garland of flowers from the head of a young girl in the middle of the dance line, and then places it on the head of a smaller dancer as the line rotates around. The crowd becomes livelier, shouting jovial praise for the dancers as more women step forward to remove decorations from one dancer to place them on another or to take them back to the crowd to adorn a spectator. Known as *tilewai*, these spontaneous transactions are highly valued public compliments, displaying admiration and pride for the performers and reinforcing important interclan relationships between admirer and performer (Weiner 1976:134–35). Referred to as "flattery gifts" (Malinowski 1929:297), *tilewai* create immediate obligations for the performers' clan members to reciprocate to the admirer a return gift—a woven mat or basket, a bunch of betel nut, a basket of yams. If the *tilewai* involves a performer from a chiefly clan rank, or *guyau*, then the anticipated return compliment is a pig.

The dancers are unflinching as they retain their somber demeanor amid the strident *tilewai* transactions. The flurried movements and raucous behavior of the admiring spectators syncopate the measured pace of the dance. The crowd's exuberance peaks when a woman rushes forward into the performance space, pulls the smallest child from the rear, and escorts her to the head of the line, crowning the small girl with a feather plucked from the hair of the lead dancer. A flutter of a smile breaks through the young child's serious expression, and her expansive pride is shared by all as she leads the line for the rest of the round. Celebrating youthful potential and regeneration, evoked by the smallest dancer taking the lead, *Wosituma* expressly connects the future to the present and the past.

Hold the image of the suspended pause between stanzas, the dancers motionless except for the smooth up-and-down movement of foot caressing leg. Now imagine a deadly virus moving imperceptibly through the cultural landscape and into particular bodies, creating the possibility of a future denied.

As a globalizing phenomenon, the HIV epidemic dominates and defines the times we live in, but HIV manifests itself differently in different cultural contexts. Starting with the assertion that "the way the epidemic is brought to people's attention will be the critical determinant of how they will respond to it" (Reid 1994:1; see also Mann and Tarantola 1998), I further consider how cultural knowledge is used to make sense of this novel and transforming phenomenon. Effective approaches to HIV communication require engagement with local ways of knowing and being in order to close the persistent gap between awareness about HIV and the preventive practices that minimize transmission. The key questions that guide the study are concerned with the articulations between the global language of HIV prevention, which speaks of abstinence, fidelity, and condom use, and local cultural meanings and expressions of sexuality. How do Trobrianders use information about HIV to evaluate their own sexual practice? How do they understand and mediate biomedical notions of "risk"? What are the gendered dimensions of these perspectives? What are the views and practices of Trobriand women and men regarding condom use to protect against HIV transmission and infection? How do Trobriand concepts of disease and illness correspond with biomedical constructions of the virus and the syndrome?

This book is based on ethnographic fieldwork from March to December 2003, after an earlier study from November 2000 to January 2001. My research process was structured around a series of community discussions and in-depth interviews in twenty-five villages on four islands. I collaborated closely with three Trobriand women who accompanied me on these visits, facilitating discussions and helping with language translation. I also conducted semistructured interviews with people in various professional and leadership roles, and elicited and participated in numerous informal conversations. The book draws on and is influenced by my experience as a long-term resident of Papua New Guinea, where I have been directly involved in the national response to the HIV epidemic since the mid-1990s. My intimate relational ties and social connections to the Trobriands as wife, in-law, mother, and grandmother for a period that spans thirty-five years, albeit residing primarily in Port Moresby, ground this anthropological study and my position as a social researcher.

The choreography of *wosimwaya* evokes the core theme of the book. Its performance is a metaphor for social bodies in motion, spiraling toward potential futures by retracing previous steps, embodying the regenerative element of social process and knowledge production in the face of uncertainty and change. The chanted appeal to ancient maternal wisdom is part of a repertoire of deep Trobriand cultural knowledge transferred and reinterpreted from generation to generation through performance. The cyclical form of the dance, shaped as a spiral, symbolizes the emergent and transformative capacity of cultural knowledge through space, time, and social interaction. The dance highlights the importance of the physical body as a "site of meaning-making" and a "tangible and substantial category of cultural experience" (Foster, ed. 1996:xi). Performance highlights how bodily knowledge and experience interact with cultural ideology, and how capacity for reflective awareness of the self is formed in relation to others. Global representations of HIV and AIDS perforce engage with local notions of the sexed and gendered body; communication on HIV prevention appeals to the embodied knowledge of lived experience and practice.

By setting in motion the ethnographic image of *wosimwaya* I aim to challenge the imposition of an imported HIV discourse onto the Trobriand cultural landscape by establishing a sense of place and demeanor that is a priori in relation to the untold present and future of an impending epidemic. I underscore how in the Trobriands, as in other places in PNG and beyond, the epidemic as a symbol of modernity and a harbinger of change paradoxically invokes the stability of the cultural landscape for mediation and appropriate response (see Setel 1999). Indeed, in discussions and interviews during my research, I was continually struck by how the popular representation of AIDS as a looming threat from beyond the islands led Trobrianders to assert cultural identity, belonging, and survival in the face of this novel threat. Katerina Teaiwa affirms that "Pacific peoples' survival strategies are found in many areas of cultural production but particularly in performance" (Teaiwa 2002:56). *Wosimwaya* celebrates the resiliency of Trobrianders in negotiating social change and reveals the importance of cultural survival for offsetting the impact of HIV and AIDS.

The measured solemnity of *wosimwaya* counters popularized perceptions of Trobriand culture as synonymous with sexual desire and abandon. Depictions of licentious islanders have been commonplace ever since the coral atolls were made famous in the early twentieth century by anthropologist Bronislaw Malinowski, who claimed that "chastity is an unknown virtue" in the Trobriands (1922:53). Malinowski's classic ethnography of Trobriand social and sexual life, *The Sexual Life of Savages*, became an essential tome in anthropological scholarship but created a sensation far beyond the academy when it was first published in 1929. His depictions titillated European imaginings of the noble savage, and popular retellings soon located the Trobriands as an idealized place of primordial desire and ecstasy—the "Islands of Love."[5] This sexualized geography is an enduring trope that continues to appear in journalistic accounts and tourism promotion (Senft 1998b; Eime 2006), and it shapes contemporary perceptions of the Trobriands among not only foreigners but other Papua New Guineans. As a young Trobriand man returning home from technical training on mainland PNG exclaimed to me, "My schoolmates over there say, 'Oh, Trobs, very sexy place!'"[6]

The expression "Islands of Love" has now found a place in the national response to the HIV epidemic in PNG, influencing popular and programmatic conceptualizations of risk and prevention that identify the Trobriands as a "high-risk setting" (Dekuku and Anang 2003; Elliot, Kitau, and Pantumari 2006). A reporter for one of the nation's daily newspapers refers to the "Islands of Love" in an article on an assessment trip to the Trobriands made by the director of the PNG National AIDS Council Secretariat (NACS), which was followed by a press release with the verdict that "the virus is spreading through cultural norms unlike in many other parts of the country" (Gerawa 2010).

It would be easy to play into this stereotype of the Trobriands with a depiction of the effusive and highly sexualized *tapiokwa* dance, also in the Trobriand repertoire, which features thrusting pelvises and ribald chanting—"Mweki, mweki, mweki, mweki" (*mweki* is a poetic synonym for sexual intercourse, or *kayta*, which literally translates "come to" or "visit"). *Tapiokwa* is known as the signature dance of the Trobriands, performed for tourists and visitors to the islands and imitated by Papua New Guineans from other parts of the country at various cultural festivals and community events. Trobriand toddlers are encouraged to mimic the thrusting movement and chant the refrain almost as soon as they take their first steps. Young children often break into spontaneous renditions of *tapiokwa* as they walk along village paths or play on sandy beaches. The dance is enacted in full costumed splendor when harvested yams are carried ceremoniously from the gardens to the yam storage houses in the villages. *Tapiokwa* is a relatively contemporary improvisation, originally created as a chant for the sport of Trobriand cricket in the early twentieth century.[7] Trobrianders often dismiss *tapiokwa* as an inauthentic representation of the cultural repertoire, regarding it as frivolous and fun but inconsequential, whereas *wosimwaya* with its deep indigenous performative history is held in high regard as a genuine expression of the Trobriand aesthetic (see MacCarthy 2010).

While my objective here is to establish a sense of cultural context with an enduring image of regeneration, I also question the depiction of "cultural practices" as causal factors in HIV transmission. The rhetorical emphasis of HIV communication on "risk behaviors" and the "cultural determinants of sexual risk" finds a ready target in cultural practices regarded as exotic, perduring, and enshrined by tradition (Seidel and Vidal 1997; Stillwaggon 2003). Such alleged risks are much simpler for interventions to name and target than are the complex aspects of social structure and the global economic and political forces that shape HIV epidemiology. In PNG, there have been repeated calls to regulate or ban cultural practices regarded as promoting sexual promiscuity or immoral behavior, including a call from a member of parliament representing a district in Milne Bay to blacklist the Trobriand *tapiokwa* dance.[8]

A significant historical antecedent to interventionist approaches to HIV is found in the conjoined projects of colonialism and Christian missionization. In the late nineteenth and early twentieth centuries, colonial administrators and missionaries in the Trobriands sought to regulate and reform what they perceived as undisciplined and immoral native bodies (Reed 1997). The transposition of Christian teachings and Western models of sexuality, reproduction, and disease were largely concerned with eradicating customs and beliefs perceived as primitive in order to rescue natives from unenlightened savagery and usher them into the modern era (Denoon 1989; Hughes 1997; Reed 1997). The pervasive emphasis on sexual promiscuity in HIV discourse is sedimented with the residue of colonial and anthropological constructions of indigenous sexuality as deviant from civilized humanity, epitomized in Malinowksi's title reference to "savages." While such depictions persist today in the popular imagination, Trobrianders tend to dismiss this racist and patronizing naming through the use of humor and riposte. In April 2003, at the height of the US invasion of Iraq, an old man approached me when I was sitting on the platform of a yam storage house during a mortuary exchange feast. Punctuating his words by hitting his fist on the timber platform, he declared, "It is savage! It is savage! It is savage what America is doing to the Iraqi people!" The old man's proclamation not only turns the imperialist label around, but also demonstrates awareness of global interconnectedness and how geopolitics position Trobrianders within wider fields of meaning, as well as how Trobrianders can reposition themselves within global events, including the HIV epidemic.

The intrusion of HIV into the Trobriand cultural landscape is but the latest wave of exogenous pathogens and frameworks of meaning from "beyond the horizon" (Jolly 2005) to interact with local ways of knowing and being. Trobrianders' assertions of place identity, or the "rhetorics of self-making" (Battaglia 1995),[9] often employ the notion of culture, or *bubuna*,[10] as a platform from which to negotiate external intrusions, accommodate change, and establish borders of difference in relation to other people and places. Trobrianders' propensity to evoke cultural reifications both among themselves and in interaction with outsiders also points to their historical relationship with anthropology and the extensive body of ethnographic accounts and theoretical analysis that the islands have generated.[11] Trobriand "borders of being" (Jolly and Ram, eds. 2001), or embodied understandings of personhood, are anchored to consistently stable notions of culture and place. The appeal to cultural boundedness and stability in Trobriand identity-making is perhaps reinforced by the finite geography of small coral atolls in the vast open sea of tremendous linguistic and cultural difference (White and Lindstrom, eds. 1993).[12] Yet the genealogy of Trobriand identity and social reproduction is not contained within impenetrable boundaries but extends beyond its named coral atolls. The orientations of place navigate across geographic boundaries in permeable ways as Trobrianders engage in interisland travel and trade, relocate to other places in PNG and to other countries, and interact with people and ideas from beyond the local horizon.

Islands of Love, Islands of Risk engages multiple voices, perspectives, and narrative styles to evoke the tensions between HIV and culture, and between interventionist ideologies for responding to HIV and the expression of cultural values through everyday practice. The use of the present tense in ethnographic description has been criticized for falsely conveying a sense of cultural timelessness, stasis, and internal coherence (see Fabian 1983; Strathern 1999). My deliberate use of this narrative style is intended to triangulate my ethnographic evidence with the interpretive descriptions of Trobriand culture in the existing literature and to vividly animate depictions of context and lived experience. Moreover, the present tense reflects how Trobrianders interpret and represent their own cultural truths in interviews and discussion.

Revered as "one of the most sacred places in anthropology" (Weiner 1976:xv), the Trobriands are emblematic of the reified field of "the Other," providing anthropology with its "mythic fieldwork charter" (Gupta and Ferguson 1997:7). The

Trobriands are renowned in the corpus of anthropological theory mainly because of the monumental work of Malinowski, who pioneered participant observation methodology during his extended fieldwork on Kiriwina early last century. Revisiting Malinowski's work some fifty years later, Annette Weiner made a major contribution to anthropological theory with her ethnographic account of Trobriand social reproduction, *Women of Value, Men of Renown* (1976). Weiner offered new perspectives on the integral position women hold in the Trobriand social universe, particularly their key role in *sagali*, the mortuary feasts that regenerate matrilineal identity and underpin the Trobriand exchange economy. While historical transformations inform my particular focus, the works of Malinowski and Weiner provide descriptive foundations and major points of reference for my ethnographic exploration.

Writing on the impact of Malinowski's intellectual contribution to social research, Eric Hirsch suggests, "Malinowski transformed the Papuan society of the Trobriand Islands into a resource with which to think through and analyse problems common to peoples throughout the world" (2002:1). This proposition that the effect of ethnographic knowledge is to transform societies into intellectual resources is debatable.[13] However, I hold to the notion that Trobriand society offers a productive site for addressing universal human problems, and for considering how local cultural knowledge might enable effective and positive responses to the global challenges of HIV and provide the requisite resiliency and cohesion to realize the future in the present.

CHAPTER 1

Models of Meaning and Ways of Knowing

HIV, the human immunodeficiency virus, is a pathogen with multiple magnifications. In microscopic imagery, HIV is a patterned geometry of interlacing circles and diamonds. Carried in the cells of semen, vaginal mucosa, blood, and milk, the virus attaches to DNA helixes and assails T-cells. HIV colonizes the most basic dimensions of human experience, exploiting our fertility and sexuality while gaining velocity through social structures and processes that map multiple routes of transmission. Far greater than a microorganism, HIV looms large in the social body as it is configured by discourses of sexuality, morality, risk, fear, and death. It is uncanny how a virus with no immediately visible manifestations has the capacity to make visible the ways people know themselves and to alter that knowing.[1]

Biomedical science has made possible an understanding of HIV pathology, how the virus damages the human immune system to the extent that infected bodies eventually die from the complications of AIDS, the acquired immune deficiency syndrome. But such knowledge has not been able to prevent the persistent spread of the virus throughout the world. Since the virus was first isolated and named in the early 1980s, the HIV epidemic gained rapid prominence as the most serious public health challenge in the contemporary world, expanding to all parts of the globe and reaching dramatic prevalence in many countries, with an estimated total of sixty million people having been infected by the virus and nearly twenty-five million deaths from HIV-related causes (UNAIDS 2010; UNAIDS and WHO 2009). This pandemic of staggering proportions has not occurred as a single global event. Rather, HIV infection proliferates into multiple epidemics within particular contexts of space and time (Mane and Aggleton 2001:23). Even as there is not one epidemic, there is not simply one virus. More accurately, complex viral strains have evolved in interaction with different biological, social, and structural environments (Hutchinson 2003; Singer and Clair 2003). The manifestations of HIV pathology are not revealed under a microscopic lens but in the way "social forces and processes come to be embodied as biological events" (Farmer 1999:14).

Concurrent with the relentless spread of the viral infection over the last three decades are multiple ways of comprehending HIV and AIDS as different knowledge and belief systems converge and interact to coproduce meaning. These conjunctions reveal how the global phenomenon is "simultaneously an epidemic of a transmissible lethal disease and an epidemic of meanings or signification" (Treichler 1999:11). Discourses of sexuality, risk, and disease influence the interpretive process of making sense of HIV and AIDS and gain currency through the public health policies and interventions that are put into place to respond to epidemics, with direct consequences for how HIV takes shape within specific contexts. Based persistently on biomedical models of disease, HIV programs infuse the language of prevention with predominantly Western assumptions and moralities about human sexuality and gender (Brummelhuis and Herdt, eds. 1995; Herdt and Lindenbaum, eds. 1992; Patton 2002; Pigg 2001b). The power of language to name and classify epidemics based on preconceived notions, and to construct categories of meaning for prescriptive responses, "is not merely symbolic, but has material outcomes that impinge on people's lives" (Seidel and Vidal 1997:59). The global migration of this discursive epidemiology (Jolly and Manderson 1997:19) potentially affects people's capacity to articulate local knowledge and form congruent links with new information to enable prevention within particular settings (see Adams and Pigg, eds. 2005:19–20).

Biomedicine, itself a cultural construction based on deeply entrenched social and historical codes (Treichler 1999:18), inextricably influences how HIV is understood and represented. Focused on the "neutral terrain of the physical body" (Lock 1988:7), the biomedical paradigm of disease causation is historically derived from Western epistemic notions about the individual as an autonomous and bounded entity of bodily elements and functions, and about sexual behavior as a naturalized human drive (see Gordon 1988; Parker 1995; and Scheper-Hughes and Lock 1987). In conjunction with this paradigm, epidemiological surveillance is used to monitor and predict HIV transmission patterns and trends by conceptually isolating sexual behavior at the individual level as an independent variable. Such methodological individualism reduces sexual acts to units of measure, disembodied from cultural meanings and lived experience (Pirkle 2009; see also Clatts 1995; Kippax and Crawford 1993; Parker 2001). Reductionism disallows that "physically identical sexual acts may have varying social significance and subjective meaning . . . in different cultures and historical periods" (Vance 1991:878). Moreover, the predictive relation between individual behavior and disease occurrence is "framed in terms of risk, an epidemiological category that plucks behavior from context" (Lindenbaum 2001:378).

As a corollary to constructions of the atomized body and the risk of disease, the majority of HIV prevention strategies employ individualist models of behavior change, which situate beliefs, attitudes, and behaviors within the psychological domain of individual minds (Kippax and Crawford 1993). These models, conventionally used for predicting and modifying behavior in relation to risk, are referred to as "social-cognitive" in the health psychology literature.[2] The "social" is generally represented as a measure of individual agency responding to various external factors, rather than the relations *between* different social actors, whereas the "cognitive" is represented as an internalized struggle between risk and reason. The emphasis of behavior change is on rational intention—the individual, armed with factual information, setting out to achieve goals.

Adjunct to behavior-change models are Knowledge, Attitude, and Practice (KAP) surveys, which use various quantitative methods to collect information at the population level. Such models and methodologies are regarded as useful for HIV interventions because they provide a means to make standardized comparisons and predictions about behavior change and they generate baseline data to monitor and evaluate the impact of awareness campaigns. To this end, paradoxically, evidence of behavior change tends to be measured as an outcome of the effectiveness of program implementation rather than as individuals acting on new information (see Patton 1990). Evidence for the effectiveness of HIV behavior change strategies remains shallow and elusive, with little robust indication of the relationship between increased public knowledge of HIV and a corresponding change in sexual behavior to minimize transmission (Campbell 2003; Kippax and Crawford 1993). What is apparent is that such individualist research methods and strategies result more readily in the externalization of risk, reinforcing the discourses of fear and blame that have dominated representations of AIDS as a "killer disease" since the beginning of the global epidemic (Hammar 2008; Treichler 1999).

The interventionist language of HIV prevention is steeped with metaphors of distancing (Reid 1994:1) that invite the externalization of risk, implicitly communicated in the epidemiological surveillance categories of "core transmitters," "risk groups," "risk behaviors," and "hot spots of infectivity" (Barnett and Whiteside 2002; Seidel and Vidal 1997). Such terms are conceptualized with quantifiable dimensions so that the relative probability of finding infection can be statistically measured (Barnett and Whiteside 2002:80). The terms assume an objective distance and stability from which to model risk factors and target interventions, providing "an illusory cartographic certainty in a turbulent terrain" (Jolly and Manderson 1997:20). The subtexts of moral and social deviancy invoked by categories of risk derive in part from historical representations of people marginalized from positions of power—prostitutes, homosexuals, the poor, and people of color (Kielmann 1997; Patton 1994, 2002; Treichler 1999). Information about HIV is thus encountered from various subject positions prefigured as "target groups" in need of transformative interventions (see Craddock 2000:154).

Behavior-change models that target individuals with assumptions about responsibility and choice, often in the guise of empowerment, belie the social and structural inequalities that contribute to the gendered vulnerability to HIV (Waterston 1997; Farmer 1999). They also obscure the dilemma of choice regarding biological and social reproductive roles, particularly for women, and the interrelated concerns of fertility control and disease prevention (Hammar 1998b:53). The biomedical paradigm for the prevention of mother-to-child transmission[3] of HIV presupposes the responsibility of individual women, which exaggerates female agency and implies that ignorance of HIV infection status is morally negligent behavior (Farmer et al., eds. 1996:182). In reality, many women throughout the world, including in Papua New Guinea, are unaware of their HIV status because testing and diagnostic services are not available or accessible, or they are uninformed subjects of antenatal surveillance in the service of producing unlinked statistical data on prevalence for the purpose of "evidence-based" HIV programming.

Whether utilizing tropes of risk or empowerment, the language of HIV prevention persistently aligns sex with deviance, disease, and death, while largely ignoring the dimensions of sexual desire, consensus, and pleasure. Such dystopic representations of sexuality pervade the standardized HIV awareness and prevention strategies pitched at individual behavior change that are promoted by international agencies involved in the global AIDS response and implemented by country programs of response (Barnett and Parkhurst 2005; Eves and Butt 2008:7–8). The standard ABC prevention model (Abstain, Be faithful, use Condoms)[4] frames sexuality in terms of risk and promiscuity in an implied moral hierarchy of behavior change, where "abstinence" and "being faithful" are preferable to condom use. Promoting condoms as protection in this lethal layering of signification reinforces a negative association between condoms, infidelity, and the spread of disease, so that protected sex is deemed morally bad and risky, while unprotected sex is held to be morally good and safe and is assumed within marriage and other intimate relationships (Hammar 1998b; Smith 2009:106). Condoms are thus inscribed with risk and danger, their use symbolizing and augmenting distrust in sexual relationships rather than negotiated consent (Bujra 2000; Sobo 1995).

The "globally circulating template" for HIV awareness (Pigg 2001a:103), preoccupied with conveying factual and consistent information about HIV while inscribing subtexts of deviance about sexual behavior, limits the application of contextual knowledge and experience that reflects the complexities and particularities of local epidemics (Treichler 1999:153). Typically, awareness sessions are held as perfunctory one-off events, and messages are delivered by rote with little or no reference to cultural meanings and lived experience. While people may readily internalize the "basic facts" about HIV, the information holds "a range of doubts, qualifications, contradictions and uncertainties, which . . . blunt the factual messages imparted" (Campbell 2003:25). The communication process seldom allows space for resolving questions that arise and for making links with social practices.

The importance of facilitating awareness about HIV and the social and structural factors that contribute to HIV susceptibility must not be underestimated for places like the Trobriands—and places elsewhere in Papua New Guinea and the wider Pacific region—where the capacity and resources to provide counseling, testing, and clinical treatments remain limited, and where even condoms are not widely available, accessible, or acceptable.[5] HIV communication strategies informed by the dynamics of place are more likely to inspire active involvement of people and communities in prevention efforts. Whether by mass media campaigns, social marketing, or interpersonal dialogue, effective communication for prevention requires an engagement of the imagination across a vast field of cultural meanings and social practice.

HIV and Culture

The *Pacific Regional Strategy on HIV/AIDS* acknowledges the challenge to develop a program of response that "feels and smells like the Pacific," representing the region's "diverse cultures and religious backgrounds, and differing national HIV epidemics" (Secretariat of the Pacific Community 2005:11). While the sensory idiom may be just a respectful gesture toward diversity, it nonetheless inspires and legitimates approaches that respect cultural ways of knowing and being.[6] Rather than simply replicating global blueprints for policies and programs designed from an outside perspective, the rhetorical ethos of the strategy encourages organic understandings of local realities as the foundation for an effective response. Appeals to

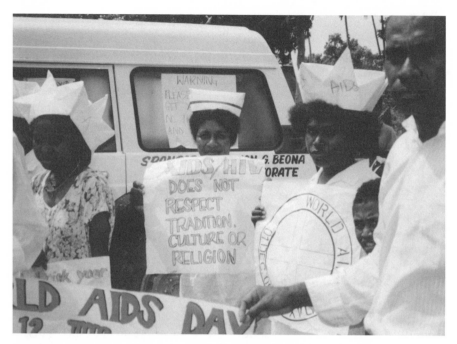

FIGURE 1.1. • Losuia District Health Center staff on World AIDS Day, 2000

cultural specificity are prominent in the Pacific, where often traditions are asserted to negotiate emerging identities and issues (Jolly 2005; Jolly and Thomas, eds. 1992; White and Lindstrom, eds. 1993). The notion of place, with its "naturalized association" with culture, operates as a key orientation for social interaction and expresses genealogical affiliation and moral location (Gupta and Ferguson 1992:7; see also Rodman 1992:646).

The importance of place in the production of knowledge invites a closer consideration of how culture is conceptualized in the language of HIV, particularly as an epidemiological variable of risk. In the mid-1990s, the awareness message "HIV/ AIDS does not respect tradition, culture, or religion" was translated into several Pacific languages on posters produced by the Secretariat of the Pacific Community to underscore the region's collective vulnerability to the impending epidemic (United Nations 1996:73, 79). The maxim quickly took hold and is recited frequently in HIV training workshops and awareness sessions in Papua New Guinea and reproduced on T-shirts and hand-drawn posters (see Figure 1.1). This rhetorical discord between culture and HIV is apparent also in the familiar assertion that "cultural taboos" do not allow open talk about sex (hence, culture negates the problem of HIV), commonly expressed in the Trobriands and many places throughout Papua New Guinea and the Pacific (Gibbs and Mondu 2010; Vete 1995).[7]

The polarity drawn here between Pacific cultures and HIV indicates a strong sense of place and a stable, rooted belonging threatened by an intrusive foreign pathogen. On the contrary, the concept of culture in the biomedical paradigm converts places of belonging into sites of the exotic "other." The global discourse of HIV persistently renders culture as a bounded and static impediment to development and behavior change. "Culture" thus easily becomes a quantifiable epidemiological variable of "risk" and disease causality (Brummelhuis and Herdt, eds. 1995; Setel 1999). Such use of the culture concept also reinforces biological explanations of sexuality in terms of instincts and corporeal essences based on essentialist assumptions about the individuated person (Jolly and Manderson 1997:1; see also Vance 1991:880). This "etiologization" of culture (Wardlow 2002:153, 154) obscures social and historical processes and the structural inequalities that produce HIV vulnerabilities, and it has the potential to thwart HIV communication by representing culture—and cultural constructions of sexuality—as pathological and in need of remedial intervention. Racial constructs of difference fold easily into notions of cultural pathology and the discordant binary between "us" and "them." Eileen Stillwaggon observes, "Persistent notions of racial difference suffused the social science literature on AIDS in Africa, especially in the first fifteen years of the epidemic. No one used the word 'race,' but it entered into the discourse as 'culture'" (2003:811–12; see also Schoepf 1995).

The totalizing view of culture perhaps is linked to seeing the spread of HIV as a singular event that manifests everywhere the same way or, at any rate, requires interventions based on standardized international best practices (UNAIDS 1999). From the initial years of the global response to the epidemic, the power of HIV to transcend borders and cultures produced an urgency to respond uniformly. In *Culture and Sexual Risk*, one of the first publications to examine the phenomenon of AIDS from an anthropological perspective, the authors observe how the epidemic "imposed upon anthropology its totalism and global effects, shattering our prior particularistic conceptions of culture and society" (Brummelhuis and Herdt 1995:xii). The gradual incorporation of culture into HIV policy and program responses largely reflects the growing contribution of anthropological research to a richer understanding of localized epidemics and the cultural constructions of sexuality, gender, and disease (Farmer 1997; Herdt 1992; Jenkins 2002; Parker 2001; Schoepf 2001). Ironically, the application of the culture concept in relation to HIV seldom draws on the vigorous theoretical critique of culture within the discipline of anthropology,[8] revealing the uneasy epistemic relations between the fields of anthropology and epidemiology (Adams and Pigg, eds. 2005; Herring and Swedlund, eds. 2010; Trostle 2005).

The notion of culture as bounded and homogeneous is increasingly destabilized by global interconnections and internal contestations of difference (Abu-Lughod 1991; Jolly and Ram, eds. 2001).[9] As the experience and understanding of HIV continues to evolve, recognition of cultural diversity and complexity *within* the different contexts of unfolding epidemics has increased. However, the behavior-change paradigm continues to perpetuate notions of culture as a racialized geography defined by "traditional" beliefs and practices, wherein discord exists between the individual capacity for change and the rigid strictures of cultural ideology (Butt, Numbery, and Morin 2002; Farmer 1997; Kalipeni et al., eds. 2004; Seidel and Vidal 1997).

The interplay between cultural beliefs and individual practice represents contentious theoretical and methodological terrain where the fields of anthropology and public health converge (Hahn and Inhorn 2009; Pelto and Pelto 1997; Yoder

1997). Individualist models of behavior change commonly used in public health interventions privilege "knowledge" over "beliefs" as the means for effecting change,
wherein knowledge pertains to people's cognitive grasp of "scientific facts" while
beliefs are rendered as the rigid set of cultural norms that dictate and constrain individual action (Kippax and Crawford 1993; Pelto and Pelto 1997). Behavior change
is deemed possible when individuals have acquired the knowledge that allows them
to transcend culturally determined practice. Paradoxically, while prevention strategies are resoundingly about behavior change, the reiterated concern that HIV communication should be "culturally appropriate" falls back on notions of cultural
determinism and stability, homogeneity, and coherence within distinct cultural
groups. Not only does the guiding principle of cultural relevance undercut the well-
rehearsed precept of individual agency acting on factual scientific knowledge, it
obscures internal contestations of difference, new expressions of emerging sexual
identities, and the fluidity of form and practice within specific cultural contexts.

There is an inverse implication in the culturalist discourse as well, which suggests that the erosion of culture and tradition, caused by rapid social change and
external forces, is the major determinant of HIV risk. Evocations of culture under
the guise of "tradition" and "custom" also provide foils for people to legitimate
harmful and unequal gender power relations and negate responsibility for action and the imperative for behavior change in response to the epidemic (Schoepf
1995:34). Such appeals to the inviolability of culture are sometimes used by Papua
New Guineans to perpetuate and exonerate forms of family and sexual violence,
and so-called traditional practices are used to punish behavior deemed untradi-
tional (Garap 2000:162; Zimmer-Tamakoshi 1997).

The National Context

The tremendous linguistic and cultural diversity of Papua New Guinea attests to
the challenges and contradictions inherent in the way culture is viewed in relation to HIV. Papua New Guinea is the largest country in the Pacific region, with
a youthful population of seven million inhabitants. The vast majority of people
maintain subsistence livelihoods in rural village communities and have limited
opportunities for participating in the cash economy. The dramatic geographic
features of the country, including mountainous terrain, isolated valleys, and numerous small scattered islands, present challenges for infrastructural development,
transportation, communication, and the provision of health and education services. The presence of HIV in PNG has been firmly established over the last two
decades, especially in urban centers where the number of deaths from HIV-related
causes has increased steadily, and the experience of living with the virus is becoming more widespread and commonplace.

Epidemiological and Social Contours

Since the first reported cases of HIV in 1987, epidemiological data have presented
an increasingly serious, if uneven and limited, picture of HIV prevalence in Papua
New Guinea.[10] My research in the Trobriands was carried out during a period that
saw a rapid escalation of the number of confirmed HIV cases at the national level,

which increased annually by 30 percent between 1997 and 2004 (National AIDS Council and National Department of Health 2004:7). In 2002, the Joint United Nations Programme on HIV/AIDS (UNAIDS) classified PNG as the fourth country in the Asia Pacific region to have a "generalized" HIV epidemic, a category based on the notion of the "general population" rather than "high-risk groups;" the classificiation is applied when HIV prevalence reaches 1 percent of women attending antenatal clinics. The evidence for this classification in PNG was limited to test results of antenatal attendees at Port Moresby General Hospital in the nation's capital (7). In 2004, the national prevalence of HIV was estimated to be 1.7 percent among the adult population (aged fifteen to forty-nine years), which represented a fourfold increase over estimates made in 2000 (7, 17). While confirmed cases of HIV infection are highest in the national capital and other urban centers, cases have been reported in all nineteen provinces, with the largest concentration in the Highlands region. Available data on the province of origin of HIV-infected persons show a distribution that includes all provinces. The expansion of surveillance and voluntary counseling and testing services throughout the country from 2005 onward produced a larger body of evidence that suggested the epidemic was moving into rural areas. However, a more adequate interpretation would argue that this evidence instead reflects increased surveillance and testing of the rural population.

The extremely high incidence of sexually transmitted infections (STI), including cases of multiple infections, in a diverse cross-section of PNG's population indicates the extent of unprotected sex and the density of sexual networks (Aruwafu, Akuani, and Kupe 2009, 2010; Hammar 1998a, 2007; Jenkins and Passey 1998; Passey 1996). Estimates made by the World Health Organization (WHO) suggest there are more than one million new STI cases in PNG every year (National AIDS Council Secretariat 2006:18). Although data on the mode of transmission are available for only 35 percent of notified cases of HIV infection, the nearly equal distribution of confirmed cases between males and females indicates the importance of heterosexual activity in HIV transmission (National AIDS Council and National Department of Health 2009:7, 9). Perinatal transmission of HIV from parent to child accounts for about 1 percent of diagnosed HIV cases where mode of transmission is recorded.[11] Although not openly acknowledged, sexual activity between men is not uncommon in PNG, and some cultural areas have traditions where intergenerational homosexual practices are integral to male initiation rites (Herdt, ed. 1984; Knauft 2003). However, same-sex practice is not generally constructed in terms of an exclusive homosexual identity and orientation, as there are strong social expectations that men will marry and become fathers (Jenkins 1996b). There is no strong evidence of drug-injecting behavior in PNG; however, the sharing of unsterilized implements for body tattoos and penile modifications is a potential mode of HIV transmission.

Available data on gender and age distribution of confirmed cases indicate an increasing gender asymmetry in younger age groups, where cumulative infection rates among girls (aged ten to nineteen years) and young women (aged twenty to twenty-four years) are three and two times higher respectively than those among boys and young men in the same age groups (National AIDS Council Secretariat 2006:10).[12] This trend points to the vulnerability of adolescent girls and young women in cross-generational sexual relations with older men who are likely to have increased HIV exposure because of their longer sexual histories. Research indicates that the average age of commencement of sexual activity for both males and females is around fourteen to fifteen years (National Sex and Reproduction Research Team and Jenkins 1994). However, for many girls first vaginal intercourse precedes first menstruation and is often a traumatic event, increasing the possibility of reproductive health complications as well as the risk of HIV transmission (Hammar 2008:61).

The most recent official HIV prevalence estimates for PNG were released in June 2010. Based on available data collected in 2009 on HIV test results among pregnant women attending antenatal clinics, the estimates suggest that the epidemic in PNG is "levelling off" at less than 1 percent of the adult population (National Department of Health 2010:1). While limitations are acknowledged regarding the quality, reliability, and scope of data used in the modeling exercises, the revised estimates are upheld by government officials and program managers as an indication of significant progress over recent years in improving the national HIV surveillance system and expanding prevention, treatment, and care efforts. However, the validity of epidemiological modeling based on limited data is problematic and holds important ethical questions about the "cultures of measurement" (Setel 2009) that dominate conceptualizations of HIV. Statistical evidence on levels and trends is privileged over qualitative methods that provide deeper analysis of the contextual factors that influence sexual practice and contribute to HIV transmission dynamics (Hirsch et al. 2009:16–18; Reid 2009).

Social research on gender and sexuality in contemporary PNG illuminates how meanings and practices are shaped by the confluence of diverse indigenous belief systems and imported ideologies in a rapidly changing social terrain (Borrey 2000; Butt and Eves, eds. 2008; Hammar 2007, 2010; Jenkins 2007; Wardlow 2006, 2009; Zimmer-Tamakoshi 1993). The benchmark nationwide qualitative study on sexual and reproductive knowledge, conducted by the PNG Institute of Medical Research (IMR) in the early 1990s, acknowledges the significant transformation of cultural constructions of sexuality and gender relations over the last several generations (National Sex and Reproduction Research Team and Jenkins 1994:76). Commenting on the historical effects of colonization, Christianity, national development, and modernization on sexual meanings and practices, the authors state: "The confusion and disturbance these shifts have caused are not trivial and have serious implications for the health of Papua New Guineans. While it may not be true that actual sexual behaviors have changed, although nearly everyone in Papua New Guinea claims they have, it is certainly true that the meanings and contexts of sexuality have changed greatly" (76).

Traditional ideologies of male dominance, female pollution,[13] and sexual avoidance common to many cultural groups, particularly in the Highlands region, continue to influence forms and meanings of gender, sexuality, and reproduction in the shifting contemporary context (Clark and Hughes 1995; Josephides 1985; Knauft 1994, 1997; Poole and Herdt, eds. 1982; Wardlow 2004, 2006). Polygamy proliferates in truncated forms under the guise of customary practice, with mobile younger men acquiring a succession of wives in different locations without the economic means to support them and their children, or to maintain the interclan exchange relations that were central to earlier marital unions.

The settings in which people engage in sexual transactions, and the identities and relationships of people associated with those settings, reflect a dynamic range of cultural meanings and motivations (Hammar 1998b; Jenkins 1997, 2000; Wardlow 2004). Urban and rural sexual networks encompass a wide spectrum of sexual transactions, from informal and occasional to commercially structured. Sexual transactions embedded in traditional exchange systems have found new expressions in contemporary contexts where the exchange of sex for money and goods occurs in multiple and fluid forms, often with serious effects on women's sexual autonomy and health (Hammar 1998b; Hughes 1997; Jenkins 1997, 2007; National Sex and Reproduction Research Team and Jenkins 1994). For example, contrary to the assumption that sex work is motivated by economic need, Holly Wardlow (2004, 2006) describes how *pasindia meri* (Tok Pisin[14] for "passenger woman" or prostitute) from Tari in the Southern Highlands engage in a form of "revenge promiscuity" out of frustration and anger that their male relatives no longer fulfill traditional kinship obligations to support them (2004:1035). This practice relates to the increasingly common view in PNG that the traditional function of bride-price in cementing relations between clans has been transformed so radically by monetization that women are now regarded as commodities to be bought and sold by their families. Wardlow (1034) reports that for many women the experience of rape and violence, and the subsequent failure of relatives to pursue justice on their behalf, often precipitates the decision to break away from their husband and kin and become *pasindia meri*.

Commenting on the sexual double standard that pervades antagonistic gender relations in contemporary PNG, Lawrence Hammar observes that "*contemporary* men still exercise *customary* sexual prerogatives to hurt women via their genitalia" (1998a:268). Acts of gendered violence involving sexual coercion, assault, and *lainap* (the Tok Pisin word for group rape or serial intercourse involving groups of men lining up to have sex with one woman) are disturbingly frequent and complicate an already challenging social environment for mediating change (Borrey 2000; Hammer 1998a; Lewis et al. 2007; Luker and Dinnen, eds. 2010; Toft, ed. 1985; Zimmer-Tamakoshi 1997). *Lainap* is highly conducive to the transmission of HIV and other STIs, not only between male and female bodies, but also between participating males (Jenkins 2007:45). The country's national strategy for responding to the epidemic acknowledges the significance of gender violence for HIV transmission and identifies "patterns of male sexual behavior," including the high incidence of sexual assault, rape, and *lainap*, coupled by weak law enforcement, as key factors in women's vulnerability to HIV (Government of Papua New Guinea and National AIDS Council 2006:10).

Papua New Guinea's contextual factors and epidemiological trends often are likened to the HIV situation in many sub-Saharan African countries (Caldwell 2000; Luker and Dinnen, eds. 2010; O'Keefe 2011; World Bank 2004). Such comparisons, stated in media reports, public speeches, and policy documents, are intended to compel an urgent response to a potentially devastating situation. Susan Craddock underscores the rhetorical urgency in the opening paragraph of *HIV and*

AIDS in Africa: Beyond Epidemiology, writing, "AIDS in Africa. The phrase itself has come to signal an almost apocalyptic level of devastation" (2004:1). More troubling in the comparisons between PNG and Africa are the implied racist constructions that collapse AIDS, Africa, and all developing countries into one homogenous pool of infectivity (Kalipeni, Oppong, and Zerai 2007; Schoepf 2004:19–22; Seidel and Vidal 1997:62, 73; Stillwaggon 2003). Comparative modeling of epidemics on the basis of trends, structural factors, and potential impact are deemed useful for formulating policy and program interventions based on international best practice. However, such comparisons have limited utility for developing responses that reflect the realities of particular contexts, and, more often than not, they carry moralistic biases and damaging assumptions about sexual practice and people's capacity for change.

There is no doubt, however, that PNG's susceptibility to HIV, or the "features of a society that make it more or less likely that an infectious disease will attain epidemic proportions" (Barnett and Whiteside 2002:71), is comparable to other countries where global inequalities and structural factors shape conditions that are conducive to the spread of HIV. A biosocial understanding of HIV highlights the interrelationships between the pathogen and the social contexts in which it flourishes, taking account of the "biological synergism" between HIV and other pathogens present in a population, and "the determinant importance of social conditions in the health of individuals and populations" (Singer and Clair 2003:428; see also Farmer 1999:5; Stillwaggon 2003:810). A biosocial understanding also reveals the reciprocal interaction between human physiology and cultural ways of knowing and being (Worthman 1998:29).

In PNG, susceptibility to HIV is compounded by endemic malaria and a high burden of other infectious diseases, including STIs, tuberculosis, pneumonia, and hepatitis, in a context where primary health care services are extremely limited and underresourced (Government of Papua New Guinea 2010; Malau and Crockett 2000). Susceptibility is also compounded by the environment in which HIV is flourishing, including high levels of population mobility, limited income-earning opportunities in the formal sector, itinerant wage labor in enclave industries such as mining and logging, and the intensified frequency of violent crime in both urban and rural settings (Luker and Dinnen, eds. 2010). The redistribution of cash in PNG's informal economy reflects reconfigurations of traditional exchange relations, the formation of new commercial and political relations, new patterns of commodity production and consumption, new desires and aspirations, as well as responses to economic hardship and increasing poverty. The flows of cash follow the routes of people's circular movement between villages and towns, between resource enclaves and urban centers, and up and down the national highway that links the Highlands to the coast, onshore and offshore, attesting to the fluid dimensions of social and sexual networks and to the connections between the local and the global. The context of rapid social and economic change demonstrates the interactive and paradoxical relationship between HIV and development (Collins and Rau 2000:35; Setel 1999:146–47). Likewise, these same factors indicate the nation's vulnerability to the impact of a major epidemic, underscoring the importance of an integrated, multisectoral response (Collins and Rau 2000:35).

The National Response

The presence of HIV in Papua New Guinea is also made known by the program of response led by the PNG National AIDS Council (NAC), in partnership with various donor agencies, churches, nongovernmental organizations, and businesses.[15] After an initial decade marked by sluggish indifference to the threat HIV posed for the nation's development (Jenkins 1996a; Ballard and Malau 2009), the early 2000s saw a groundswell of popular and political interest as more resources were committed and mobilized to implement the country's multisectoral strategy.[16] The tempo of the accelerating response in large part reflects the dynamic and changing nature of the expanding epidemic and the degree to which its presence is being felt. The invigorated attention to the challenges of the epidemic has produced a virtual industry of interventions as different international and local agencies and groups claim areas of special interest and expertise, and attempt to collaborate and coordinate efforts in areas of common concern.

Despite the structures and coordination mechanisms that were put in place with the establishment of the NAC Secretariat (NACS) and its network of provincial committees, program activities for HIV have been highly contested and variable, and implementation has been uneven and sporadic (Aggleton et al. 2010; Ballard and Malau 2009; Hammar 2010; UN/USAID Review Team Mission 2002). Responses are not always amenable to the "international best practices" advocated by UNAIDS and international development agencies, nor do the global mandates fit neatly into the PNG context. To some extent, competing perspectives and priorities and the uneven coordination of the overly bureaucratized national response reflect local resistance to the predominance of overseas technical advisers and specialists who arrive with their own ideas and agendas about what constitutes appropriate action (see Haley 2008). There is now a growing call among Papua New Guineans involved in HIV work for local success stories and achievements to be documented and shared so that "PNG best practices" can guide the national program (NAC and UNAIDS 2006).

Spreading Awareness and Talking about Sex

Setting the pace for the accelerated response in PNG during the early 2000s was a nationwide media campaign orchestrated by NACS with support from the National HIV/AIDS Support Project (NHASP).[17] The phased campaign employed a range of popular media to convey information and key prevention messages, including pamphlets on the "basic facts" of HIV and AIDS, comic books, posters, newspapers, community awareness theater, and radio and television. Ubiquitous throughout the country are large billboards and signs in the national colors of red, black, and yellow, erected at government offices, airports, markets, and on public transport, which bear the key message of the campaign in English or Tok Pisin (see Figure 1.2). Derived from the ABC slogan, the message instructs: "Protect yourself from AIDS: Don't have sex, be faithful, or always use a condom." The Tok Pisin translation assumes the individualist focus of the targeted message, using the singular pronoun for "you": "Lukautim yu yet long AIDS: Noken koap, stap wantaim wanpela tasol o usim kondom."

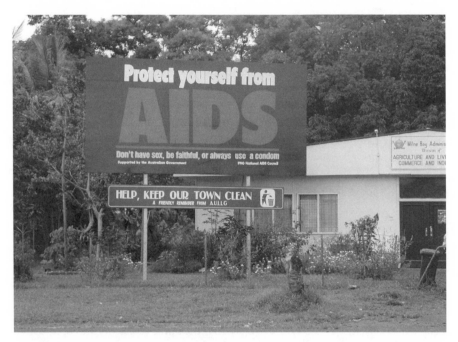

FIGURE 1.2. • AIDS awareness billboard outside provincial government offices in
               Alotau, Milne Bay Province, 2003

The sign in English is displayed at the entrance of the district government office
in Losuia. As one person observed, "The sign is so big it can't hide itself."[18] While
marshaling the symbolism of national identity, some signs also delineate the imagined protective borders of regional identities. Travelers in the departure lounge at
Gurney Airport in Alotau, the provincial capital of Milne Bay, encounter a sign
that implores: "Don't bring AIDS back to Milne Bay."

The first stage of the media campaign, launched in 2001, deployed a biomedical
representation of the epidemic. Posters and newspaper advertisements showed a
photograph of the founding director of NACS—Dr. Clement Malau, a prominent
PNG public health specialist—in white medical jacket beside a microscope and
laptop computer, looking straight into the eyes of viewers. The accompanying text
imparted basic facts about HIV and modes of transmission. Television and radio
spots featured the director addressing the audience in a direct and frank tone, re-
iterating the ABC slogan in Tok Pisin and encouraging the use of condoms for
protection. The strategic intention was to establish the epidemic as a serious health
and development issue for the country, requiring open, forthright talk about sex.
Along with tropes of "bush fire" and "time bomb" that warned of the impending scourge of the epidemic, the campaign created controversy with the Tok Pisin
word *koap*, meaning "go up" or "fuck" in its direct English translation, which was
used in the ABC imperative "Noken koap" (Don't have sex).

The disease control officer for Milne Bay Province summarized the public's response to the media campaign in the provincial capital, where the images and messages were received with a mixture of curiosity, keen interest, and civic acceptance:

People are hearing the message everywhere, everyday. We've never seen such things before—billboards with health awareness messages about sex and condoms—but we are used to it now. The big billboard outside government offices has been up for eight months now and still there has been no stone, no spit, and no graffiti. People don't spoil it. When Dr. Clement Malau comes on the TV, everyone rushes to watch. People are starting to call condoms "*kalementi* things," or just *kalementi*, ever since an old woman referred to them as such during a community awareness session. *Kalementi* is the Milne Bay way of saying the name Clement. In Milne Bay, we don't like the word *koap*. We find it offensive because we don't speak pidgin, so when we hear this it is like hearing the English word "fuck." It is better for the messages to say "have sex" or "sleep with." [Interview notes, 9 April 2003]

The key objective of the second round of the NACS campaign, launched in September 2002, was to encourage normative condom use by emphasizing protection through the notion of individual choice: "If you choose to have sex, condoms provide the best protection from HIV, other sexually transmitted infections, and unwanted pregnancies" (NACS 2002). The campaign specifically targeted young people in an attempt to foster a "positive, cognitive link" between proposed sexual activity and condom use, and "to increase target group negotiation skills, confidence and build hope with young people to be able to make the desired changes toward abstinence, monogamy, and safe sex practices" (NACS 2002). In addition to distributing free condoms in generic packaging, the social marketing campaign launched the branded commercial condom *Karamap*, Tok Pisin for "cover up," in packaging that featured a photo of a young, modern couple in an affectionate embrace, both wearing fashionable clothes. The name for the new condom ignited another controversial debate, expressed primarily in a rash of letters to the nation's daily newspapers, because *karamap* is the word used in the New Guinea Islands region for small packets of food cooked in earth ovens. In 2006, a new packaging design for the issue of free condoms was introduced in conjunction with the establishment of a number of voluntary counseling and testing (VCT) facilities throughout the country. Once again deploying nationalist symbolism for the purpose of social marketing (see Foster 2002), the small square black boxes, about the size of a pack of playing cards, each contain three condoms and a packet of lubricant, and bear the term *kondom* (the Tok Pisin spelling of condom) in bold yellow lettering underneath the image of the national flag.

With activities geared to different levels of participation, PNG's multisectoral strategy provides the framework for working closely with local communities. In partnership with NACS, various nongovernmental organizations and churches have conducted numerous training workshops and peer education activities in workplaces, schools, and churches in urban and rural communities. Although these activities have been instrumental in imparting information and raising awareness, the preponderance of AIDS in the interventionist language of prevention has eclipsed communication about HIV and the multilayered factors that shape vulnerability to infection. Militaristic metaphors about waging a battle against the "killer disease," which feature prominently in the global discourse on HIV (Treichler 1999:31–32;

Waldby 1996), have found popular expression in PNG, including tropes about the "AIDS war" and awareness posters that depict traditionally clad warriors bearing shields in the shape of condoms (see Wardlow 2009:145).[19]

AIDS is a dominant theme in popular commentary about PNG's fate as a young nation, featuring alongside other negatives in narratives of development unrealized—corruption, crime, lawlessness, gender inequality, violence, the breakdown in government services—and is represented not so much as the consequence but the cause of such doom (Luker and Dinnen, eds. 2010). The epidemic has been cast as a security issue in assessments of PNG's political and economic viability, highlighted by some commentators as a major factor in a "failed state" prognosis (Windybank and Manning 2003:11). For many people, apocalyptic Christianity with its promise of cure through conversion provides the most meaningful framework for making sense of the epidemic, especially in areas of the country where Pentecostalism has a strong following (Eves 2003). Much of the talk framing HIV and AIDS is beset by the perceived threat of sexual deviance, sin, and the punishment of God, which inculcates a dreaded connection between sex and death and promotes fear as the prime motivation for behavior change (see Keck 2007:51). Such associations have intensified moralistic social responses in which stigma, shame, and blame are persistent expressions. The prevailing tone of "fear and loathing" (Hammar 2008) is increasingly punctuated by media reports and anecdotal accounts of witchcraft accusations and violent treatment, including banishment, of women and men living with HIV and AIDS, or believed to be HIV positive or sick with AIDS, by relatives and community members.[20]

The catchphrase "reaching down to the village level" is a common expression in Papua New Guinea, reflecting the "top-down/bottom-up" rhetoric of interventions that endorse participatory approaches to HIV prevention and care, meeting the willingness to take action with the promise of providing services. However, this hierarchical metaphor of intervention and service delivery tends to overlook the social connections and interactions that operate *within* local communities and existing networks of communication and knowledge. Recommendations from the PNG National Summit on HIV Prevention, held in March 2006, called for intergenerational and intergender community conversations about HIV and AIDS to help people overcome fear and confusion, to diminish the reactions of stigma and blame, and to create supportive environments for behavior change.[21] The then minister for community development, Dame Carol Kidu, stated: "The challenge now is to move from generalized awareness to specific and focused community engagement so that communities become better equipped to respond to the emerging crisis in their families. We must now personalize the epidemic and bring the national response right inside our communities and homes" (NAC and UNAIDS 2006:12).

Increasingly, approaches to HIV prevention in Papua New Guinea reflect the growing consensus that the national response lies at the community level, grounded in local understandings and experiences. Over recent years, important work on HIV prevention and care has been implemented through a number of community-oriented projects that draw on shared values and relationships of identity and belonging (see, for example, Reid 2010). The development of the *National HIV Prevention Strategy, 2011–2015* (NAC 2010) involved many people and organizations in PNG that support communities to generate their own responses to the presence of HIV in their lives. Yet the power of quantitative models of meaning to determine what constitutes the "evidence base" for an effective response persists in tailoring approaches toward measurable outcomes, with little consideration for the complexities of context and place or for the unpredictabilities of implementation (see Merry 2011). Resistance to utilizing qualitative knowledge for strategy development reflects the position that such evidence is merely anecdotal and too complex and messy for monitoring and evaluating against standard indicators (Setel 2009). As principal author of the *National HIV Prevention Strategy*, I encountered such views from various technical advisers during the process of drafting the strategy. A comment on the first draft stated that incorporating qualitative evidence would open up a Pandora's box that would make the strategy too unwieldy. Finding a complementary balance between standardized strategies advocated at the global level and approaches that reflect local realities is one of the key challenges for responding to HIV.

CHAPTER 2

"In the Process of Knowing"

You know, we Trobriand people are not like other parts or places, our customs are different, about love and all this; they are really different from other places. If we, if the sickness comes—or maybe it is already here—and we are not faithful or honest to each other, then some years' time it will be a very big problem. Because what I heard from a health worker, there is no treatment and no cure and whoever is sick will die. I think we might have only a few people left.

—Elizabeth, aged early thirties, 29 July 2003

Because we are living in this place, we believe in our traditional customs. We are still believing.

—Amanda, twenty-year-old Trobriand woman, 24 June 2003

Custom is very, very important on Trobriand Islands. Through custom come realities. Belief becomes reality.

—Ethel Jacob, community leader, 23 September 2003

These three statements by Trobriand women of differing generations distill the central question of how HIV and models of prevention are understood in relation to cultural knowledge, sexual values, and practices. Generalized assumptions and moralities about sexual behavior and the risk of disease, which permeate global HIV prevention orthodoxy, are both contested and incorporated into local models of meaning as Trobrianders contemplate the presence of HIV in their lives.

As in other parts of rural Papua New Guinea, estimates of the number of people living with HIV in the Trobriands are highly speculative, given limited primary health services and the absence of HIV voluntary counseling and testing facilities (VCT).[1] At the time this research was undertaken in 2003, only a few Trobrianders had direct experience with the clinical and social manifestations of diagnosed HIV seropositivity. There were several unconfirmed reports of people returning home to the Trobriands after having tested HIV-antibody positive in urban centers, and there were a few anecdotal reports of people dying from HIV-related illness. AIDS was speculated to be the probable cause of death in a number of instances, especially if the deceased suffered prolonged, degenerative illness after having traveled or resided outside of the islands. Speculation was based as well on the numbers of deceased arriving in coffins from other parts of the country for burial at home.

In 2001, the first confirmed case of HIV was reported by the Losuia District Health Center after serum testing was conducted at the Central Public Health Laboratory in Port Moresby. The district health extension officer (HEO) requested the test after the patient failed to respond to drug treatment for diagnosed tuberculosis. The HEO called this the "first homegrown case" because the patient had never traveled outside of Kiriwina (T. Elliot, HEO, pers. comm.). Only seventeen years old, the female patient died at home in the village within six months of confirmed diagnosis. A further confirmed case in 2004 involved a pregnant woman in her early twenties, diagnosed during routine antenatal testing while residing in Port Moresby. Her baby died at three months of age and the young woman died a month later after returning home to the Trobriands to bury the child.

Notwithstanding the indeterminacy of HIV prevalence in the Trobriand population, the discursive presence of the epidemic is palpable. The islands are inundated with the paraphernalia of the national awareness campaign—caps, T-shirts, posters. AIDS awareness stickers are used to decorate schoolbooks and betel-nut lime containers, and they appear on house walls and doors. Talk about HIV and AIDS has also gained prominence through various community-based awareness activities and the informal exchange of information. The last several years have seen an increase in HIV training workshops for health workers, teachers, local government officials, and church and community leaders, organized through the provincial and district governments and the churches. Prior to my research in 2003, awareness activities were a component of two separate research projects conducted by the PNG IMR.[2] The Trobriand paramount chief has consistently endorsed the various activities over the years, reinforcing support and interest among community and church leaders.

A main channel for HIV communication in the Trobriands has been the village birth attendants (VBA) program. Established in the early 1990s with funding and technical support from UNICEF, the VBA program involves more than 140 women volunteers who have received basic training in clinical birthing procedures and reproductive health, including HIV awareness. Every village in the Trobriands has at least one trained VBA, and several villages have built birthing houses where the VBAs assist with deliveries. The VBA program also serves as a condom distribution network in the Trobriands. The volunteers collect free supplies of male condoms from the district health center and provide them on request to both males and females in their villages. The effectiveness of the VBA program in providing information on HIV and distributing condoms varies from village to village and largely depends on the commitment of individual volunteers, their status and recognition in their respective communities, and the ongoing support they receive from program management.

The process of engendering awareness about HIV, and making sense of its invisible presence in the Trobriands, is succinctly described by Diana Siyotama Lepani, one of the three Trobriand women who collaborated with me on my research.[3]

"Awareness." We use this word for its English meaning when talking about HIV/AIDS. Those not used to hearing this word think of it with AIDS, like "AIDS awareness." The two go together. We should think of it as still in the process of learning. Also, it tells how people are accepting something, taking the knowledge with them. The Kiriwina word is *nikoli*, knowledge, or *bitaninikolisi*, we are still in the process of knowing.[4] But using the English "awareness" captures it the best. It highlights it because it is English. This sickness is a new thing so a new word can be useful for thinking about it. [Interview notes, 29 August 2003]

In awareness about AIDS in Trobriand Islands it's a good thing because people come to realize the bad side of behavior—the outbreak of the virus. It is a learning point, a turning point. Knowing about sexual organs, knowing about personal feelings, keeping these things in mind. Turn back, look at the back and see what we have done, and look forward and be careful. [Taped group discussion, 19 September 2003. Translated into English.]

Diana made the first statement to me during one of the many conversations we had sitting on a pandanus mat on the concrete floor of her cookhouse, which she fashioned out of a disused shed at the Oiabia United Church mission station. At the time, Diana and her family lived at the old station, a vestige of colonial years, where her husband managed the church canteen. In addition to the basic food provisions sold at the canteen, Diana sometimes had a supply of generic-brand condoms available free of charge on request.[5] The second statement is a translated excerpt from Diana's concluding remarks during a village group discussion. Diana was speaking to a group of over seventy men, women, and children assembled in the church building in Kuruvitu, an isolated village located on the swampy northwest side of Kiriwina.

Diana's explanation about the meaning of AIDS awareness in the Trobriands alludes to the reciprocal ways in which different knowledge systems interact and inform one another. She explains how "awareness" is a new concept that encapsulates the new phenomenon of AIDS, yet she draws a meaningful parallel to the Trobriand concept of knowledge production. She also hints at the confrontation that results when cultural understandings of sexuality are recast by introduced moral constructions. Behavior assumes a "bad side" in terms of the consequences of a viral epidemic. Most significantly, Diana's insights are instructive for what they reveal about pace and temporality in the production of knowledge, how we continually engage in acts of accepting and taking new knowledge with us as we turn reflectively back and look forward. Awareness, or the ongoing process of knowing, is a directed movement made visible by purposive activity that is socially constituted, relational, and evaluative. The transformation of behavior is an ongoing process, not a one-time event, and it takes varied directions for different people in diverse contexts. Diana's articulation of "knowledge-in-action" is akin to anthropological insights for public health interventions that emphasize "the situated and constructed nature of knowledge as it is used in social interactions" (Yoder 1997:141). Facilitating conceptual connections between ideas and actions requires sustained communication to illuminate the social structures, processes, and practices that create pathways for HIV transmission.

Diana's observations about the process of knowing also call to mind the dialectics of ethnography: "the knowledge process must be initiated by confrontation that becomes productive through communication" (Fabian 2001:25). Ethnographic research elicits and productively sustains the dialogic exchange of viewpoints. In my research process, the invisible presence of HIV in the Trobriands was the prompt by which communication took place in an interactive, reciprocal way. Information about HIV initiated a process of reflection on cultural meanings and embodied experience, and cultural knowledge in turn provided the medium for clarifying information about HIV prevention. The process was charged with articulations of fear of an unseen and impending sickness, ambiguity about the likelihood of a full-scale epidemic, and a fervent readiness to "turn back," as Diana puts it, in order to effect change toward an uncertain future. As people collectively and individually contemplated and talked about the causes and effects of a looming epidemic in their lives, and as they confronted their own selves as readily as the abstract notions of an invisible virus, the process revealed how different ways of knowing converge and interact to coproduce meaning.

Making HIV Visible

When we got the awareness, we are all afraid of AIDS, so we are asking, do you have any ideas to help us see this thing, to help us with our feeling about AIDS, to help us understand about AIDS so we won't be afraid? [Taped group discussion, 19 August 2003. Translated into English.]

This statement about fear of the unseen and unknown qualities of HIV was one of the most supplicatory questions that confronted me during fieldwork. The speaker was a middle-aged woman who actively participated in a group discussion in Kiriwina language with about twenty women of mixed ages, all seated on a large communal platform next to the church deacon's house in their village. The woman's question demonstrates how important dialogue and social interaction are to the production of knowledge. The question is a provocative reminder of the significance of emotional understandings in the process of knowing. The question also is an example of how perfunctory "awareness" information typically invokes fear about AIDS without supporting conceptual connections between viral transmission and the manifestation of illness. It underscores the need for sustained communication, once initial "awareness" is delivered, to enable the ongoing process of knowing.[6] On a more troubling level, the woman's question confronted me with the ethical responsibilities of ethnographic engagement, the imperative "to consider a way of understanding that values the ethical and emotional responses invoked by our participation and observation" (Mallett 2003:244) and the obligation to answer questions and not simply ask them.

The woman's question was voiced midway through our open-ended discussion when the observation was made by one participant that because AIDS has no cure, *kariga* (death) will surely come from it, making it distinctly different from other *katoula* (illness) that can be treated and cured. The comparison made about treatment shifted the focus to *sovasova*, the illness caused by the breach of the Trobriand incest taboo, when members of the same clan have sexual relations (see Chapter 6). The women explained to me how clear signs and symptoms herald the onset of the illness—weight loss, nausea, and malaise—and how affected people use various herbal and magical treatments to effectively manage *sovasova*. They also reflected on the sexual practice that brings about *sovasova* and how people can avoid the illness altogether by simply not having sex with a fellow clan member. The relative visibility of *sovasova* as the certain outcome of sexual transgression makes prevention a viable option—disclosing clan identity to a potential sexual partner is straightforward. Available treatment allows potential breach to become a safe possibility, albeit socially undesirable. Our ensuing discussion teased out broad comparisons between *sovasova* and HIV as sexually transmitted infections, and between the similar signs and symptoms of *sovasova* and AIDS, demonstrating how established cultural models of disease etiology provide interpretive frames for making sense of new phenomena (see Farmer 1990). But the discussion came up against the standard slogan used in HIV awareness in PNG at the time—"AIDS has no treatment or cure"—and that was when the woman posed her question.

How did I answer the request for help to see the invisible virus and understand it so that fear might be transformed through insight? My immediate response was a hesitant pause, and I began rehearsing in my mind a battery of my own unanswered questions. How can HIV awareness draw on cultural constructions of illness to better enable prevention? How can awareness shift from a preoccupation with the signs and symptoms of disease, inciting responses of fear and dread, to focus instead on sexual practice and HIV prevention? And most pressing, how do I ethically respond with an answer that exposes the inadequacy of HIV awareness when it is not met by services? In fact, there *are* treatments for HIV infection, but the treatments, particularly antiretroviral drugs, are not readily available in PNG, where the national health system struggles to provide the rudiments of primary health care and where even basic supplies of antibiotics are chronically lacking in rural health facilities. Such an admission brings into sharp relief the global and local inequities of access to knowledge as well as resources, where information is negated by the inability to act.

The anxiety of knowing that resources are not yet in place to deal with an impending epidemic was expressed candidly to me by Ridley Mwaisiga, a health extension officer at the district health center: "With concern from a health point of view, I don't feel secure or confident that we can handle HIV positives or AIDS cases. It is very difficult to say that we can manage. We have no equipment to receive any patient; our health facilities cannot cater for full-time care of patients. We rely on guardians to look after their relatives in the wards. We are lacking on HIV counseling, no skills, no training" (Interview notes, 10 December 2003).

The disparities in resource distribution that affect local capacities to respond to HIV intensify the ambiguities that pervade HIV communication. As happened at other times during the course of my research when such questions were posed in interviews and discussions, I found myself trying to match information about HIV with contextual realities—indeed, the quandary between information and access to available resources and services is commonly encountered in rural Papua

New Guinea. Our discussion touched on these disparities, but my answer to the woman's question involved what may have seemed like circuitous logic. Reflection on sexual practice makes the virus visible and helps redirect fear toward prevention. Once the virus is conceptually visible, no longer abstract, then possibilities for prevention become viable. Diana encouraged the women to "turn back" and to engage in *nanamsa*, or reflection. Our discussion was then recharged with more talk about *sovasova* and notions of risk, sexual liaisons, infidelities, and ambivalent feelings about condom use.

The process of knowing reveals that meanings and practices can be "modified and transformed in reflection on past events" (Kippax and Crawford 1993:257). Reflective evaluation is also a key empirical concern for research on sexual behavior, where methods for obtaining and validating information rely almost exclusively on people's verbal statements, evaluations, and self-representations (Friedl 1994:834). The confrontational prompts and the reflexive process of research create opportunities for people to reconsider what is often taken for granted on an experiential level.[7]

The recurring strand of uncertainty about the presence of HIV was expressed in nearly every interview and group discussion during the course of my research. People repeatedly confronted me with the question, "We don't know what HIV looks like, so how do we know if it is really here in the Trobriand Islands?" This conundrum points to the paradoxical nature of the virus, particularly in places like Papua New Guinea where the burden of other infectious diseases is already significant. HIV is symptomatically invisible because its debilitating effects on the immune system are masked by the familiar illnesses of tuberculosis, pneumonia, and malaria. HIV is diagnostically invisible because confirmatory testing is not a readily accessible option throughout much of the country. HIV is officially invisible to assure confidentiality to protect against stigma and discrimination.

To an important extent, the uncertainty expressed by Trobrianders as they consider the biomedical representations of HIV and AIDS relates to the ontogeny of the virus and the perplexing length of time it takes—anywhere from two to ten years—for the effects of its presence to become apparent in a human host. The invisibility of HIV and the temporal hiatus between initial infection and manifest illness does not easily support a conceptual link between sexual practice and viral infection, nor does it necessarily compel immediate action to minimize and prevent potential transmission. Fear of the manifestation of AIDS has been widely induced by the language of prevention, yet this fear intersects with an equally unsettling ambivalence about the urgency of the problem. Trobrianders find it hard to conceptualize a manifestation of illness as something that has no treatment or cure, either medical or magical. This is tied in with complex questions of cause and effect, whether explained by witchcraft or germ theory or a combination of both, and questions of agency, how bodies are subject to the intentions of others, and the appropriate social responses to the consequences of social action.

HIV's invisibility holds the challenge of compelling action before the foretold problem has announced its presence in a way that demands an immediate response (see Pigg 2001a). The challenge calls for the productive interaction of different ideas and values to make visible the possibility of preventive action. Community-based

HIV awareness activities in the Trobriands typically rehearse the standard epidemiological checklist of sexual risk behaviors: early onset of sexual activity, multiple
and concurrent sexual partners, high prevalence of sexually transmitted infections,
and low levels of condom use. Less often do such exercises move out from the standard model of risk to consider the "biological synergism" between HIV and other
pathogens, and how they interact with the social environment (Singer and Clair
2003:428). In the Trobriands, this involves immune systems compromised by endemic malaria, high rates of pneumonia and other respiratory infections, increased
cases of tuberculosis across all ages, and limited infrastructure and resources for
the provision of integrated primary health services (see Stillwaggon 2006). Less
often, as well, does awareness about HIV attempt to identify structural factors
that create potential pathways for HIV transmission, such as increased mobility
between the Trobriands and urban centers, intensified commercial trade networks
through maritime travel, limited income-earning opportunities within the local
economy, and greater population pressure on a finite resource base.

Yet, as Elizabeth's statement in the epigraph indicates, many Trobrianders
readily identify aspects of "custom" that might facilitate viral transmission: the
sexual freedom of young unmarried men and women, which for many involves
having multiple sexual partners; the period of abstinence during pregnancy and
lactation, when women acknowledge that their husbands are likely to have other
sexual partners; the mutability of marital status; the mobility of exchange relations,
including the traditional Kula trade ring, which hold opportunities for expanding
sexual networks; and *milamala*, the annual season of yam harvest festivities when
ancestral spirits return to the world of the living and sexuality is celebrated.[8]

In spite of the ready indictment of the role of culture in contributing to HIV
transmission, the specter of AIDS as a "killer disease" wrought by sexual excess
and transgression is not easily accommodated by Trobriand models of sexuality
and disease. Talking about HIV prevention through reflective evaluation is fraught
with contradictions when practices defined by cultural values are held against morally inflected discourse that frames sexuality in terms of "risk," "promiscuity," and
the imperative for behavior change. Trobriand mediations of HIV prevention involve reconciling the fear of sickness and death, and the behaviors attributed to
HIV transmission and infection, with sexual practices that are culturally valued as
life-affirming acts that build and reinforce social relations.

Countering the epidemiological framework of risk are aspects of Trobriand society that may serve to allay the potential impact of HIV. Social cohesion, principles of reciprocation and consent, and the overall level of societal wealth are key
variables in diminishing a society's susceptibility to HIV infection (Barnett and
Whiteside 2002:88–96). How might the ideology of matrilineal kinship and social
regeneration that avows gender equality, and a particular history that has engendered a resilient cultural identity, provide Trobrianders with a strong collective position from which to mediate new phenomena? How might a sexual culture that
values consensual, pleasurable sex as part of a young person's physical and social
development into adulthood provide the basis for HIV prevention? Exploring these
dimensions of the Trobriand ethnoscape provides a critical standpoint for making
visible the interactions between culture and HIV.

"Everything Has Come Up to the Open Space"

I think that to our culture . . . it is really *tambu* [taboo] to talk about sex. And sitting with men and women together, especially with men and women we cannot talk about it. Unless there is only women around or there is only men then they can, you know, talk about it in their way. But times have come and passed and I feel now it is open, it is already open to anybody or everybody who can sit down and talk about it. To me, what I see and hear, it's already open. But now, open space, how will I say this? Yes, maybe, yes, the time when the change takes place. Because what our sister has said, that is one part of this, unless you sleep with the man you won't get your period and the other one is when you sleep with the man then you will have your *nunu* [breasts]. Everything has come up to the open space. Words and actions and all these things. That's why things have already changed, a very big change. Now it is twelve years of age, a kid can have sex. Before, no. Taboo. But I heard from my granny, it was about that age, too. It's the natural feeling, how will I explain? [Bomi, age late thirties, taped group discussion, 24 November 2000]

The metaphor of "open space" is useful for describing a mutual site of interaction for translating different models of meaning and for consolidating collective knowledge and action for HIV prevention. The metaphor suggests a multivocal common ground for talking, listening, and exchanging points of view. In a group discussion on sexuality with about twenty women of mixed ages, Bomi evoked the metaphor to describe how social barriers have been broken, issues have come into the open and are no longer hidden, and people are able to sit down and talk about sex.

In the Trobriands, and elsewhere throughout PNG, kinship and gender relations influence ways of talking and listening and determine who can or cannot talk in the presence of whom and in what context. These sensitivities and protocols have implications for how to approach communication about sexuality and HIV in different settings (Vete 1995:136–37). At times customary protocols silence particular voices and perspectives and inhibit the sharing of information and knowledge between different social categories of rank and status, men and women, and elders and young people (see Brison 1992). For some people, religious doctrine impedes the ability to discuss sexuality openly in relation to the HIV epidemic. Yet the efficacy of imparting information and knowledge in open space—whether the small intimate spaces shared by peer groups or the large spaces of public meetings—draws on long-standing traditions of collective gathering, witnessing, and storytelling. Talk actively constructs social reality and has the power to reproduce or alter beliefs and social relations (Brison 1992:5).

Bomi also uses the metaphor to consider the transitional phase of puberty in relation to a Trobriand belief that sexual activity helps young girls grow and mature into fertile women. She then explains her view that young people in the Trobriands are engaging in sex at an earlier age, inferring that social change has accelerated the transition from puberty to adulthood.[9] Open space is transitional and transformational; it exposes what was previously discreet and concealed, it brings together what was previously distinct and separate, and it symbolizes the factors of development that influence people's behaviors and the cultural meanings attached to behaviors. The dynamics of open space induce change, transforming the landscape with new opportunities, risks, and desires.

After pronouncing that "everything has come up to the open space," Bomi hints at a cultural conundrum—Trobriand society is experiencing a period of great change, yet maybe things have not changed all that much. Maybe part of what is being experienced is the way cultural meanings are measured against—and safeguarded from—the factors of change, including new ways of talking—"It's the natural feeling, how will I explain?" An initial interpretation of Bomi's difficulty in explaining the early onset of sexual activity falls back on the universalist notion of sexuality as a "natural" bodily function. Sex is something that people *do*, not something about which people talk.[10] By inference, the problem of explanation also suggests that other pedagogical forms, such as stories, jokes, chants, and dance, more readily explicate sexual desire. The taboo regarding talking about sex does not preclude other modes of communication (Vete 1995).

A second reading of Bomi's statement underscores how the specter of AIDS confronts people with moralistic and authoritative judgments about their lives and ways of being. She hints at the difficulty of talking about sex when the prevailing discourse undercuts cultural meanings and delimits the acceptable truth value of articulated beliefs. At times, perhaps, equivocation is a better recourse than exegesis, insulating cultural consciousness from exposure to contradictory moral codes. Bomi's hesitation to elaborate also suggests that, "although subjective and personal, sexuality remains beyond the capacity of individuals to define at will in terms of identity and consciousness" (Setel 1999:16). The layered sedimentation of patterns of practice inhibits attempts at exegesis even in times of great transition and transformation. The language of HIV has the potential to rupture these deep layers of cultural meaning and expose established forms of sexual practice to new, potentially negative, evaluations. Philip Setel's ethnography of HIV in northern Tanzania demonstrates how "the disordering effects of the epidemic are simultaneously creative of new meanings and revealing of long-standing values which surround social reproduction" (1999:16). Encountering HIV prevention messages that construct sexuality in terms of risk may prompt resistance to such distancing rhetoric, or may simply lead to avoidance and disinterest rather than promoting dialogic exchange of information and reflective evaluation of practice (see Herdt 2001).

Both cultural continuity and change inhere in the process of knowledge production. People's perceptions and understandings of HIV and AIDS change over time with direct exposure to the virus and the changing experience of living with the effects of an unfolding epidemic (Farmer 1990, 1992b). Knowledge is not accessed evenly or conclusively but takes differential forms and tempos depending on social position and historical context. Yet the pedagogy of HIV awareness assumes instantaneous cognitive assimilation of the information by everyone in the same way, with little consideration given to the divergent local phases of an emerging epidemic.

Moreover, the timing of qualitative research affects the eliciting of perspectives on HIV. It "calls attention to the problems inherent in studying cultural meaning while it is taking shape" (Farmer 1992b:287). Research activates the process of mediating new information within existing frameworks of meaning, and in doing so creates moments of disjuncture and incoherence, as well as moments of clarity and revision.

Knowledge as Social Process

Sociality, or the "creating and maintaining of relationships" (Strathern 1988:13), is a salient aspect of knowledge production in the Trobriand cultural context and throughout Melanesia and the Pacific, where social relations centered on kinship and networks of exchange shape personhood and form the basis for action. Such constructions of relational personhood, where persons are "the plural and composite site of the relationships that produced them" (Strathern 1988:13), are made visible and activated in multiple ways by culturally constituted forms of practice.

Situating knowledge in the social person brings into sharper focus the values and practices of sexual expression and embodied experience. The concept of "sexual culture" has been used productively in social research on HIV to underscore the diversity of ideologies that construct the social and personal experience of human sexuality across cultures and over time, and the life processes through which shared beliefs and values are reproduced (Herdt 1997, 1999; Parker 2009; Parker and Ehrhardt 2001; Parker and Gagnon, eds. 1995). More specifically, the concept brings into focus the interaction between cultural discourse and lived experience (Tuzin 1991:872), the connections and disjunctions between people's idealized statements and what they actually do.

But what of the singular sexed and gendered bodies that *koap*, the bodies that put on condoms (or not), the bodies that abort, give birth, get injected with Depo Provera contraceptive every three months, the bodies that test positive or negative for HIV?[11] Questions of embodied practice bring to the fore the "living, palpitating flesh and blood organism," which Malinowski (1934:xxxi) urged students of anthropology not to lose sight of in their interpretations of culture. The embodied self is the "existential ground of culture" (Csordas 1990), reproducing, resisting, and transforming established forms of practice through routine performativity or deliberate actions (see Ahearn 2000; Butler 1995; Ortner 1996). Agency locates the self in relation to others, elucidating how knowledge-in-action is contingent on social interaction.

Viewing agency in terms of relational personhood contrasts with models that "firmly anchor the self to a body" (Becker 1995:4–5), the autonomous individual who acts on self-interest, independent of mutual social relations. In this formulation, agency becomes a central concept for apprehending the behavior-change model for HIV prevention, which locates the individual moral actor as the site of public health interventions—the body that chooses to abstain from sex, be faithful to one partner, or use condoms. But not only singular bodies take in and act on information. Communities of bodies, which share collective identity and purpose, also act as key mediators between the social actor and the structures that shape arenas of action.

A distinctive feature of the HIV awareness sessions held as part of my research in the Trobriands was how the whole village—women, men, and children of all ages and social positions—gathered together to host the visit and collectively participate in the exchange of information. Such collective engagement to enable individual and interpersonal activation of knowledge about HIV prevention underscores how the process of knowing is inherently social. Approaches to HIV prevention that recognize the potency of place in mediating knowledge and behavior, and that ensue from a common ground of social relatedness, have far greater potential to turn the process of knowing into the practice of knowing and doing.

CHAPTER 3

Connections to Place

Research journal, 28 November 2000

My first day in the field.

Igau! [Wait!] This calls for an aside. Look how easily a tired formula fixes itself on paper. Who do I think I'm writing for anyway? "The field," indeed! This is the Trobriands. This is Orabesi village. This is my mother-in-law's house. I am at home with *yawagu* [my mother-in-law] Sarah. Since when did the Trobs become "the field" in my sense of place and positioning? Since I became a student in the field of anthropology?

I am overwhelmed by a rush of familiarity and I find myself looking for nuanced change. What I see and hear is measured by recall, by sensory memories, by relationships already established and sustained, by perceptions already elaborated in reflection and interpretation. There is one significant difference to this re-entry: of all my prior trips this is my first time to come on my own. I have arrived with notebook in hand.

"*Ambesa vivila latum, kasusu?*" [Where is your daughter, your last-born child?] The disappointment expressed by all who come to greet me is persistent, an incredulity that demands an explanation. Bubu Sarah went to the airstrip to welcome her eight-year-old granddaughter. I was pleasantly surprised to see her when I stepped down from the plane, not expecting her to have made the twenty-minute drive on the back of the truck to be there upon my arrival. She greeted me with affection, a soft embrace and deep inhale with her nose rubbing against my cheek. "Oh, *yawagu, yawagwe, kapisi!*" [Oh, my daughter-in-law, daughter-in-law (emphasis), I am sorry for you!]. But her disappointment was not concealed. Where is Veitania? How can I travel here without her, arrive home on my own?

In important ways, this solitary arrival carries a clear message: I am here to do my work. *Ulo paisewa ginigini* [my writing work]. In a society where productive labor is given form through social relations, where people are defined by their relationships, where I have always been defined by my children and the father of my children and my in-laws, I have been given leeway to be defined by my work. This is significant and it is a privilege. My presence takes on a different meaning—a different status, perhaps—and people are making space for me. I am being accommodated in a new social space. So, this is the field, this "spatial practice of dwelling."

Affinity in the Field: Doing Research as an In-Law

My connections to the Trobriands have been woven into the lineage of place since 1978, through marriage, childbearing, and my position as *vevai*, or in-law. In the early years of marriage, my learning about Trobriand culture was through attentive watching and doing, not questioning. To question felt like second-guessing, an intrusive and objective interrogation of what I thought should become apparent through passive absorption and mimesis. Increasingly, I became interested in turning my embedded familiarity with the Trobriands into a relationship defined by research and to shift my position from passive participant to active observer.

My sense of solitariness as I reentered the familiar field of my chosen research site functioned as a form of spatial distancing to allow my work to redefine my presence, with the objective of translating "ongoing experience and entangled relationship into something distanced and representable" (Clifford 1997:57). The conspicuous absence of my children and husband on my arrival gave heightened clarity to the reconfiguration of my relational field. Transforming my sphere of accustomed relationality into a site for focused study did not suspend or transcend established social relations. Rather, embarking on ethnographic fieldwork, and this new "spatial practice of dwelling" (Clifford 1997:57), gave fresh contours to well-defined relationships. As a transient member of a household in which I had ongoing personal and social investment, I was critically aware of the newly drawn distinctions inscribed by my role as researcher.[1]

Papua New Guineans commonly declare their marital status and affinal ties by referring to place rather than by naming their partner. "Mi marit long Trobs" (I am married to the Trobriands) is how I avow my status in Tok Pisin, situating myself and asserting my identity in the social landscape of belonging. The value of connections to place, and the social relations that make these connections apparent, generates credibility and legitimacy for conducting social research on HIV. Many of my PNG colleagues involved in the national response to HIV regarded my decision to do research in the place of my affiliation as both intuitive and commonsense. The engagement of *asples* researchers[2] in HIV-related research is viewed as pragmatic and principled, cognizant of the diversity of languages and cultures in the PNG context and the need to work collaboratively with communities through established social networks.

The assertion of social relations as a methodological principle in social research collapses the bifurcation of home and field (Visweswaran 1994:113). My scholarly work transposed a new spatial delineation onto familial space, yet this reconfiguring of the Trobriands as the research "field" had an interdependent and complementary effect. Concurrently, my research connected both the home and field of Port Moresby with the Trobriands, drawing in and on my established familial and professional networks in the urban center. This translocal orientation is a patent reminder that neither the geography nor the cultural world of the Trobriands— nor the ethnographic process—is located in an isolated, closed, or distant field (Peirano 1998).

My interest in social research on HIV stems from my experience as coordinator for the development of Papua New Guinea's first national HIV/AIDS multisectoral strategy in 1997. Since then, my ongoing personal and professional involvement in HIV policy and program development at regional, national, and local levels has provided grounding and orientation for pursuing research, and contributes to the validity of my ethnographic purpose. Moving in and out of different fields of engagement in HIV work—between formulating strategies, reviewing projects, and facilitating workshops—and the fields of engagement in research—between ethnographic emplacement and academic distantiation—has productively sharpened and moderated multiple perspectives and positions, my own as well as those of others.

The subject of HIV itself challenges the schisms between different sites of knowledge, competence, and capacity for action. Not only do the movement and transmissibility of the virus, and its multiple representations, transcend demarcations of place, but the actions required to respond comprehensively to the epidemic, where local capacity is intimately tied to technical support, resources, and services that come from national and global sources, also collapse the distinctions between inside and outside. Dichotomous representations are exposed as well, not only in anthropological framings of self and other, but in the epidemiology of risk and the persistent othering in discourses of vulnerability, stigma, and presumed responsibility for viral transmission, or what Paul Farmer has termed the "geography of blame" (1992a). The distancing between authorized strategies and informally scripted responses has made me acutely aware of the discursive power of HIV to discredit and harm people and communities when the language of prevention fails to connect with the complexities of lived experience. The well-intentioned strategies that call for community-based, participatory approaches to HIV prevention and care are eclipsed by interventionist models that circumscribe sites of risk as somewhere out there and other than, beyond the familiar spheres of relationality. Social research brings us back into the shared, open spaces of mutual accountability.

Shared Presence

Just as home and field are malleable and transposable, the multiple subject positions and lived connections that inform ethnographic research unsettle the dichotomous configuration of insider and outsider. In an oft-cited essay that questions "the fixity of a distinction between 'native' and 'non-native' anthropologists," Kirin Narayan argues for textual enactments of hybridity, or the multiple identities and situated knowledge that reveal how ethnographers belong "simultaneously to the world of engaged scholarship and the world of everyday life" (1993:671–72). Narayan asserts that "the issue of who is an insider and who is an outsider is secondary to the need for dismantling objective distance to acknowledge our shared presence in the cultural worlds that we describe" (680).

One of the most valued aspects of my ethnographic research was my extended shared presence in the daily life of the household of my widowed *yawagu* (mother-in-law), Sarah Watson, who was in her mid-seventies at the time.[3] *Yawagu* also valued this continuity of presence, as she herself expressed to me frequently. "Saina bwena yokwa bogwa bukusimwa baisatuta" (It is very good you stay this time). Being part of the world of everyday life in my mother-in-law's home enriched my ethnographic perspective in untold ways. The routine of my work fell into rhythm with my mother-in-law's daily routine, imbued by our reciprocal understanding of purpose and need, and mutual respect for *kaisisu*, our respective habits and daily concerns. My work was facilitated by the care and attention *yawagu* gave to my comfort and well-being. In turn, I supplemented the household provisions with additional resources and helped her attend to day-to-day obligations in a complex network of exchange relationships. I also was directly involved in supporting her preparations for numerous *sagali* throughout the period of my residence. I came to understand firsthand how the work of *sagali* is perpetual and passionate. "Sagali, sagali, sagali," *yawagu* often would sigh with resignation, patting the pile of folded pieces of material she was busily preparing and leaning back against the wall to rest and chew betel nut.

Living in Sarah's household at the time were two adult grandsons, a sixteen-year-old granddaughter, enrolled in grade 9 at Kiriwina High School, and the fifteen-year-old grandson of a neighbor, who was enrolled in grade 8 at Losuia Primary School. Throughout the period of my residence, various circumstances, events, and itinerant visitors reshaped the household composition. At one time during a *sagali*, the number of people eating and sleeping under the one roof swelled to twelve for several days; at other times there were just *yawagu*, my niece, and me. Members of the household were all aware of the purpose of my extended visit, but for personal and ethical reasons they did not directly participate in the study as discussants or interviewees.

Yawagu maintained tactful discretion in discussing the details of my research, but she was generous with her insights when asked. Often our quiet conversations at night would segue into long soliloquies and she would pour forth with memories or wonder philosophically about the unknown future. She would often end these conversations with an apologetic appeal that I forget everything she had just said and not write anything down in my notebook. Her request gave distinct clarity to what I saw as the permeability between home and field, but I was obliged to honor the division that she drew. However, the intimate interactions that defined our shared space and time together provided me with an empathic frame of reference to guide my understanding and representation of the broader field of interactions and articulations elicited in the course of research.

Scholarly work provided me the purpose of not just visiting but *living* in the Trobriands for a sustained period. It became apparent to me that many Trobrianders perceived and evaluated my extended presence not in terms of my research agenda but rather in terms of my demonstrated practice of a valued form of relationality. The work of sustaining affinal relations defined my identity and subject position foremost; my role as researcher was secondary. People would often express appreciation that I had come to live in the Trobriands, and they qualified this by saying, "Gala dimdim, yokwa yakidasi" (You are not a white person, you are one of us). As my work took me around the islands on foot, by truck, and by boat, strangers often greeted me with a praise of acceptance, "Eh, gala dimdim, yokwa kwaka-tubaiasa numwaiya Kiriwina!" (You are not a white person, you present yourself as a mature Trobriand woman), and they would admire the long, full, brightly colored cotton skirt I was wearing. My skirts were lovingly crafted by *yawagu*, sitting on the floor in the front room of her house, turning the crank on her old hand-operated Singer machine. As I moved about the islands doing my work, my public presence in these skirts projected the care and attention *yawagu* provided me as a member of her household. My embodied presence affirmed the productive value of affinal relations.

My presence also carried with it a constant social identifier that erased my *dimdim* otherness as a white foreigner. Everywhere my research activities took me in the Trobriands, I was recognized, welcomed, and introduced as Modudaiya *lakwava*, the wife of Charles Lepani, who lives with her mother-in-law, *nakakau* (widow) Sarah Watson, in Orabesi village. Calling Charles by the Lukwasisiga clan name his father, Lepani Watson, gave him—Modudaiya—evoked the legacy of *tomwaiya* (old man) and the important relationship Charles and his father shared in the domain of politics and public service.[4] Often when walking along village paths, I would overhear young children say to each other with aplomb, a flick of the eyebrows and heads nodding in my direction, "Numwaiya Modudaiya lakwava" (The married woman is the wife of Modudaiya). Young ones who had never seen Charles and were not even born when he returned home in 1994, to make *sagali* for his deceased father, reaffirmed through social recognition my sense of connectedness to the genealogy of place. Their assured appraisal of who I was securely emplaced me in the field of belonging.

My own children provide the essential pivot for my sense of belonging and social attachment to the Trobriands. This is not only because I am an outsider "marit long Trobs." The more I understand Trobriand society through sustained social attachment, the more apparent it becomes to me that offspring provide an essential basis for mediating and justifying social action. Children are the embodiment of the links between clans. I was adopted into my father-in-law's clan, Lukwasisiga, because of the imperative that my children have clan membership to give them identity and place of belonging, to guide their social obligations, and to carry their future. My children's clan membership activates my own affiliation as *vevai*; not only am I an in-law through marriage but I am an in-law through my children. Children expand the important network of *tabu*[5] interdependency in the reproduction of social relations (Weiner 1979:333) and provide motivation for acting with others in mind (Strathern 1988:272).

My daughter, Veitania, did indeed follow my solo arrival by several weeks in 2000, and then in 2003, when she was ten years old, she lived in the Trobs for the first three months of my residence. My daughter's presence added an important dimension to my own subject position and the way others viewed my presence. Through Veitania's experience and perspective, I gained experience and insights that would not have been accessible on my own. Her presence opened up conversations and allowed for interactions that would not otherwise have happened. In a collection of essays by various ethnographers who reflect on the experiences of having their children with them during fieldwork, Joan Cassell notes the effect of children's presence on ethnographic encounters: "The relationship between those who study and those who are studied becomes less interrogative, more dialogic. This mutual disclosure, where each is encouraged to observe, judge and interpret 'the other,' can lead to more profound understanding" (1987:259).

Enrolling Veitania in grade 5 at Losuia Primary School brought me into the classroom and into conversation with the teachers as a parent, not as a researcher.[6] Taking her to the crowded outpatient clinic for antibiotics when a small cut turned into a tropical ulcer, where we sat with other parents and sick children waiting for the health worker to call our ticket number, disclosed a different perspective on the health center from that which I had come to know as a researcher. I gained entry into the exclusive realm of childhood as the only adult tagging along with a group of twelve boys and girls from Orabesi, aged three to sixteen years, who took turns poling an old leaky dinghy up the coast to a secluded beach for an impromptu picnic outing. I watched in subdued appreciation as the girls set to work domesticating the sandy space, competently constructing temporary shelters out of gathered sticks and coconut fronds, and starting a fire from dried tinder to cook yams and bananas. The boys speared fish and impressed the girls with their abundant catch while vying for a glowing ember to start their own fire. I watched a ritual feat of negotiation that involved much teasing and cajoling before both sides mutually agreed to exchange fish for yams and cook the food all together in the one fire. With stomachs satisfied, the girls and boys having eaten at separate spots on the beach, they shared a dessert of betel nut and then challenged each other to diving feats and played flirtatious tag on the beach and in the bush. They huddled together during a sudden downpour, the older children attentive to the little ones, keeping them warm with T-shirts and towels, wiping their runny noses. I listened as their conversation turned to a hushed recounting of the recent deaths on the islands and speculations about cause and consequence. I listened as they embellished well-known ghost stories and then exchanged information about a recent episode of witchcraft at the high school involving spurned love, the boy suddenly struck by sickness in the classroom after a night visit from a young witch who fancied him.

Here was Malinowski's "Children's Republic" in action, as vibrant as ever, the collective agency and sociality of young people independent of, yet emulating in fine detail, the world of adults.[7] There was perhaps no other time when I felt more like an outsider than on this picnic, age setting me apart as well as an awkward self-consciousness that I was the only parent present because of some displaced sense of protectiveness I had about my daughter's safety in an unknown environment. My estrangement from my daughter and her new social world cast me as the maladroit *dimdim* observer, accommodated good-naturedly by my young companions—who perhaps even viewed me as a captive audience of one. But my presence was inconsequential. It was only during the long return trip home at twilight in the leaky dinghy—when my lap provided comfort for one of the tired little ones, her timidity replaced by unquestionable trust—that my sense of displacement faded and I felt intrinsically connected once again.

At Home in the Field

Indeed, children often unquestioningly reaffirmed my sense of connection to place. Once during a group interview with four mature-aged women at a village some distance from Orabesi, I was introduced to a three-year-old girl who was sitting in the lap of her mother's maternal aunt, a middle-aged woman who had adopted and weaned the young child, not having had children of her own. Told that I came from Orabesi, which was her father's village and where her parents were currently residing, the young girl's face lit up and she said to me, "Ikapisi lopogu! Orabesi mavalu!" (My belly is sorry for you! Orabesi is our [dual inclusive] place!).[8] The idiomatic expression of emotional affinity drew appreciative laughter from all of us sitting together on the shaded platform. While the adoptive mother expressed pride in her daughter's verbal alacrity, I felt the pride of emplacement disarmingly affirmed by the child. Such sentiments from one so young indicate how the value of place identity and connection develops early in life and carries with people as they move to different locales, shaping their social worlds.

My dwelling space in my mother-in-law's house in Orabesi village was a visual metaphor of the intrinsic yet partial connection I had to the field of home. Soon after my arrival in 2003, I arranged for the construction of my own room as an extension to my mother-in-law's house. Made from bush materials with coconut frond siding and sago palm roofing brought by Tomwaiya Lepani's relatives from Dobu,[9] the little room was a lean-to appendage on the front side of the main house. Even before the room was built, I had commissioned the carpenter at Kiriwina High School to make me a table. Apart from being a practical and indispensable furnishing for the embodied work of research, the table was a symbol of how home was also the field, demarcating my place of work in the shared domestic space.

Trobriand *bwala*, or family dwellings, are by design small and intimate enclosures of only one or two rooms, used mainly as private spaces for storing material possessions, resting, sleeping, taking shelter from inclement weather, and retreating from the activity of village life. The houses are raised on posts a meter or so above the ground, with pole steps leading up to a small veranda at the single entrance. The square or rectangular dwellings are constructed with sapling frames and rafters lashed together with split bark and vines; the walls and roof are made of pandanus or coconut-frond matting or, alternatively, woven sago bark. The diminutive houses are built close together in residential clusters called *katupolusa* (hamlets), based on *dala* groupings. Covered or open-air cooking areas are usually adjacent to the family *bwala*, although some houses have an interior hearth. The sitting platforms on food storage houses, also built next to family dwellings, are the shaded communal spaces where people gather informally to socialize.

Most villages have a communal water tank for rainwater catchment, or they have manual or solar-powered pumps that feed water from underground wells to a series of communal taps. Latrines are uncommon in villages, and people use the bush or mangroves for their toilet. People bathe with water from underground springs or in the coral pools along the shoreline that fill with fresh water during low tide. The separate male and female bathing pools for Orabesi are sheltered by the mangroves in the lagoon, located across the gravel road from the village down a path that cuts through a block of bush land that people refer to with euphemistic humor as *Igidimati* (literally, "they [singular] are busting!").

Orabesi is nestled between the old Methodist mission station at Oiabia and Kiriwina High School, on the southern coast of the main island of Kiriwina. It is located just off the western end of the main coastal road, which connects the two neighboring coastal villages to the west—Mulosaida and Kavataria—to Losuia (see Map 2). With a fluctuating population of approximately three hundred people,

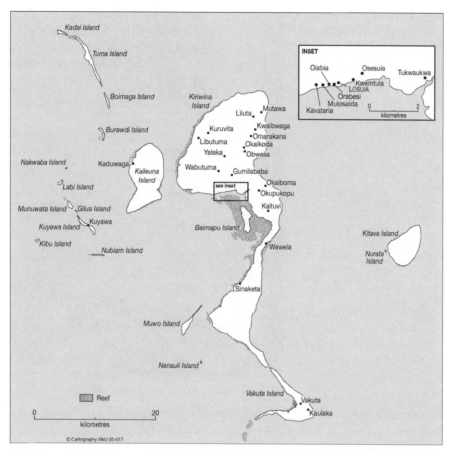

MAP 2. • Trobriand Islands showing villages visited during the course of research.
Courtesy of Cartographic-GIS Services, The Australian National University.

and forty-eight households, Orabesi was established by the first generation of retired Trobriand Methodist missionaries and parishioners in the early 1960s, on
land previously used for gardening. My mother-in-law's house is set back from the
main road at the entrance to Orabesi, adjacent to the church building on the path
leading into the center of the village. Known locally as Kountryside (spelled with
a K) because of its proximity to Losuia, the area encompasses several hamlets and
extends down to Kiriwina High School and the two main trade stores located opposite each other on the road. The grassy expanse of land where *yawagu*'s house
stands is affectionately called Kaugere, a nostalgic reference to the Port Moresby
settlement established during the colonial administration in the 1950s to accommodate the first generation of indigenous public servants. Lepani and Sarah Watson resided in Kaugere for a number of years when Lepani was a government clerk
and welfare officer, and their house was a focal point for the Milne Bay migrant
community living in Port Moresby at the time.

My mother-in-law's three-room dwelling, with an attached interior cooking
area, is spacious compared to most Trobriand houses. Raised on stilt posts and

FIGURE 3.1. • Sarah Watson sitting on the front steps of her house in Kaugere, Orabesi village, 2003

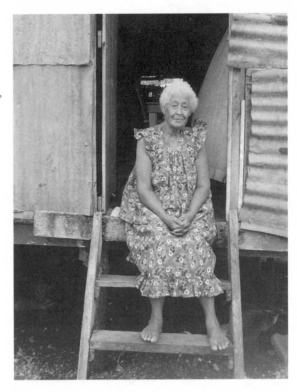

made from a combination of sawn timber and woven sago bark with a corrugated iron roof, it has a high ceiling and enough floor space in the front room to lay out a spread of food on the mat and invite a dozen people to sit around comfortably and share a meal. Three flat timber steps lead up to the entrance, which is always wide open during the day, making the interior a welcoming space. Just as the Kaugere house in Moresby was always open to the community, so too is the Kaugere house back home in the Trobs. This is Sarah's way of being, her *kaisisu*, and the legacy of her deceased husband. In my mother-in-law's house there is a continual flow of people dropping in for a chew of betel nut and a cup of sweet tea, and to exchange information and the latest news. Women in mourning will arrive at the doorstep and lean against the frame in deep sorrow, releasing an extended lament for their deceased relative—"This is the house that my loved one would always come to visit." On Saturdays, relatives come from distant villages laden with garden produce, and they sit and rest in the house before returning in the late afternoon after a good meal, never leaving empty-handed. And always there are the simple, mundane requests made at the doorstep—for an ember from the fire, a spare betel nut or two, a coconut to scrape for cooking the evening meal, some sugar or tea, a small amount of kerosene to light a lantern.

The physical location of the house on the main road gave me a unique vantage point to observe much of the pedestrian life of the village and the surrounding area. One of four communal water taps for the village is located on the side of the yard, and there is a steady stream of people throughout the day, mainly young girls, coming to fetch water in bottles, buckets, and large plastic containers. In front of the house is a large thatched roofed platform where people gather to talk, relax, and pass time together. The big grassy yard invites a host of communal activities, including impromptu ball games in the late afternoon, "Bring and Buy" fund-raising events organised by the OKO (Oiabia, Kountryside, Orabesi) Women's Fellowship, and *sagali* distributions. *Yawagu* and I would joke that the large door frame was like a TV screen—although I thought it offered better viewing.[10] Sitting inside the darkened house, we could look out the door and have a vivid picture of the world going by—the perpetual daytime pedestrian traffic on the main road, people walking on the track into Orabesi village, children playing, torpid dogs and petulant pigs, all set to the backdrop of lofty coconut palms fringing the lagoon.

Aesthetics of Belonging

Dawn arrives swiftly in the village and stirs into motion the routine of early morning activity. A succession of sharp clangs on the rusty metal bar hanging from the church roof beam declares the new day, the first of "three bells" marking communal units of time. Kaugere, our household pig, agitates the dawn with her distressed squeals of hunger, prodding us into the new day from under the house. Bosewaga rubs open her eyes, roused from her sleeping mat. The ten-year-old stands and straightens her twisted skirt, grabs the bucket of vegetable peelings and coconut gratings from the corner by the hearth, and releases the wooden door latch with her elbow. The door swings open and the sun spills in, cutting a sharp line of light across the timber floor. Bosewaga pauses at the steps to survey the morning. She looks across the grassy stretch and over the road to her parents' dwelling in Kountryside for a hint of her little sister already awake and playing on the veranda. Dawn enlivens the road with young boys from Mulosaida and Kavataria hastily carrying poles on their shoulders strung with the night catch of small reef fish. Young girls follow the sunrise with lilting song, walking in twos and threes down the pathway to the tide pool, balancing dirty cooking pots on their heads and toddlers on their hips. Small siblings traipse alongside them, trailing their towels. Girls and women gather at the communal tap, the bubbling flow of pumped water filling an assortment of plastic containers and buckets. Bosewaga sings out the morning greeting to them, "Bwena kaukwau!" They return smiles and nod, "Bweno!" Kaugere clambers at the steps, frantic for her feed. Bosewaga jumps down nimbly to the dewy grass, kicking the pig out of her way as she pours the slop into the giant clamshell by the house post. Inside, *yawagu* squats at the hearth, squinting as she stirs the cold ashes to recover a smoldering ember. With deft efficiency, she adds dry kindling, blows the ember into a brisk fire, and sets the kettle to boil for our breakfast tea. The acrid smoke curls into the morning sunbeam and hangs languidly, a translucent curtain dividing the small front room.

One morning at dawn, a man from a neighboring village—someone I did not recognize—arrived unexpectedly at the doorstep of my mother-in-law's house, carrying on his shoulder a large metal dish filled with ten massive coral trout freshly caught during the night. Standing at the steps, he lifted the heavy weight off his shoulder, placed the dish on the floor, and pushed it forward into the house. Without coming inside to sit down for conversation and a cup of tea, he perfunctorily spoke a few words to *yawagu*, cast a nod of acknowledgment in my direction, and then quickly departed, cutting back across the path toward his village. This utterly unexpected display of abundance dazzled me. "Your *wotia*," *yawagu* announced matter-of-factly, her eyes indicating the fish to me. She appeared unabashed but her seemingly nonchalant manner could not conceal a hint of satisfaction, almost glee.

I was nonplussed. Part of our early morning routine was to watch out for the young boys passing by on the road with a fresh catch of fish. We would call out, "Louisaula yena?" (What is the price for the fish?), and they would come to the doorstep and sell us our choice, K2 each or three for K5, depending on the size.[11] If the Orabesi men went out fishing, *yawagu* would receive a large fish or two as her share in the distribution of the catch. There were also times when a relative or in-law from a fishing village would arrive at the house and present *yawagu* with several *yena*, and the visitation would invariably include reciprocated hospitality— a meal of hot food and tea followed by a chew of betel nut. Other times I would head off to the market at Losuia in the late afternoon, accompanied by my nieces, to purchase fresh fish from the boats when the fishers returned from a day at sea. However, to receive unsolicited a dish brimming with ten prime fish was not an ordinary occurrence and certainly beyond my comprehension. *Amakawala besa?* (What is this?) My *wotia*? What did *wotia* mean? *Avakapela?* (What for?) What could I possibly do with all those fish!

Yawagu said, "Wotia, besa kaula pela kabiyamati" (This food is offered as a request for a return favor). She added, "When there is a death in the family, you carry a basket of yams piled high, or plenty of fish, to someone who can help you prepare for *sagali*." *Yawagu* impassively explained that the man wanted me to have the fish so I could help him with some money in return for his hard work. He was busy preparing for *sagali* and needed cash to buy trade-store goods—rice, sugar, tea, and *karekwa* (fabric). The man's effort of labor at sea rewarded with a plentiful catch, he decided to use the fish for *wotia* and presented me the challenge to reciprocate with what I determined was appropriate remuneration. In turn, I would have an abundance of capital to put to work within my own network of exchange relationships. I could redistribute the fish as the means to subsidize my outlay of support, or, alternatively, I could use the distribution to my advantage by creating debts that I could draw on in the future. In effect, *wotia* obliged me to act as an investment banker for the donor's enterprise.

Wotia literally means a catch of fish strung together on a rope. *Wotia* is a pragmatic way to transform resources through transactions of indebtedness. Increasingly, cash is the sought-after commodity in *wotia* transactions, over that of clay pots, *doba*, and other *sagali* exchange valuables. The challenge of *wotia* confers trust and social status, and proceeds on the premise that the recipient has the means to reciprocate immediately, either through accrued resources or because of the capacity to activate a line of ready support. However, there is an element of risk in *wotia* for both donor and recipient—the risk of shame in not achieving the desired effect. If the recipient were to reject the challenge or not meet the call because of inability to respond accordingly, *wotia* would not take its anticipated form and could potentially disrupt social relations.

Sitting on the floor, dazzled by the fish glistening in a beam of sunlight cast at an angle through the slats of the roof, I felt affronted, distrustful of the figure

I assumed from the donor's perspective. Did I appear as an easy catch, a *dimdim* researcher with disposable cash? Perhaps I was simply a proxy for my husband in absentia. Why did this impressive display of *wotia* appear to me like a contrived imposition? Then I suddenly recognized that there was nothing contrived about the plenitude of freshly caught fish, redolent with anticipation, impatiently eyeing me from the dish. I knew it was imperative for me to act.

Yawagu coached me on my next move, how to proceed with distributing the fish and how much money I should give in return. Word about the *wotia* went out to the other households in a tactful relay of information, and one by one, electively, people came to the house to collect a fish. As they appeared at the doorstep, people expressed muted praise for the munificent display and appreciation for my generosity, but there was no discussion of what each transaction entailed in terms of reciprocity. Negotiations were implicit and I did not ask for or expect cash in exchange. When the dish was empty, Bosewaga rinsed it at the tap and carried it upside down on her head back to the man's village, my *wotia* cash payment in an envelope discreetly carried in her hand.

Disturbed by my conflicted emotions and skeptical response, I retreated to my books in an attempt to locate an ethnographic reference to *wotia*. I could find nothing at all, not in Malinowski, not in Weiner. Instead, I found assurance in Mary Catherine Bateson's words about the need to untangle conflicting reactions in ethnographic research and her observation that "discomfort is informative and offers a starting point for new understanding" (1994:17). Marilyn Strathern observes that ethnographic fieldwork involves "yielding to the preoccupations of others" (1999:6). The commitment of immersion is at once totalizing and partial as "the fieldworker enters into relationships with people for which no amount of imagining or speculating can serve as advance preparation" (6). Strathern uses the word "dazzle" to describe the mesmerizing effect of "ethnographic moments," or those points in time of revelation and perception when what is analyzed at the moment of observation is joined to what is observed at the moment of analysis (6). In a deliberate twist of form, Strathern demonstrates how the work of ethnography is homologous to Melanesian sociality, where people act with others in mind (16). The actions of a fisherman who arrived early one morning with a load of fish on his shoulder made the convergence of these forms apparent to me, representing a turning point in my sense of identity and belonging. The man appended his exchange network to mine and the newly forged link turned around immediate benefits for him to meet obligations for an impending *sagali*, while offering me the benefits of redistribution. The incident gave me fresh appreciation of how "the effectiveness of relationships thus depends on the form in which certain objects appear" (16). The man chose neither to take his abundant catch to market to sell for cash nor to distribute the fish in his immediate village network in exchange for future in-kind payments. Rather, he put the rewards of his efforts to strategic use as *wotia*, an aesthetic form that represented the value of his purposive labor while activating a new relational link that yielded concrete results.[12]

Wotia gave me a new frame of reference for observing the power of agency and how intentions are visibly communicated, compelling others to respond. *Wotia* was a direct lesson on the etiquette of persuasion and negotiation, and how display and concealment, appendage and detachment, are strategic moves in the choreography of exchange relations. I also understood in retrospect that the challenge to me was an endorsement of my extended presence in the community as a capable, contributing member. *Wotia* firmly located me in the convergence between home and field.

Fidelity in the Field: Trustworthiness and Dialogue

Fidelity, a quality widely mobilized in HIV prevention discourse, simultaneously points to the partiality of ethnographic engagement in communities of belonging and to the ethical rigor of trustworthiness in guiding the qualitative research process.[13] Ethnographic objectivity and adherence to detail emerges from relations of rapport and empathy, engendering an ethics of mutual trust through the convergence of different perspectives (Abu-Lughod 1991; Behar and Gordon, eds. 1995; Fabian 2001).

Stepping into the field of home revisited gave me a passport to new forms of social engagement. I welcomed the mobility that came with my new position as researcher. For the first time, I was able to traverse a wider spatial field in the Trobriands, to move beyond my well-defined relational sphere and expand an independent network of acquaintances and friendships. Additionally, my mature age and reproductive status as *numwaiya*, an older woman with children, helped legitimize my research activity and allowed encounters with a diversity of people. Mindful of how my status offered a particular route of access into the field of inquiry, I found new confidence in activating established rapport to explore previously unquestioned terrain. The privilege of being free to ask questions, inexhaustibly, one after another—the probing why and how of anthropological inquiry into cultural meanings and practice—was what I welcomed most about being a researcher. I came to appreciate how "home once interrogated is a place we have never before been" (Visweswaran 1994:113).

Yet I was also aware of the potential of the research process to either enhance or deplete local meanings and significance (Mallet 2003:114). I valued the opportunity to move beyond seeking explanatory answers to a battery of questions. While the practice of dwelling defined for me the contours of ethnographic homework, my research was concerned principally with facilitating participatory processes of knowledge exchange on sexuality and HIV prevention. I was interested in observing the ways people engage with and mediate new information, shifting my perspective "from participant observation to the observation of participation" (Tedlock 1991:82). The emergent and transformative capacity of ethnographic research guided my methodological approach (Mannheim and Tedlock 1995:9), based on the understanding that the exchange between researcher and participant is a *dialogic process* within which interactive learning takes place (Page 1988:163).[14]

The ethnographic method facilitates passage into a reflective space where the work of articulation coproduces new ways of knowing through critical exegesis. The open-ended questions of my research prompted dialogue that reasserted cultural ideals and aesthetics and revealed direct experience. Standpoints shifted frequently and fluidly between speaking for the collective and speaking for the self.

Personal desires, intimate revelations, and imagined futures were expressed, while other enunciations were simply descriptive of practice, the discourse of day-to-day living and materiality. When discussion broached the intersections between bodies of knowledge and participants considered the phenomena of HIV in relation to what is known and experienced, at times there were uncomfortable pauses and confusion as well as moments of great lucidity.

Collaborators in the Process

The people who selected to be actively involved in the research project, either participants in discussion groups or individuals who volunteered to record their stories on tape, had a direct effect on how it unfolded, the directions it took, and the incremental and iterative process of data interpretation.[15] The collaborative efforts of three Trobriand women, Diana Siyotama Lepani, Florence Mokolava, and Ethel Jacob, significantly contributed to the participatory structure and process of the research, including the willingness of others to be involved. My presence in the field as an observer of participation was largely defined by the complementary presence of these women, jointly or individually. They made contact with potential research participants and arranged visits to village communities to hold group discussions and impart information on HIV; they served as language translators between Kiriwina and English; they provided germane and insightful information on the physical and social landscape; and they gave me feedback on interpretation and analysis. The women brought to the study their own experiences and understanding of the issues explored. While their individual comprehension of biomedical information about sexual and reproductive health and HIV varied, and influenced their approach to imparting information, each of the women was a competent facilitator of group discussions. Their willingness to put themselves in positions of public view demonstrated confidence and leadership.

Ethel Jacob is a widow in her late forties and mother of four children. Ethel returned to live in the village when her husband died from lung cancer after working as a printer in Port Moresby for twenty years. I first met Ethel through her daughter, Buna, whom I befriended during my first period of fieldwork in December 2000. Buna identified herself as "a town girl, born in Port Moresby, raised up in Moresby, my first nineteen years of life spent in Moresby." When her father died in 1996, she went home to the Trobriands with her mother "to help her get over her sorrow." Ethel easily joined in the conversations I had with Buna when I returned in 2003 and offered to help with my research through her position as secretary for the United Church Kiriwina Circuit Women's Fellowship. In 2002, she became one of the "24 Wise Men and Women," the term used for the community leaders nominated as "agents of change" in the community-based HIV awareness project conducted by the PNG IMR and UNICEF.[16] She attended a leadership-training workshop on HIV and AIDS, which included developing an action plan for awareness activities at the village level. During 2003, Ethel resided in her home village of Kwemtula, about a ten-minute walk east of Losuia on the lagoon side of the island. At the time, two of her grandchildren, aged three and four, were living with her, as was her last-born son, who was a grade 8 student at Losuia Primary School.

FIGURE 3.2. • Ethel Jacob at
                    Osesuia village,
                    November 2003

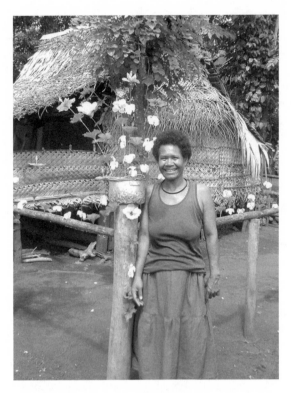

Florence Mokolava is a professional nurse and midwife with extensive work experience in the PNG national health system. In her early fifties, Florence retired in 2001 after working in Port Moresby for many years and returned home to the Trobriands with her husband, who had also retired from a senior management position in banking. The daughter of the late Chief Pulitala, Florence is well known and respected throughout the Trobriand Islands and continues to practice nursing and midwifery in the community. At the time of my fieldwork, Florence was actively engaged in HIV awareness work as a health worker and was one of two field coordinators for the IMR project. Florence and her husband built a house near Wapipi on the northern side of Kiriwina, where they live with their three youngest children. Florence's medical and clinical knowledge, combined with her intimate cultural knowledge, gives her a distinctive perspective on the challenges of HIV communication.

Of the three women, Diana Siyotama Lepani was most directly involved in the research in terms of the time we spent conversing and reviewing the taped recordings and transcripts of discussions and interviews. We became friends during my first period of fieldwork when she approached me to express interest in the study and to volunteer her participation. I still remember vividly our first conversation and Diana's directness in explaining her reasons why she wanted to be involved. As we sat on the floor in my mother-in-law's house, the wind picked up and there was a sudden downpour. The din of the rain pounding on the corrugated iron roof granted an unexpected intimacy to our conversation. Although we had to raise our voices to hear each other, the noise allowed for a candidness that might not have come so easily in the sluggish heavy heat before the clouds broke. Diana explained

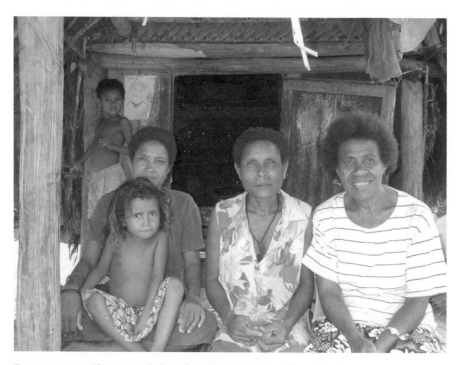

FIGURE 3.3. • Florence Mokolava (far right) at Mutawa village, October 2003

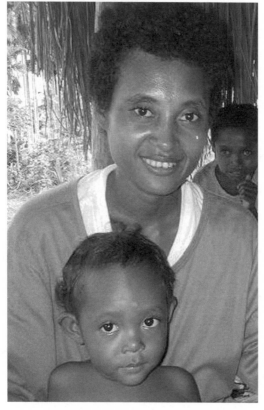

FIGURE 3.4. • Diana Siyotama Lepani with youngest son, Dopato, October 2003

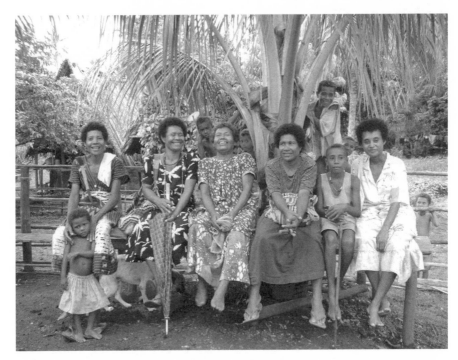

FIGURE 3.5. • Ethel and Diana with women from Tukwaukwa village, December 2003

that she became a mother and wife at a young age and consequently was not able to pursue her education beyond lower secondary school. She said she desired new experiences that would allow her to explore different ideas and gain new knowledge. She told me she had the right personality to ask people questions because she is not the kind of person who holds "grudges," that is, she accepts what people say and does not gossip or judge. She said she worries about young people and their ability to manage social change, and she wants to guide them and give them information to live a good life. A graduate of grade 10 at Kiriwina High School, Diana is actively involved in various community activities. She is a youth leader in the Orabesi United Church, she is a volunteer religious instructor at Kiriwina High School, and she helps manage the OKO women's soccer team. Diana turned thirty years old in 2003. She and her husband are both from Orabesi and live at the Oiabia mission station with their four children, aged twelve years, ten years, five years, and eighteen months. Her youngest child was still breastfeeding at the time and often came with us on our visits to villages around the island.

Village Visits

The major component of fieldwork during 2003 involved visits to twenty-three villages on four of the six islands for group discussions and interviews followed by HIV awareness sessions (see Map 2). The islands are laced with myriad walking tracks that connect villages and garden sites, and there are three main unsealed roads transecting Kiriwina, from Losuia in the south to Kaibola on the north coast, and to Gilibwa on the southern tip. To reach villages located over an hour's walking distance from Orabesi, I booked transportation through one of three local trade stores or from the local government council. With only a dozen operational vehicles on the island, including one large flatbed truck that operates a public transport service, several utility trucks, and one minivan, the availability of reliable transportation is limited. Travel to the three outer islands was by motorized dinghy.

At least one of my collaborators accompanied me on the visits to help with group discussions and to facilitate the information sessions. After initial introductions, people were invited to organize themselves in discussion groups according to their preference for participation, whether mixed or separated by gender and age. Groups ranged in size from ten to fifty people. In most villages, people chose to remain in a large mixed group for the duration of the session. Discussions typically lasted ninety minutes, followed by half-hour information sessions in a question-and-answer format. The village visits established opportunities for follow-up interviews with smaller groups and individuals, which were scheduled for separate times and locations if they did not take place on the same day. I also conducted semistructured interviews with people in various professional and leadership capacities—health workers, village magistrates, church leaders, teachers, village birth attendants, and local government officials. Most discussions and interviews were recorded, and in all cases participants gave their informed verbal consent.

The women's fellowship network of both the United and Catholic churches provided the initial contacts for many of the village visits, which were usually scheduled for Wednesday mornings, the standard weekly meeting time for the groups. This had implications for male participation during these morning sessions, but the women's groups also provided contacts for scheduling alternative times for small group discussions and interviews with older and younger men. Other visits were arranged through the village birth attendants, as well as local government councillors and village church deacons, who are all men, and these sessions tended to have greater male participation. Most group sessions and interviews took place inside the village churches or on large communal platforms on the church grounds. The church building is a prominent structure in every Trobriand village. The majority of churches are made of permanent building materials—concrete, timber, corrugated iron roofing—and their durable physical presence represents communal enterprise and social stability. The large, open-air structures with an expanse of cement floor are ideal spaces for a range of community functions, including meetings, village court sessions, maternal and child health clinics, training workshops, and social gatherings. In the Trobriands, as elsewhere in PNG, the church network is an important channel for mobilizing local resources for various endeavors and for disseminating information on a wide range of topics, including HIV awareness.[17]

Collectively, villagers received the visits with interest, curiosity, and anticipation, matched by generous hospitality.[18] Of the twenty-three villages visited, seven had not participated in any prior awareness activities on HIV. Some of the sessions began with welcoming songs and speeches, setting a convivial tone of oratorical formality. The initial attendance was always overwhelming, often over a hundred people, but numbers would adjust as people made the decision whether or not to participate after introductory statements. There were always a few disengaged but inquisitive onlookers, often young men and boys, peering over the ledge of the church walls rather than coming inside. Young children, both girls and boys, were always present, often rapt in attention, and were never shooed away by the adults. I would bring an ample supply of betel nut and pepper sticks for participants to chew during discussions and would make a contribution of biscuits, tin meat, rice, sugar, and tea for follow-up refreshments. The visits would usually finish with a communal meal prepared by the hosts, followed by a guided tour of the village before departure.

In some ways, the sessions assumed a format that was antithetical to the interests of ethnographic research—arranged in advance, not impromptu, enthused by anticipation of a set agenda, and moderated by the protocol of community representation. However, engaging with groups of people in this way had important epistemological and ethical advantages for exploring how HIV information is mediated collectively. The prevailing ethos of hospitality and reciprocity invariably generated a productive exchange of information and perspectives, where the dynamics of interaction were decidedly egalitarian and open. The inclusivity demonstrated in attendance and participation and the collective encouragement given for each person to speak if they so desired were impressive features of the proceedings. The assembly of women, men, adolescents, and children, representing all ages and social positions, was a powerful image for how collective engagement enables the potential for turning knowledge about HIV prevention into practice.

There were delightful moments when mirth and candor would ease my tentative concern about a presumed code of behavior, and I came to appreciate more fully the expressive potency of a community of belonging. I remember vividly one such moment in the Catholic Church when the discussion with a group of twenty women turned from infidelity to the various forms and effects of *kwaiwaga*, or love magic, and how the Sri Lankan nun kept popping her head in the door to see what the peals of laughter were about. I asked for assurance from the women that it was OK to talk about these things inside the church. They dismissed my concern emphatically, saying, "Of course it is OK! *Mokwita!* True! This is our church where we come together to share. *Makala* [like], it is not as if we are doing these things right here—we are just talking about them!"

Kiriwina Language

The dialogic process calls into question issues of language and translation. During my research, I relied on my collaborators to translate for me when discussions and interviews were in the vernacular. My linguistic competency in Kiriwina language remains limited even after many years of passive language immersion. The spoken, sung, and chanted sounds of Kiriwina, the intonation, pitch, and modulation of voices, solo and in unison, have long surrounded me in household conversations, at community gatherings in Port Moresby, and during visits home to the village. The sounds of the language have settled permanently in my subconsciousness like a much-loved musical composition. However, while I have acquired a relatively extensive lexicon of key words, terms, and definitions, I do not have conversational fluency. I am better at listening to Kiriwina than speaking it. Trobrianders, many of whom are multilingual and proficient English speakers, amiably accommodate my lack of confidence in speaking their language.

I acknowledge an obvious contradiction between the shortcomings of my language acquisition and my theoretical argument for the importance of the vernacular in mediating HIV information. The effect of my limited linguistic skills on participating in dialogic exchange was to some extent balanced by the predominant use of English in HIV awareness materials used by health workers and community leaders for training and dissemination, not only in the Trobriands but in other parts of PNG as well (Gibbs and Mondu 2010:18). Indeed, research participants often expressed a preference for the use of English as the starting point in communicating about HIV and AIDS as a perceived measure of assurance that the information imparted is consistent with the language of biomedicine. This preference for English reflects perceptions about the pedagogical authority of the biomedical model in explaining novel and exogenous disease phenomena (see Pigg 2001b). To an important degree, the expectation that my sources of knowledge about HIV were legitimate and trustworthy defined my role as researcher. People viewed me as a reliable link to outside information, and in this regard my dependence on English was compensated. Yet I was troubled at times by what might have appeared to be my complicity with hegemonic Western medical discourse, especially in perpetuating the dichotomy between traditional and modern, and the assumed efficacy of a biomedical approach to HIV prevention.[19] Although my reliance on English at times impeded the flow of communication and delimited my interpretive field, the process of intercultural communication nonetheless involved productive tensions that forged significant links between spoken words, ideas, and meanings.

Fidelity to Purpose and Process

In addition to my established relationship as *vevai*, my marital status, age, and maternity contributed greatly to generating the trust and rapport that made research on intimate matters possible. Being *numwaiya* proved to be a practical and unambiguous qualification for engaging people in discussions about sexuality and HIV and AIDS, and this was true for my collaborators as well as for me. Moreover, our teamwork approach reinforced the position of trust and authority that the social category obtains. Nonetheless, the intersecting variables that constitute sexed and gendered subjectivities, such as age, ethnicity, kinship, and socioeconomic status, influence the relational terms of engagement, the dialogic process, and the interpretive outcomes of any research undertaking. Casting these variables into the dynamics of research on sexuality perhaps sharpens the contingencies of consent, affect, and discovery. Specifically, the sexuality of the researcher as expressed and experienced in the field is a critical component of the ethnographic encounter (Bell, Caplan, and Karim, eds. 1993; Markowitz and Ashkenazi 1999; Kulick and Willson, eds. 1995).[20]

To this extent, my affinal status was perhaps the main variable that defined unambiguously my sexed personhood in the field. I was aware that people's willingness to approach the topic of my research and talk openly with me about sex was an extension of respect for my relatedness as *vevai* and, reciprocally, my self-conscious demonstration of faithfulness to my affinal relationship. There was an apparent contradiction between the general protocol in PNG that restricts interactions between in-laws and people's openness to discuss sexual matters with me during fieldwork. This points to the semantic use of the terms "taboo" and *tambu* and how in Tok Pisin the meaning of "that which is forbidden" is extended to the relationship term of *tambu*, or "in-law," to reflect the special observances maintained in affinal relations. Talking about sex is commonly regarded as "taboo" throughout PNG, and, as a corollary, in-laws talking about sex is particularly forbidden out of mutual respect for maintaining relations of difference and, more tacitly, to safeguard against the potential power of intimacy to disrupt kinship alliances. While this sentiment is somewhat modified in the Trobriand context, where the pidgin gloss is less salient, the likely tensions that my research subject posed were in fact mediated by the respect people accorded me as an in-law. Additionally, my status as in-law was qualified by the prominent social standing of my husband and his family, which no doubt influenced the reception I was given wherever I went and contributed to the readiness of people to participate in the research. That said, however, I also acknowledge that people's willingness to overlook the conventions of taboo was a measure of the importance with which Trobrianders regard the topic of HIV.

While fieldwork opened up for me a new sense of social freedom, I was neither able nor inclined to transcend my affiliation as a fixed condition of fieldwork. My method of participant observation largely involved a self-imposed regimen of deportment as an expression of fidelity to purpose, within the dimensions and limitations of my sexed and gendered personhood. It was important to me that my movement in the wider social sphere carried respect for my embedded social connections. In my choreography, I imagined myself striding confidently with a large basket of *doba* balanced on my head, a public and visible display of capacity and intentionality. Everywhere I walked, I made apparent my purposive mobility, mindful of how my public conduct was scrutinized by others. I did not want my demeanor to communicate ambiguity, indecisiveness, or carelessness. Nor did I hold expectations that fieldwork would gain passage for me into realms not otherwise accessible because of my gender, age, and marital status. Because of selective restriction, I did not accompany young women and men on their nocturnal trysts in the bush, nor did I go to the wharf at night to observe firsthand the sexual consort between visiting boat crew and young women. In this sense, my work in the field was not "deep hanging out" (see Clifford 1997:56; cf. Bolton 1992). Rather, I limited my immersion to areas of inquiry that felt appropriate and responsive to the ways people viewed me and to how research participants chose to accommodate my presence. Consequently, the scheduled interviews and discussions during village visits primarily involved female participants, while informal conversations with men and young boys were more opportunistic as social situations allowed.

The dialogic process also brings into focus the power relations intrinsic in research encounters (Wolf 1996). The politics of speaking for others has become a central theme confronting and redefining social research over the last four decades, with feminist theory providing much of the momentum for reexamining the ethics of ethnographic representation.[21] Much of the debate concerns the differentials of power between the researcher and the researched, the process by which knowledge is produced, and the purpose to which it is applied (Wolf 1996:2). Feminist standpoint theory advocates amplifying the voices and experiences of those whose subject positions are marginalized or rendered invisible by the structures of power. However, the act of "giving voice" most often takes place in the researcher's textual retellings, in the translation of experience through a process of distantiation and objective detachment from the moment of exchange, underscoring how movement out of the field of encounter is regarded as indispensable to the interpretive process. Catherine Reissman cautions about the aim of empowerment in such representations, stating that as researchers, "we cannot give voice, but we do hear voices that we record and interpret" (1993:8). To hear, record, and interpret voices involves a reciprocal relationship. My textual strategy is to retain the tenor of the conversations, monologues, reveries, and narratives elicited in interaction, as well as my own voice and location. My position is not to speak for but on behalf of, to represent voices and viewpoints by being faithful to the dialogic process and context.

I recall how one of my earlier research collaborators came forward to tell her story. Daisy organized several life-history interviews with women from her village and helped me with translation. She surprised me one day when she arrived at my doorstep and announced, "I'm here for my turn." "Your turn?" I asked. "To be interviewed, of course," she said. "I want to tell you my life history." So we found a quiet place and I turned on the tape recorder and she spoke for nearly ninety minutes nonstop. No random sample this. Through the act of telling, lived experience is given new meaning.

Through the act of retelling, the empirical issues of truth and validity come to the fore. The dilemmas of representation are perplexing—how to portray the intimate and familiar without betraying confidence and identity, how to honor the richness of personal statements without reproducing them verbatim, how to generalize from multiple voices without essentializing the particular. Riessman states that "trustworthiness" and not "truth" is the critical issue for validation in qualitative research: "The latter assumes an objective reality, whereas the former moves the [validation] process into the social world" (1993:65).

As I traverse the particular field of my research and the broader field of HIV policy and program implementation, I am troubled by how the extended tempo of ethnographic engagement is seemingly discordant with the urgent imperative to respond to the growing epidemic.[22] How do I reconcile the dissonances of pace and position? The purpose of my research in the context of an imminent epidemic requires an awareness of how my position and approach contribute to and affect the exchange and interchange of information and knowledge. By being attentive to the quality of relations with the people whose lives I represent in ethnographic text and to my concurrent commitment to field and home, I resolve my position as one of interconnectivity in an ongoing process of knowing.

The shift from passive participant observation to structured research and textual representation was not as seamless as I had imagined it would be. The position created new social demands that would not otherwise have confronted me— perceptions and expectations that I could provide access to resources and services beyond the reach of most villagers, including better health services. Of course, I was also drawn into situations and events because of my prior relationality, irrespective of my position as researcher. I had to know when to put away the notebook and engage experientially and emotionally without an objective standpoint.

As well, I knew that I had the means to depart the field, leave behind the materiality of life in the islands, and return to the familiar comforts of another home in another place.

The escalating HIV epidemic in PNG gave fresh purpose to my long-held interest in observing and representing lived experience. My research proceeded on the understanding that my affinity to the Trobriands shaped and influenced the opportunity to study the intimacies of people's lives, offering me access to social dimensions that might not be available to others. However, my particular subject position as *vevai*, and as Modudaiya *lakwava*, also posed tensions and restricted lines of pursuit and inquiry that might otherwise be open. Partiality is intrinsic to affiliations of all kinds, influencing how the research process unfolds. In a vital sense, all ethnographic research is about affinity in the field and fidelity to home revisited, about the sympathies marked by a community of interest and belonging.

CHAPTER 4

"Because We Can!"
Gendered Agency and Social Reproduction

I was visiting my good friend Buna in her village shortly after the birth of her third child. We sat together on the raised veranda of her one-room family dwelling, and I cradled her newborn while she and another young mother chewed betel nut. Two playful toddlers and a crawling baby animated the small space, moving between our laps and outstretched legs. Our casual talk turned to questions I posed about pregnancy and childbirth when an older woman, a mother of five whose last-born child had just turned one year old, ambled over to ask for betel nut. She paused to listen to the thread of our conversation and then suddenly turned to me and said, "Do you know this picture, *In a Savage Land?*"

"Yes, I do, I have seen it," I answered.

"So, what do you think of it?" she asked.

In a Savage Land is an Australian feature film shot on location in the Trobriands in 1998. Billed as "a sweeping romantic adventure set at the outbreak of the Second World War," the film depicts in sepia tones the story of a husband and wife, both anthropologists, who follow Malinowski's footsteps to study Trobriand sexual customs. The film explores colonial gender relations through a range of stereotypical characters—anthropologist, missionary, colonial administrator, merchant trader, beachcomber—and their competing agendas in the "Islands of Love."

I sensed that the woman had a strong opinion about the film and asked if she had been involved in the production, knowing that although it generated some welcome income on the islands, the film also provoked considerable controversy as Trobrianders vied for participation or protested the filming for aesthetic and political reasons.[1]

The woman answered my question with an emphatic, "Ga!" (No!), she was not involved. Her face wrinkled with disapproval. "Sainagaga!" (Very bad!), she said.

"Avakapela?" (Why?), I wanted to know.

"Because the picture made Trobriand women say the wrong answer to the wrong question!" was her definitive answer.

"And what was the wrong answer to the wrong question?" I was eager to know.

Her response was delivered in mockery. "Why do Trobriand women have so many babies? Because we love so much having sex with men!"

"So what is the right answer to the wrong question?" I probed.

Standing tall with uplifted arms, a self-evident gesture of exasperation as much as affirmation, the woman projected her full stature to the relentless gaze of an imagined audience. "Because we can!" she declared. "Because we are old enough to go with the men! Because we are old enough to have babies!"

"So what is the right question?" I asked with tactful reserve, feeling restrained by the seeming indiscretion of ethnographic inquiry.

The woman hit back without missing a beat—"I'm tired of questions!"

A Question of Embodied Capacity and Potential

The impromptu conversation in the vignette noted above agitates the tensions between Trobriand assertions of cultural identity and the colonial and anthropological representations of Trobriand sexuality as casually excessive and wanton, representations that persist in contemporary depictions and parallel the discourse on sexual risk and promiscuity that dominates HIV communication. The conversation offers a framework for exploring cultural constructions of gender, sexuality, and reproduction, and how meanings are activated in embodied practice. As an expression of sociality, sexuality is a productive resource in relationship building. In particular, the period of youth sexuality represents a fertile field of possibilities as the arena for demonstrating capacity and potential for social reproduction.

In the storyline of *In a Savage Land*, the woman anthropologist protests her husband's disregard for her own theoretical quest and criticizes his methodological bias in not paying attention to what Trobriand women do and say. Then in one of the few scenes in Kiriwina language with English subtitles, the woman anthropologist sits with a small group of Trobriand women on the beach and questions one of them about conception beliefs. In response to the explanation that *baloma*, the ancestral spirits from Tuma, impregnate women by arriving on sea foam or driftwood, the anthropologist asks, "Avakapela kukwekaytasi?" (Why then do you copulate?). The woman answers, "Pela dikwadekuna" (For pleasure).[2]

The question asked by the woman anthropologist captures the perceived anomaly of Trobriand conception beliefs that has "long excited Western observers" (Strathern 1988:235) and that sparked relentless debate on the notion of "virgin birth" following Malinowski's initial account of Trobrianders' purported ignorance of physiological impregnation and paternity (Franklin 1997). Edmund Leach (1967) first used the idiom "virgin birth" to argue that the Trobriand belief in parthenogenesis reflects a cosmological dogma about metaphysical incarnation rather than biological ignorance of conception. It is not my intention to rehearse the debate here or further employ "virgin birth" as an analytical construct.[3] What is at issue is conception without paternity, not conception without sex. As Malinowski himself categorically stated, in a sentence that stands alone as a paragraph, "A virgin cannot conceive" (1929:153). Analysis of the so-called doctrine relies heavily on the universalist assumption that kinship is predicated on biology (Franklin 1997; Montague 1971; Loizos and Heady 1999; Schneider 1984). Mark Mosko argues that the virgin birth construct "smacks of Western ethnocentrism," based not on Trobriand beliefs and practices but on "a distinctly Western notion about reproduction" (1998:687; see also Mosko 2005). Indeed, the perennial theoretical preoccupation with Trobrianders' supposed ignorance of physiological paternity remains unsatisfactorily answered because the question itself "has been misconceived" (Delaney 1986:494). As the Trobriand woman made abundantly clear to me, the wrong question yields the wrong answer.

Putting aside explanations of either cognitive ignorance or cosmological dogma, what is important to distill from the ethnographic accounts and various interpretations of Trobriand conception beliefs is the core significance of sociality and interclan relations for procreative potential. Fertility signifies the strength and potency of matrilineal identity. *Buyai* (blood) and *nunu* (breast milk) are the inalienable resources of matrilineal *dala* substance that contribute to the viability of new life. One person explained their *dala* identity to me by stating, "I have every right to be part of my *dala* because I was breastfed by that *dala*."[4] However, the making of new life requires the complementary mixing of inalienable matrilineal substance with a consistent source of paternal form through ongoing social acts of nurture and support, ideally sustained by an exclusive conjugal relationship (Weiner 1979:332–33). The complementary social contributions of intimate bodily contact, food, and material support given by the father—and by extension, his *dala*—to the mother during pregnancy form the gestating fetus in the image of the father. The distinctive agency of Trobriand paternity is a process of "feeding and forming" to grow a social being (Mosko 1995:768, 1998:685). The development of a newborn's social identity by paternal nurture is a continual enterprise that involves sustained contributions of physical, emotional, and material support from the father and his *dala* members, particularly his mothers and sisters, throughout lactation and into childhood and adolescence. Paternal efficacy in shaping the social identity of the child is indicative of *dala* fulfillment of reciprocal obligations and continues throughout the life course with ongoing investments of *dala* resources given by a man to his children (Weiner 1976:125).

A statement made during an interview with a married couple, both in their early thirties, directly reflects the cultural value of women's reproductive capacity and men's paternal contribution to child development. We were discussing *meguva*, or magic, and the man was explaining how the specialized knowledge of protective magic passes along two paths, either between members of the same *dala* from one generation to the next, or from a father to his children. Then, in what for me was an unexpected punctuation in the flow of the conversation, the man suddenly turned to his wife, pointed at her pubic area, and declared, "In Kiriwina, we men have high feelings for the lady. The private parts of the lady are a treasure. That's why fathers want their best things to go to sons and daughters, because they came from that treasure."[5] The woman was unfazed by her husband's graphic gesture, and without pause he continued his explication about *meguva*, expanding on the use of protective magic to ward off witchcraft and sorcery. Perhaps his overt aside can be interpreted as a claim to male ownership of the "treasure" of women's reproductive capacity or perhaps as a sentimental adoration of maternity influenced by Christian religiosity (the man was a pastor). My reading, however, suggests that the man's statement is direct evidence of the value ascribed to paternal nurture, which a father demonstrates by bestowing highly valued knowledge on his children.

Children learn from an early age the premium value given to the embodied effect of paternal agency in their gestation and development. The greatest compliment that a Trobriand child can receive from others is the indisputable recognition of the father's features in their own face. People say that the father's face is *migila inini wala*, literally "peeled off" and molded onto the child's face. A common contemporary idiom is that the child is a "photocopy" of the father, and young mothers in particular will proclaim this semblance with proud humor. While such compliments implicitly acknowledge paternal efficacy, praise extends to the child for actively assuming the countenance of the father through responsive love and respect; agency, thus, has a mutual and reciprocal effect. On the contrary, to suggest that a child looks like his or her mother, or any other matrilineal relative, is an intolerable insult that causes great offense and shame (Malinowski 1929:174; Weiner 1976:123, 1988:58). This was one of the first cultural principles I learned as an in-law through the trial and error of faux pas. The reaction to my naive comparison between the facial features of a young child and his mother was immediate and palpable; the people who heard my comment literally shuddered with acute embarrassment. My mother-in-law swiftly corrected me with a gravity reserved for the most serious of oversights. Stern and shameful reprimands inculcate the rule at a young age when a child innocently makes such comparisons. When I pressed for the reason why such a similarity is so unthinkable, especially given the indelibility of matrilineal identity, I was told that it is not something people give much thought to; rather, it is *lumkola*, something that is felt emotionally. To paraphrase a consistent explanation, "It feels like a shameful thing because maybe it is just like saying the father is not a good gardener; he does not care for the child."

This strict social protocol likely reflects the uncertainty of biological paternity in a sexual culture where unmarried women enjoy the same rights as unmarried men, multiple partnering is the norm before settling into a steady relationship, and women have the social power to control their fertility. Young Trobriand men, in particular, are wary of claims that an unmarried pregnant woman might make in naming the father of the baby she carries. A young boy in his late teens, speaking inclusively during a group discussion with his peers, explains the commonly shared concern among men: "If only we know the relationship is just between the two of us, then we would feel right to look after the child. But if it is not a steady friendship, we want to see the face first. OK, if we see our face, then we know, yes, I am the father of this child" (Taped interview, 19 August 2003).

A further interpretation would point to the exogamy taboo of *sovasova*, which forbids sexual relations between members of the same clan. Comparing a child's appearance to the mother implies a breach of the proscription. However, my particular focus here is concerned with how the differential effects of maternal and paternal reproductive contributions bring to the fore the significance of sociality and interclan relations in cultural constructions of sexuality. The rejoinder, "because we can," shifts the analytical lens to consider the importance of gendered agency and how sexuality is a productive resource in relationship building. Perhaps the "right question" to ask Trobriand women about their sexual and reproductive agency might be something about embodied capacity, regenerative potential, and efficacy. Posed in this way, procreation is "known and understood by its effects"

(Mallett 2003:130), including viable pregnancy, childbirth, and the social integration of new life. The volition expressed in the woman's straightforward answer to the wrong question speaks directly of the potency of sexual practice to make visible the capacity for social reproduction. Sexual relations form and transform larger social networks, including networks of exchange. Questions of sexuality are not simply about the "itch," or pleasure, of individual sexual acts but should seek to explore the meanings produced on the collective scale by intimate desires and pleasures (see Tolman and Diamond 2001).

Philip Setel's insights on "sexuality as the cultivation of embodiment and personhood" are instructive here, illustrating how sexual activity takes meaning in relation to shared understandings and "commonly held categories of social persons and the life course" (1999:140–41). In this sense, I suggest that the link made between desire and being "old enough," as expressed by the woman in her answer to the wrong question, is not evidence of a Trobriand understanding of an axiomatic or biologically determined faculty of reproductive nubility, but reveals a distinctively Trobriand framework of social reproduction that includes the social category of *tubwa*, or age group. *Tubwa* affiliation nurtures personhood and makes apparent a young person's sexual readiness and capacity for social reproduction within a recognizable social unit. The commencement of sexual activity is directly associated with the onset of puberty and is culturally valued as a critical transition in the physical and social development of a young person. Being sexually active is a prerequisite for growth into healthy, strong adult women and men. While there are rules and restrictions about whom one can couple with and where encounters take place, young people enjoy considerable sexual freedom before marriage, rehearsing their future economic roles as married adults by forging the potential alliances that will sustain the relations of social reproduction.

Kiriwina language does not have a linguistic concept of "virginity" that associates sexual inexperience with chastity and virtue, equating the commencement of sexual activity with loss of innocence, or that conveys a social value concerned with preserving a young woman's hymen for marriage. In fact, the cultural expectation for youth sexuality carries a value judgment about girls and boys who do not actively exercise sexual freedom—"They are not worth anything if they don't go out. That's one thing about Kiriwina."[6]

> *Nakumakala*, a girl who does not go out. And for boy—*tokumakala*. If people say this name during a quarrel it is very shameful. Women in the village will know that this girl hasn't started going out and the mother gets shame when other women talk. Everyone is encouraging her [to go out]. [Interview notes, 11 December 2000]

Women told me that when a young girl has her first flow of *kabuyai*, or menstrual blood, it is the sign that she is ready to start having sexual intercourse. Some women contradict this view and say that intercourse brings on menstruation, and they encourage their young daughters to become sexually active so they will start menstruating. Other women told me that when they learn a young girl has reached menarche, they will say knowingly to each other, "Oh, yes, she has started going out with boys."

In custom when girl gets *nupisi* [budding breasts], the mother says, 'Hurry up and go sleep with boys so you will hurry up and get your period.' When she gets her period then women know she is sleeping with boys. The mother sees she has her period and she will go and tell her aunties. They are happy because the girl will bring presents from the boys." [Interview notes, 11 December 2000]

These explanations provide evidence of the interconnected meanings of sexuality and fertility in terms of desired effects, and are consonant with the generalized understanding of physical development as a product of social relations—how the body comes into a new life stage in response to the cultivated effects of social interaction. The urgency to bring about the physiological transition indicates the value placed on sexual activity as a means to generate exchange relations within a broader sociality.

The interactions and transactions of social reproduction illustrate how Trobriand sexual and reproductive agency is a composite of complementary personal capacities and intentions made apparent in relation to social others. Agency thus comprises the physical, social, and symbolic attributes of personhood activated through relations of exchange. Strathern's notion of "partible personhood," where capacity represents the generalized sociality contained within persons who are comprised of multiple parts of social others (1988:13, 185), is germane. Capacity becomes evident in social interactions and the exchange of substances and objects between people, primarily between people representing difference, such as clan identity or gender. Weiner's analysis of Trobriand exchange contextualizes agency in relation to the reproduction of persons, objects, and relationships, or "the regenerative aspect of sociality, wherein exchange is the *modus operandi*" (1980a:72). Individual agency is situated within differential social relations, where "one's self, one's position, and one's potential as a reproductive agent depend on relations with 'others'" (Weiner 1980a:82).

Sameness of Substance and Mixing of Difference

At this point, it is helpful to review the basic elements of Trobriand social reproduction that uphold the principle of maintaining reciprocal relations of difference, including sexual relations. In the Trobriand matrilineal clan system, *kumila* define the broadest distinctions of sameness and difference between people. *Dala*, the subclan lineages, are the operative groupings from which people create and reinforce exchange relations both within and between clans. Together *kumila* and *dala* comprise the incontrovertible and regenerative substance of matrilineal identity. *Veyola*, or the "sameness of substance" (Malinowski 1929:422), is the general term for clansperson, or "people like us," as opposed to "people different from us," who are referred to as *tomakava* (Weiner 1976:52–54). The process of reproduction throughout the life cycle is socially viable when investments of nurture and material support for matrilineal substance channel through exchange relations with *tomakava*, established primarily through conjugal partnerships and through children's relational ties to their father's *dala*. These pivotal connective relationships, called *keyawa*, ensure the optimal flow of resources between different *dala*. They are achieved primarily through marriage and affinal ties, particularly when sons marry into their father's clan and daughters marry into the clan of their maternal uncle's wife, which ideally is their own father's clan as well.

The ideal marriage partner for a young man is his father's sister's daughter; likewise, the ideal spouse for a young woman is her mother's brother's son. The pool of suitable partners is inclusive of the offspring of the parents' classificatory siblings (Malinowski 1929:86; Weiner 1976:53). The term *kaytabula*, a compound of the word *kayta* (sexual intercourse) and the kinship category *tabu* (see note 5 in Chapter 3), signifies the ideal sexual partner and potential spouse for reconnecting members of the same clan through pivotal affinal exchange relations. The *kaytabula* partnership represents what Trobrianders call a "crisscross" strategy for reinforcing affinal exchange ties and ensuring that *dala* resources stay between two lineages linked by *tabu* relations (Lepani 2001:59). Weiner (1976:53) reports that both men and women laughingly told her this strategy was a "trick" because marrying *tabu* serves as a link for creating "significant and long-term exchange relationships with members of one's own clan." *Kaytabula* reflects the premium placed on the corporeal mixing of difference in heterosexual partnering and suggests how sexuality is a productive resource to build and reinforce exchange relations between people of different clans and lineages.

The activation and maintenance of interclan relations is an ongoing process throughout the life course, valued as an expression of personhood and social identity. Sexuality is a positive component of personhood, registering the efficacy of consensual and pleasurable practice in building and reinforcing exchange relations.[7] The transactional aspect of these valued relations symbolizes the capacity for social reproduction. The power of sexuality to demonstrate capacity and potential is true for women and men, young and old, but holds particular salience for adolescents. The collective term for unmarried male and female youth, *kubukwabuya*, also connotes "freedom," representing the extended life stage when young people enjoy unencumbered scope for pursuing their own social activities without the responsibilities of adulthood. In English, Trobrianders refer to *kubukwabuya* as "single boys and girls," or "young boys and girls," basing the age distinction on marital and reproductive status.[8] *Ulatile* and *kapugula* are the gendered terms for sexually active unmarried males and females, respectively, which describe both the subject and act of being mobile in pursuit of sexual liaisons. Both terms also signify the "prime of life," reflecting the cultural value placed on this life stage. Youth sexuality embodies the autonomy to pursue one's desire, to attract the desire of others, and to test out successive partners for potential conjugality. Sexual autonomy is exercised equally, although differentially, by males and females. Young girls express confidence in their sexuality and have the right to reject the advances of suitors they find undesirable. They encounter few societal restraints on their sexual behavior and are "accorded full respect for the power of their sexuality" (Weiner 1976:193).

That sexual relations incorporate the value of exchange is expressed by *buwala*—the requisite gifts of betel nut, tobacco, clothing, or cash—which men give their sexual partners after lovemaking and which girls and women anticipate as a respectful gesture of protocol and a symbol of mutual pleasure. *Buwala* is evidence of a young girl's ability to attract partners, and it indicates the "fitness" of a potential husband to help grow the woman's *dala* and expand the relational network between clans.[9] The importance of mutuality is reflected also in the term *bilamapula*, which describes the physically reciprocal movement between partners during sexual intercourse that results in orgasm, when semen and vaginal fluids, both referred to by the single term *momona*, effect the corporeal mixing of clan difference (Malinowski 1929:285).

However, consent and mutuality are not without contestation in the exercise of personal desire. Both males and females use *kwaiwaga*, or love magic, to demonstrate their power to seduce and attract potential partners and to cause "love" to overcome the chosen partner, thus making visible their efficacy in another person's embodied desires.[10] The use of *kwaiwaga* is the primary means to secure fidelity and pave the way for the bond of marriage. In this way, the efficacy of *kwaiwaga* shifts the pleasures of intimate sociality from the private domain of desire into public purview, where sexual alliances serve the larger social networks within which they operate (Weiner 1988:71, 1992:76).

The intimacy of a sexual encounter invariably extends beyond the union of two bodies and ultimately represents the relationality between two clans. For this reason, the strict decorum of *katupwana*, or concealment, retains the autonomy of youth sexuality and prevents activation of the social obligations that commence when a relationship is formally recognized through marriage. Young people take great care to be discreet and hide their sexual liaisons from public view until they enter into a steady partnership and seek endorsement from their respective families. Specifically, a young girl conceals her sexual relations from her father, who represents the key social link to another *dala*—a link that takes on new significance through marriage, when a sexual relationship is transformed into a publicly acknowledged interclan exchange relationship. *Mosila*, or shame, motivates secrecy to ensure sexual relations do not become public. "Feeling shame," as people refer to the sensation in English, is not associated with sexual activity as such but rather its concealment.[11] Shame affords privacy and discretion in sexual encounters until a steady partnership is formed and both parties are ready for the relationship to be recognized socially by their respective families and clans.

Of fundamental importance for both males and females is the concealment of their sexual activity from cross-sex siblings by strictly adhering to avoidance taboos. Young girls in particular take extreme care not to be seen by their brothers, or to see them, when they are with their respective sexual partners. Avoidance between cross-sex siblings is related to the "supreme taboo" of *sovasova*, which prohibits "any erotic dealings . . . between brother and sister," and, by extension, between any male and female of the same *dala* or *kumila* (Malinowski 1929:437). Characterized by Malinowski as the "most important and most dramatic feature" of Trobriand society (1929:451), deeply ingrained in the collective psyche, the *sovasova* taboo is an "inviolable law" of primeval ordination, "tokunabogwa ayguri" (of old it was ordained) (1929:462).[12]

A Broader Question of Pleasure

Returning to the wrong answer to the wrong question as scripted in the film *In a Savage Land*, I want to explore a further inference about the significance of sociality in gendered expressions of sexual and reproductive agency. I find it noteworthy that the woman heard the question about "copulation" in terms of fecundity—

why do Trobriand women have so many babies? Not only does this hearing indicate something about the effect of preconceived meaning on the interpretive process, but the rephrasing draws attention to the continuum of meaning between sexuality, fertility, and social reproduction. I suggest that "having babies" is not simply a euphemism for sexual intercourse, nor a veiled assumption that all sexual activity has a reproductive imperative, but rather an indication of the complementary, relational link between intimate desires and pleasures and a broader sociality.

The move in feminist and social constructionist theory over the last several decades to separate analytically the concepts of sexuality and fertility represented a significant shift, challenging biological determinism by exploring the diversity of meanings and expressions within distinct domains of experience (see Tolman and Diamond 2001). Importantly, analysis moved beyond the sex/gender and nature/culture binaries, which positioned women in a passive biological role as bearers of children, and men in an active productive role as bearers of culture (see Mallett 2003; Strathern 1988; Vance 1991). However, these theoretical moves have tended to dismiss the relationality of meanings that inhere between sexuality, fertility, and social reproduction in different cultural contexts (see Manderson and Jolly, eds. 1997). Setel argues that in an attempt to subvert "outdated essentialist views about the very nature of sex" (1999:14), new agendas for the study of sexuality as distinct from reproduction actually conceal the complementary and dialectical interactions between these domains of meaning and their influence on embodied experience and expressions of agency and desire in diverse cultural settings.[13] Margaret Jolly also acknowledges the theoretical intention to free sexuality from "the sclerotic presumptions of a constrictive, normative reproductive heterosexuality" (2001a:176) and to rupture the gender binary that holds men as sexual agents and women as reproductive objects. However, she suggests that such theoretical moves are problematic for Melanesia, where "desire and fertility are very intimate partners, and both homosexual and heterosexual practices are focused on conception, growth, and health" (176–77).

The efficacious pronouncement "Because we can!" is testament to the social links between sexual practice and its promised and achieved effects, which manifest on a continuum of interrelated, not separate, meanings. The assertion indicates how "sexual desire is entangled with broader questions of pleasure," such as the "pleasures of . . . collective sociality" and the "pleasures of fecundity" (Jolly and Manderson 1997:24; see also Rival, Slater, and Miller 1998). In the Trobriand context, the intimate pleasures of corporeal contact and the desired mixing of sexual fluids merge their effects with the regenerative investments of nurture and support, which register collectively in intergenerational and interclan ties and in the larger networks of exchange that maintain social cohesion. Additionally, the regulated periods of sexual separation and abstinence are synonymous articulations of the cultural values that define sexuality and fertility, and are linked to the safety of the mother in childbirth and the healthy growth of the baby. As Jolly notes, by "privileging restraint rather than excess," such regimens of practice serve to "heighten desire and to secure vitality, fertility, and health" on a collective scale (2001a:200).

In the Trobriands, a couple observes a period of sexual separation and abstinence during the last months of pregnancy and throughout lactation, particularly for the firstborn child. Women describe the practice in terms of their dedicated respect for the baby's well-being. Diana explains, "When we are mothers, we concentrate on pregnancy and breastfeeding. It is respect for the child that we are not sleeping with our husbands before and after giving birth."[14] Lisepa Tony, the coordinator for village birth attendants, explains, "Abstinence is more about the focus on the baby so it will grow properly. Sex will spoil the milk that is for the baby."[15]

Around the fifth or sixth month of pregnancy, the in-laws of an expectant woman escort her back to her natal household, carrying baskets of yams, mats, and other gifts for her family. Although marriage is clan-exogamous and virilocal, with the woman moving to the husband's place of residence, many couples are from the same village or neighboring villages, so in fact the move back home during pregnancy may only be a short distance.[16] However, it represents a significant spatial reconfiguration in the process of generating new life. The woman will remain "under the parents' roof" for childbirth and until the baby is weaned or has started to walk and eat solid foods (Lepani 2001:78). During this time, the father of the child will visit daily, bringing garden produce and firewood for the mother and her family, demonstrating that he is working hard for his in-laws. The husband may take up residence in his in-laws' household, but the couple does not resume sexual activity for several months after birth. The spatial practice of separation and seclusion has significant social and symbolic effects. The nestling of the maternal body in her natal household secures reproductive viability and health through intergenerational support from her female *dala* relatives and from her father and his *dala*, while reinforcing the important affinal exchange relations with the child's father's *dala*.

The social practices that herald a marital union in the Trobriands do not involve elaborate ceremonies in the public domain, unlike in many Melanesian societies where bride-price ceremonies are key social institutions. The act of marriage is an inconspicuous event, occurring when the young couple shares a meal of yams together for the first time at the husband's parents' dwelling. The meal signifies the marital bond, and for the first time the couple is seen together in public. The husband's female relatives tie a new long skirt around the bride's hips and then cut the frayed banana fibers into a clean hemline at the knees, the length that signifies adult womanhood. The length also symbolizes the end of the young woman's sexual freedom and mobility, for marriage is said to *katupwela kaikela*, or "fold the legs" of a woman. The marriage is then publicly formalized by *katuvila* (literally, "turn around"), a series of reciprocal exchanges of yams, cooked food, clay pots, and shell valuables between the two immediate families, with support from their respective *dala* relatives.

The Trobriand mother's return to her natal home during pregnancy and lactation, the Trobriand father's devoted physical and emotional attachment to his offspring, shared breastfeeding of babies among women of the same *dala*, the adoption[17] of children for weaning and early socialization within a different household from the natal family—these are the regenerative aspects of sociality that attest to the connections between sexuality, fertility, and social reproduction. They are the intimate practices of collective enterprise that associate procreative capacity with sedentary dwelling—a sharp contrast to the mobility that expresses the sexual capacity and reproductive potential of unmarried youth. But these intimate practices are aspects of regenerative sociality that are accounted for in the larger domain through public demonstrations of capacity, potential, and acting with others in mind.

Sagali, the collective enterprise of mortuary exchange that ensures regeneration in the cosmic realm through the combined effects of corporeal work and pleasure, profoundly demonstrates the constellation of interrelated meanings of sexuality, fertility, and reproduction. Weiner (1976:61) calls *sagali* an event of "spectacular visual communication" of the matrilineal system and the reproductive power that women embody. She argues that the materiality of *sagali* distributions—the banana-leaf bundles called *doba*—reflects the enduring ideological concerns of matriliny and human reproduction in Trobriand society, ensuring intergenerational social stability (Weiner 1976, 1980b). The ephemeral bundles of dried banana leaves are the durable material of cultural resilience and continuity.

The mortuary exchange rituals of island societies throughout the Massim are infused with symbolism of fertility and sexuality, representing the vitality and health that restores social balance after the disruptive effects of death (see Damon and Wagner, eds. 1989). Frederick Damon suggests that the regenerative symbolism signifies how "the dependencies created by the production of children are being paid back at death, and the conditions for the reproduction of children in the future are being established" (1989:18–19). I turn now to *sagali* to illustrate how embodied capacity and potential, and the pleasures of generational fecundity, are expressed on a larger social scale. As a ritualized practice of social cohesion, *sagali* offers insights into the sociality of communication and exchange relations that hold crucial relevance for enabling HIV prevention and care.

"Going Inside" *Sagali*

Small groups of women and girls began arriving at Orabesi village just after daybreak, balancing huge baskets of *doba* on their heads, many of the younger women counterbalancing the baskets with babies on their hips. As the sun ascended the morning sky, the grassy expanse in front of my mother-in-law's house steadily filled with people arriving for *sagali*, some having walked the length of the island—over three hours—to reach this destination. The women set down their baskets, brimming with bundles, skirts, and brightly colored fabric, and arranged themselves in recognizable *dala* groupings around the central clearing under the blue tarpaulins that the young men of the village erected for shade.

The atmosphere is that of a festive bazaar, set into motion by colors and sounds and the breathtaking bounty of goods on display. Some women have come to *valova*, or increase their own supply of *doba* for future *sagali* commitments by trading in a range of consumable items: lollipops, packets of chips, and balloons for the kids; sticks of tobacco and strips of old newspaper for rolling cigarettes; betel nut and pepper; empty plastic water bottles; kerosene in old beer bottles; baked scones and boiled shellfish. Men mingle and children play along the periphery, a pedestrian thoroughfare congested with onlookers attracted to the spectacle. In the distance under the lofty mango tree, other men are busily tending the earth oven and stirring taro puddings in large clay cooking pots, preparing the feast that will feed hungry participants after the day's proceedings. The sound of pigs' anguished squeals, which cut through the stillness of the early morning, lingers in memory as the smell of roasted pork wafts from the earth oven.

With the scorching sun at its highest peak, hundreds of people are now congregated at Kaugere hamlet, an undulating swarm of activity encircling the open space where *sagali* transactions take place. The sixteen *sepwana* piles of *doba*, symmetrically stacked on flat woven baskets, tower impressively over the seated women, heralding the key relationships that are on display. The women sort through their massive baskets of *doba* as the pre-*sagali* lobbying intensifies with much shouting, swearing, and cajoling. Arguments erupt and then crescendo into hoots of laughter and congenial backslapping. Finally, one of the *sagali* organizers peers up at the sun, high in the expanse of blue cloudless sky, and announces that it is time to begin. Her forehead sparkling with sweat, she smacks the red betel-nut paste on her lips, turns to me and exclaims with jovial zest, "We want our skin to be on fire!"

To observe and partake in *sagali* is dazzling to the senses. I have been witness to countless *sagali* over the last thirty-three years, yet each new event fascinates me.[18] Strathern notes that the effect of being dazzled by social phenomena, or being "on the threshold of understanding" (1999:11), draws ethnographers to "arenas of social life where people appear to be reflecting on their practices and often seem to be 'revealing' to themselves facts about themselves not always immediately apparent" (10). During one of the first *sagali* I experienced, held at our house in Port Moresby in 1982, with over three hundred people in attendance, I received a revelation that continues to provide me with an important frame of reference. My own fascination for the ardent proceedings was echoed in sentiment by one of my husband's cousin-brothers,[19] who undoubtedly sensed that I was overwhelmed and disoriented by the engulfing activity. The in-law quietly confided to me, "*Sagali* is amazing, isn't it? But the key to *sagali* is to know who you are and how you fit in." For me, this succinct statement not only offered guidance on the terms of engagement in *sagali*, it also yielded an insight on the way embodied practice ensures the continuity of social forms from one generation to the next. Trobrianders themselves are dazzled by the dynamic complexity of *sagali*. Perhaps the seductive spectacle of *sagali* guarantees continued enactment through people's ongoing desire to make known their revelations about themselves—how they fit into the web of social relations on display.

Knowing who you are and how you fit into *sagali* begins with how you are related to the deceased. The members of the deceased's *dala* are the *sagali toliu'ula*, or organizing sponsors, responsible for distributing the exchange items. Malinowski and Weiner both gloss *toli* to mean "owner." However, Edwin Hutchins's translation of *toli* as "a relation of social responsibility" seems more apt (1978:55). *U'ula* means the core or foundational reason or purpose of something. To assume the sponsorship of *sagali* entails responsibility toward a common social good. On the receiving end of *sagali* distributions are the *toliyouwa*, or workers, people from other clans who actively mourned for the deceased and supported the deceased's relatives with food and *doba*. The central and most important *sagali* distributions are in the name of *kakau*, the deceased's spouse, and *kapu*, the father and his line, which represent the primary social ties between clans. The female relatives of the bereaved spouse and father are the ones who go into the central clearing to collect the *doba*.[20]

People talk about "going inside" *sagali* as the orientation for their active participation. There are two main ways to go inside *sagali*. *Veyalela* is working *sagali* for one's own *dala*, or the mother's side, and *litulela* is working *sagali* for the father's side. As verbs, these terms describe how one participates in *sagali* and contributes to the distributions; as nouns, they describe the particular form a distribution takes. The women who bring massive amounts of *doba* to *sagali* are from the *toliu'ula dala*, or they are the daughters of the male members of the *toliu'ula dala* who "go inside" *sagali* to work for their fathers. Women are always compelled to do *sagali* for their father's *dala* because, they say, "He was the one feeding me when I was a child." One woman explained it this way: "When it comes to *sagali* for the father's side, we can feel the difference between our mothers and our *bubus* [father's sisters]. Mothers have nothing to do with it. That's the time we feel the separation from our *dala* and we feel closer to our father's relatives" (Journal notes, 9 September 2003).

Behind everyone working for *sagali* are the people who provide support, and every contribution reflects yet another layer of support. Contributions come from many directions and people are able to activate multiple exchange relationships concurrently during a *sagali*. Fathers help sons to support their mothers and sisters; sons support fathers by providing food and giving support to their father's sisters through their own wives. Women might work as *veyalela* while also providing support in the name of their spouses. For example, women from the same clan as the *toliu'ula* might go inside *sagali* in their capacity as in-laws, supporting the wives of their husbands' brothers, who are also their own kinswomen. In this way, *sagali* provides people with unlimited opportunities to reinforce and expand important social ties with *keyawa*, or those people with whom one has ongoing exchange relations. People who provide support will be reciprocated at *sagali*, and in turn they will redistribute the *doba* they acquire within their own network of relationships.

The sponsors of *sagali* refer to carefully compiled written lists of recipients' names to account for all required transactions, and distributions proceed through several distinct stages to cover various categories of mourning that require repayment (see Weiner 1976:107–15). The stages generally follow an established order, although this is not fixed but can vary according to preference or circumstance. Some *sagali* are combined efforts to meet the obligations of more than one death in the clan, and may include a separate form of exchange called *lubwau*, literally meaning "soup," which acknowledges the work of those who brought food and provided care for a person suffering from a serious illness.

Immediately prior to the commencement of distributions, a parade of support takes place, which demonstrates the importance of *vevai*, or in-laws, in the work of *sagali*. Referred to as *kabiyamala*, the female in-laws of the *toliu'ula* line up in single file and walk to their brothers' and uncles' wives to give them several bundles of *doba* or pieces of material to publicly acknowledge the yams they have received from their male relatives throughout the year. *Kabiyamala* is described in English as "helping hands," representing the reinforcement and supplementary support given to *sagali* sponsors even though they have accumulated sufficient stores of *doba* to "stand on their own." The first set of *sagali* distributions is called *kauwela*, which repay the people who provided food and support throughout the mourning period. The main segment of *sagali* involves distributions called *kaimelu*, which acknowledge the work of all male clansmen who provide yams for the current and previous *sagali* that the *dala* has sponsored. As a senior member of the *toliu'ula dala* calls out the names of male relatives, several women move swiftly to the woven mat that marks center stage and throw down bundles of *doba*, folded pieces of cloth, and at times coins or paper notes. As they retreat to their baskets on the sideline and prepare for the next round, the wives or daughters of the men whose names were called rush into the clearing and collect their piles of *doba*. With the transactions lasting from three to four minutes, *kaimelu* can take the entire afternoon to complete. Thousands of bundles of *doba*, as well as hundreds of pieces of cloth and cash amounting to several hundred kina, will change hands. By the end of the day, the women will have walked in and out of the central clearing many hundreds of times (see Figure 4.1).

Sagali culminates with the distribution of large bunches of betel nut, raw food including yams and other garden produce, packets of rice, flour, sugar, tea, tobacco, and pieces of uncooked pork. Also called *kaimelu*, this distribution is made in the name of the participants' residential hamlets and is the responsibility of the male relatives of the deceased, whose wives have already received *doba* from their

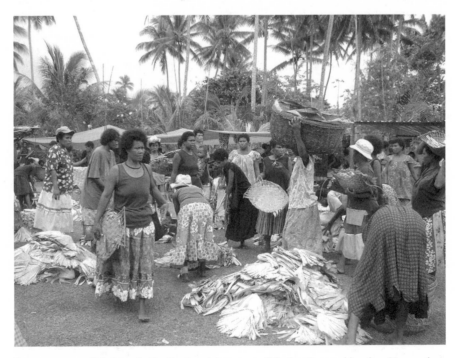

FIGURE 4.1. • Ethel Jacob distributing *doba* at a *sagali* for her deceased brother, Kwemtula village, 18 July 2003

sisters-in-law during the earlier stage. The event then finishes with a feast of cooked food prepared by the men of the organizing *dala* for their female relatives and all the participants.

Trobrianders often refer to the activity of *sagali* as *mwasawa*, or game. They joke that they are playing cards or trading in shares on the floor of the stock exchange. With a competitive passion similar to Kula trade and *kayasa*, or yam harvest competitions, which are the dedicated pursuits of Trobriand men, the game of *sagali* compels Trobriand women to throw down as much *doba* as possible to assert the vitality and renown of their *dala*. The *doba* that *toliu'ula* women distribute in *sagali* unties the deceased from all worldly obligations and is a direct statement about the strength of the *dala*, as demonstrated by mutual support between siblings and women's exchange relations with their husbands' *dala* and their fathers' *dala*, members of which were mourners and supporters throughout the mourning period. In effect, *sagali* distributions represent a temporal process of "de-conception" where the loss of a clan member is deliberately dissipated and then transformed by the "expansive creation of new persons and relations through new or additional exchanges" (Mosko 2000:383; see also Mosko 1983). In this sense, *sagali* serves the interests of the living as much as it resolves the interests of the deceased.

Growing *Dala*

Trobrianders speak with great affection and passion about *sagali*. They say, "*Sagali* is in our blood, we can't give it up. *Sagali* is too close to us." The fundamental importance of *sagali* factors strongly in women's reproductive decisions. Women speak with assuredness about their regenerative power to "grow" their *dala*—to have large families—to be strong for *sagali* (Lepani 2001:56). *Bidalasi*, the active verb for reproduction (third person), derives from the core concept of matrilineal source and substance. The following statements made by older Trobriand women illustrate the importance of *dala* in relation to the value of *sagali*, and the synchrony between biological and social reproduction.

> If a girl is going around with a man and they know that man is from a strong *dala*, her mothers and aunties will want her to marry him because he will bring them good support for *sagali*. Same for boys, the mothers will tell them to go for that girl because she is from a strong *dala* and will work hard for *sagali*. On both sides, boys and girls, it is the same. [Taped group discussion, 11 December 2000]

> It is through the ladies where we have the *dala* growing. So when one lady gives birth, if she has a daughter, and that daughter gives birth then the *dala* goes on and it becomes bigger. So that's what happens with the culture. In having a lot of people they would be making a lot of gardens, more food. And if somebody has to die then they would have the number of people to make *sagali* for that person. [Taped group discussion, 12 January 2001]

The collective congregation of *dala* members working to lift the period of mourning following the death of a clansperson is a powerful image of fecundity, an event where the important ties of social support are on display. The enactment of

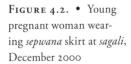

FIGURE 4.2. • Young
pregnant woman wear-
ing *sepwana* skirt at *sagali*,
December 2000

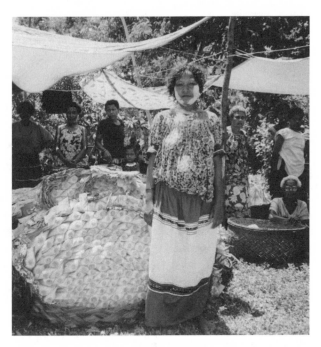

sagali makes visible the complementary values of fertility and sexuality in numerous ways. At one *sagali* I attended during fieldwork, the clanswomen of a young
pregnant woman selected her to wear the long *sepwana* skirt, the special mourning
skirts made and worn by clan members of the deceased's spouse and father (see
Figure 4.2).[21] This was a notable choice. Not only was the young woman in the last
month of pregnancy with her firstborn child, she was her mother's firstborn daughter, and, significantly, she married into the *dala* of the deceased, which was also
her father's *dala*. It was a stunning display of the permeability between persons
and things and how social relations are made visible in objects of exchange (Strathern 1988:181). The young woman's personhood quite literally embodied matrilineal
identity while simultaneously being projected onto the objects of exchange. The
"aesthetics of generational fecundity" took center stage in the public realm (Jolly
and Manderson 1997:24).

Working for *Doba*

The durability of *sagali* as a distinctive Trobriand social form is apparent in the
dedicated time and effort women invest in making and acquiring *doba*. The materiality of *doba* is a patent and ever-present feature of the Trobriand landscape.
Along tracks and roadways and in the villages, the ubiquity of *doba* production
will strike even the most casual observer: Women cutting and scraping banana
leaves on the incised *kaidawagu* boards to remove the outer layer of skin and make
patterned textures on the thin strips. Rows of banana-leaf strips, imprinted with
designs, lying on the ground, bleaching in the sun. Women alone or working in
groups tying the strips into bundles. Women with large baskets of *doba* balanced
on their heads, walking purposively to *sagali*. Huge baskets of *doba* stored in the
recesses of the small residential dwellings.

Women refer to *doba* as their *paisewa*, or work. As objects of exchange, *doba* signify the value of women's labor in the wider domain of social relations. The act of mourning is also work—observing food taboos, wearing black clothing, restricting mobility and usual activities. Organizing and participating in *sagali* is also the embodiment of labor. Mortuary exchange is a continuum of hard work, from the moment of death, to the planning and mobilizing of resources during the prolonged period of mourning, to the culminating event of *sagali*. Work is valued for its performative effects and is continually on display through the production of goods and the efficacy of exchange. Productive activity creates social value; the objects people produce and exchange assume the embodied value of their labor, serving as a measure of their social relations and interconnectedness and a public reckoning of personal agency and acting with others in mind. Weiner observes, "the production in yams and *doba* is always being evaluated and calculated in terms of effort and energy expended" (1976:282). The work of exchange is a moral duty, a sign of respect, and evidence of the strength of a person's character.[22]

Shortly after the death of a clansperson, women begin the work of *sagali* by making and accumulating *doba*, purchasing material, and sewing cloth skirts. Women receive contributions of *doba* from their in-laws and friends, and they take careful note of who supports them because these people will be the recipients of *doba* during *sagali*.[23] Small transactions involving the exchange of various commodities—food items, firewood, kerosene, and betel nut—for *doba* bundles are a daily occurrence as women work to build up their *doba* reserves. Called *valova*, these exchanges illustrate how *doba* as a unit of value is converted to other commodities. Women will use cash to purchase goods from the store and then exchange those goods for *doba*. Through *valova* exchanges, men also become directly involved in supporting their mothers, sisters, and wives in working for *doba*. Women would never make *doba* just to sell it for cash. When women *valova* they are building their supply of *doba*, not getting rid of it. The exchange process works only one way; it is driven by a demand for *doba*, not a demand for cash. Women can acquire *doba* with cash in one particular way—giving a cash donation to the women's fellowship at church obliges members to reciprocate collectively by contributing a commensurate amount of *doba* to the donor.

Trobrianders often speak of the process of accumulating *doba* by using the verb *nene*, meaning "to search," which evokes the effort that goes into mobilizing resources through established exchange networks. Rather than talking about *doba* as something one makes, searching for *doba* suggests that productivity is inherently social and not something achieved in isolation from other people's efforts. The search for *doba* often is the reason for increased mobility beyond the islands. Men will talk about their reasons for traveling to Alotau or Port Moresby as being to "search for *doba*" to help their mothers or wives with the work of *sagali*. The *doba* they find are not banana-leaf bundles, but rather the bolts of material purchased at shops with money acquired through other forms of labor or by activating exchange relationships with people who have sources of cash income.

The continued participation in *sagali* among Trobrianders who reside in Port Moresby and other areas in PNG attests to its importance as an integrative force in their social and economic life and its essential role in regenerating matrilineal identity. During my fieldwork in 2000 and 2003, three separate *sagali* took place in which the key sponsors were Trobriand women who live and work in Port Moresby. Arriving back home with impressive amounts of material and cash, these women invested many months of dedicated planning and preparation toward the events. Even women who have married outside of the Trobriands and reside overseas will return home when the obligation to make *sagali* calls them. The *sagali* these women are able to sponsor, with their inputs of material and cash, are highly praised in the Trobriands and draw huge numbers of participants and crowds.

It is a matter of speculation whether the further incorporation of cloth and cash will put unsustainable financial pressure on the stability of *sagali* as a key integrative event in Trobriand social life. One man in his forties told me, "Money is part of custom now. Everything is money now. It would be hard to *sagali* without money. We need money for *doba*, money for *sepwana* and *deli*."[24] *Sagali* places significant demands on resources, and consequently it is the source of concern and ambivalence for women and men who feel the constraints but also say that they cannot "give it up" because "*sagali* keeps calling us." One village on Kiriwina made the collective decision a few years ago to give up *sagali* because it was getting too expensive and kept people from other activities. Yet people from the village routinely attend and participate in *sagali* in other villages through their clan affiliations. The decision to cease *sagali* activities within the village has affected how the young girls there view marriage options. As one woman explained to me, "Our girls don't want to marry here because no *sagali*. They want to marry other places so they can go there and *sagali*."

Most people cannot imagine dealing with death without going inside *sagali* and working for *doba*. As a nondurable exchange item, *doba* continues to represent a deep genealogy of belonging and it holds potency for future possibilities. In making a social prognosis about the stability and continuity of *sagali*, it is important to bear in mind that the compulsion and imperative to work for *doba*, and to demonstrate *dala* capacity and vitality through investments of labor, endure as key motivations.

For me, the dazzle effect of *sagali* continues to yield insights on its social and symbolic significance. An older man made the following unsolicited observation to me in the aftermath of a *sagali* I attended in 2000: "There are two English words to describe *sagali*: connection and communication." When I asked him which two Trobriand words best translate those concepts, he told me that translation is not important. "We don't need words to describe *sagali*. We *do sagali*," the man emphasized, and then laughed heartily at his retort.

The observation provides important insights even if the English gets lost in translation. Connection speaks of relational ties, of *sepituki* (joining or uniting), or, figuratively, of *seluva* (tying together the banana-leaf bundles). *Doba* is the binding social fiber that connects people through exchange, reinforcing social relations. Communication speaks of the importance of bringing exchange relations into public view, or *saimatala*, which means "to put into public view" (*sai-*, do by putting; *matala*, eye), to make intentions visible and publicly accountable. Communication also suggests how acts of labor, or working for *doba*, symbolize people's capacity and vitality, as well as their social embeddedness. Connection and communication are relational concepts; it is important to pay close attention to *sagali* transactions for the information they communicate about future obligations and reciprocations. Connection and communication also evoke the collective ethos of *sagali*, that of *kabiyamala*, or contribution, the reinforcement and extra support people give to one another even when they can stand on their own.[25]

Of course, it is pretense to suggest that *sagali* is never a hotly contested site of interaction, an event of fierce competition and emotional intensity. At times the performative aspects of *sagali* yield unilateral expressions of personal autonomy. I vividly recall one *sagali* held for a middle-aged man who died from tuberculosis after a prolonged, debilitating period of illness. During the proceedings, a woman stunned the large crowd of more than one hundred participants into absolute silence when she contested a particular transaction that she believed was her right to receive. She stood defensively next to the pile of *doba* in the central clearing as other women tried to take their share and, thumping her chest, she yelled out, "Yeigu! Yeigu wala!" (Me. Me only). She then confidently collected the *doba* and strode to the sideline. At stake was her claim that she, more than others, had devoted time and resources to the care of the deceased.

Sagali is a system of transparent scrutiny and accountability. As a collective enterprise conducted in the public arena, *sagali* brings into the open the complex social ties—at times contentious and tenuous—that hold Trobriand society together. As a robust cultural form, *sagali* is responsive to the exigencies of circumstance and is able to withstand impassioned disputes and provide resolution for contested interests.

Social Connection, Communication, and HIV Prevention and Care

> News about *sagali* always spreads like bush fire from one end of the island to the other. News about important information like HIV/AIDS travels very slowly. Meanwhile, if we are not careful, the virus will spread like bush fire! [Florence Mokolava, 15 July 2003]

As metaphors for the regenerative capacity of *sagali*, connection and communication represent the continuity of form and function and the ability of culture to respond to social change while maintaining stability and cohesion. Clearly, *sagali* as the cultural form for resolving the disruption that death brings to a community has important implications for how Trobrianders will respond to the potential impact of HIV on their ways of knowing and living. What is patently at stake is the continued capacity of people to cope with the demands of social obligation in the face of overwhelming illness and death, and whether the system of *sagali* will be able to absorb increasing demands. There is likely to be an increase in *lubwau* obligations, the form of *sagali* that acknowledges people's support during times of prolonged illness. An increase in obligations will put constraints on limited resources. It is possible that there will be an easing of expectations to more efficiently make use of limited resources. As a precedent, people refer to a malaria epidemic in the mid-1990s, when scores of people died within a period of a few months. In response to the overwhelming loss, which in retrospect people generally accepted as having been caused by malaria and not the scourge of sorcery or witchcraft,[26] there was a collective agreement among affected communities to ease *sagali* obligations. Although *sagali* provides an effective system for resource mobilization, the exchange relations that support *sagali* efforts and the relations acknowledged in *doba* distributions link directly to the cycle of yam cultivation. In subsistence economies, it is manifestly clear that food production and food security are affected by the toll HIV takes on the productive members of society. The potential effects of HIV on the sustainability of the Trobriand exchange economy are issues and concerns that Trobrianders themselves must confront by bringing together cultural knowledge with newly acquired knowledge about HIV.

The insight about connection and communication offered to me by the old man provides a way of thinking about the social process of knowledge production in relation to HIV prevention and care. The deep-seated sense of social obligation instilled by the ethos of *sagali* is a valuable cultural resource for cultivating a positive collective response to the challenges HIV imposes on communities. Rather naively, I once proposed to my research collaborators that *sagali* might be a possible forum for communicating about HIV—an open space for dialogue—given that it brings together large numbers of people focused on collective enterprise. I was told politely that my idea was probably not feasible; it would not "feel right" to use *sagali* for talking about HIV. Besides, my friends explained, people are too busy at *sagali* to think about anything other than *doba* and knowing that they will be enjoying a meal of pork at the end of the day. True, feelings are high at *sagali*; there is a great festive atmosphere, it is a place to rendezvous with others, and young people meet potential sexual partners and make arrangements for nighttime trysts.

The fit between *sagali* and HIV communication activities may not be practicable or appropriate. Nonetheless, *sagali* offers insight into the sociality of communication and how exchange networks represent important social connections for mobilizing resources and responses, for reinforcing a sense of community responsibility and commitment, and for ensuring social cohesion in times of great stress and sorrow. These are the cultural resources needed for responding to HIV. The social networks that spread news about *sagali* are the same channels that can be mobilized to facilitate communication about HIV prevention and care.

Trobrianders often speak of the work of *sagali* in affectionate terms, using the word *bobwailila*, which translates as love, gift, generosity, or contribution. Florence, as well as many other people, often expressed to me the sentiment that the Trobriands is a "sharing and caring place." Indeed, when I asked people what they thought the "Islands of Love" signified, without hesitation the answer almost invariably would be, "Trobriands is a sharing and caring place." Whether this is a rehearsed counter to the imposed reputation of sexual extravagance, whether it has become rote platitude imbued in part by Christian values and biblical sayings, or whether it expresses the deep-seated cultural ethos of *bobwailila* is perhaps irrelevant. What does hold significance is the embodied capacity and potential to act with others in mind.

Constructions of Gender and the Gendering of HIV

I now shift perspective to consider how the use of "gender" in the language of HIV risk and prevention interacts with Trobriand constructions of gendered agency and complementarity between sexuality and fertility as exemplified in procreation beliefs and the values of matrilineal social reproduction. In making this shift, I take guidance from Strathern's analytical strategy in *The Gender of the Gift*: "The task is not to imagine one can replace exogenous concepts by indigenous counterparts; rather the task is to convey the complexity of the indigenous concepts in reference to the particular context in which they are produced . . . by exposing the contextualized nature of analytical ones" (1988:8).

The standard usage of the concept of gender, defined as the socially constructed roles and responsibilities assigned differentially to males and females within a given cultural context, has gained currency in development policy over the past several decades and in the global response to HIV more recently (Carovano 1991; Gupta 2000; Heise and Elias 1995; Long and Ankrah, eds. 1996; Reid 1996). This trend is apparent in Papua New Guinea as well. Gender terminology is widely applied in social-sector development policies and programs, largely at the behest of international donors, with emphasis on the principles of women's empowerment and equal rights.[27] Most development projects routinely incorporate gender as a crosscutting theme, with the aim to "mainstream" gender issues into all project activities. The concept is written into school curricula and training manuals for community health workers, the police constabulary, and agriculture extension workers. The public-sector planning cycle incorporates gender analysis, using the concept as an evaluation tool and as a variable in needs assessment and problem solving. The gender concept is also folded into a cluster of other reified development principles, such as "community participation," "empowerment," and "ownership," and is prominent in the United Nations Millennium Development Goals (Overseas Development Institute 2008).[28] The PNG government's *Medium Term Development Strategy, 2005–2010* prioritizes both gender and HIV/AIDS as crosscutting development issues (Government of Papua New Guinea 2004). In 2006, the National AIDS Council commissioned the development of a National Gender Policy and Plan on HIV and AIDS with the stated purpose "to strengthen the integration of gender into all aspects of the National Strategic Plan, in recognition of the key significance of gender factors in shaping PNG's epidemic" (National AIDS Council 2006:2).

The use of the gender concept in PNG has created tensions regarding the seemingly disproportionate emphasis on women's issues in isolation from social and cultural context, a focus perceived as privileging women rather than redressing inequalities between women and men. Nationalist rhetoric about the purported egalitarianism of traditional social structures, and the complementarity of traditional male and female roles and responsibilities, is often used to assert that contemporary gender inequalities are simply the product of colonialism, not of deeply rooted cultural ideologies, and that, regardless of the colonial legacy, everyone stands to benefit equally from independent nationhood and development (Macintyre

1998:222–23). Convergent with this line of thinking is the notion that the post-colonial urban economy has transformed gender relations to such an extent that women are no longer acting like women but assuming individuated autonomy in relation to traditional male authority (Macintyre 1998:223).[29]

Before I commenced my first period of fieldwork, several PNG women colleagues cautioned me about using gender to frame my exploration of cultural meanings and lived experience, urging me instead to look more closely at family and clan relationships. Although not articulated as such, I believe my colleagues' concern related to the way the static categories of "male" and "female" occlude the more salient kinship relations that comprise sociality in Papua New Guinea (see Jolly 2003:135). Related to this, I suspect, was apprehension about how the discourse on gender rights tends to emphasize the public domain of social life for measuring equality of opportunity and participation, thereby implying that domesticity makes women less than full persons, denying them their unrealized potential as individuals in the broader world (see Sepoe 2000:68–69).[30]

The tension between Trobriand constructions of gendered agency and analyses of gender based on the dichotomous alignment of male/female with public/domestic are reflected in the views of Lisepa Tony, the coordinator for the village birth attendants program in the Trobriands, who is familiar with the gender concept as an aspect of development work. During one of many conversations with Lisepa, we talked about the gender division of labor in the Trobriands and I asked her how she saw gender roles in *sagali*. Lisepa paused before answering, the assumed model of binary difference not immediately translatable or relevant to the dynamics of *sagali*.

> Maybe we don't see it along those lines. The roles in *sagali* are the *dala*, the clan, and how you go into it, working for the father's side or working for our mothers. One word to describe the status of women in Trobriand society: *sagali*. I say it again: *sagali*. That is the value of women here. Women are valued because it is a matrilineal system. In the VBA program, we do role-plays and we talk about these things. I have covered all the islands with workshops. Most men realized that it would be true—we opened the eyes of men to see that the work of women is more than men. We did an exercise to scale the workload. Gender relations are unbalanced because men regard women as the laborers. The only pay packet for women is to say "thank you," but many times they don't even get that pay. But labor is valued. *Paisewa*. *Sagali* is *paisewa*. That's how it is viewed. Fitness is important for both men and women. You will be ignored if you can't work hard. Nobody wants to be thought of as lazy. [Interview notes, 20 December 2000]

When talking about gender in relation to VBA work, Lisepa's description illustrates how the concept is generally applied in development work to focus on the differential roles and status of men and women, and it suggests how gender is viewed as a novel foreign notion aligned with development in opposition to "culture."

> We have been using the word "gender" in the VBA program. We have learned about the work of women, work of men, time spent in work. People are aware of workload but because of the culture there is a fight in their mind all the time

whether we believe the new things coming in or we stick to our culture and that's why there is no development. The roles of men, that's garden work, but most of the time is spent chewing betel nut with friends. Carrying firewood, jobs in the house, these are women's jobs. Mind you, when we launched the gender program, we brought in all the heads of districts plus chiefs, and then the Paramount Chief cried tears, and also the police sergeant. The PC said, "You know, when I heard that message I started helping out in the house." This is gender. [Interview notes, 23 October 2003]

The contrasting views that Lisepa presents resonate with the concern expressed by my colleagues about preconceived notions of gender. Women and men are daughters and sons, sisters and brothers, wives and husbands, mothers and fathers —often mothers and fathers before they are wives and husbands—aunties and uncles, grandmothers and grandfathers, members of clans and in-laws. People do not act as "women" or "men" as much as they act as gendered persons in complex sets of relationships, which are realized in a vast field of social interaction. Furthermore, these multiple roles and relationships are constructed, acted upon, maintained, and altered throughout the life cycle. In the process, they configure social status and shape the differential experiences of males and females. Gender takes form and meaning in relational difference, not categorical difference (Moore 1994:28). As Strathern (1988) consummately demonstrates for Melanesian sociality, gender is not simply a question of gendered domains (domestic or public) or gendered roles (making babies or making "culture"), but is embodied in a multiplicity of forms and positions that activate relational personhood.

Gender and the Feminized Persona of HIV

Since the mid-1990s, the global response to HIV has increased the policy and program focus on the gender dimensions of HIV epidemiology and the differential impact of the virus on men and women, particularly in the context of the growing incidence of HIV infection in young girls and women, or the so-called feminization of the pandemic (UNAIDS 2004). Gender has become a major conceptual tool for illuminating how HIV is socially structured and signified (Dowsett 2003:21).[31] Frequently, the gender concept takes a reductionist line, where "gender equals women equals mothers" (Luker 2002:1).[32] The maternal image of gender draws heavily on the dualisms of sex/gender and sexuality/fertility, essentializing women's reproductive biology and collapsing women and children into an inseparable category of vulnerability. This equation not only lumps all women together under universal assumptions about sexless maternity, it obviates the importance of men and masculinities, reinforcing a parallel conflation of men with sexuality but not paternity, and it diminishes the diverse spectrum of gender identities and sexual desires.

In the early years of the global epidemic, the biomedical model of HIV maintained that the virus could not penetrate the "rugged vagina," which was "designed to withstand the trauma of intercourse as well as childbirth" (Treichler 1999:17).[33] When enough scientific evidence accrued to determine that HIV *could* be transmitted during vaginal sexual intercourse and during childbirth and lactation, constructions of risk hardened around the image of the female sex worker as the vector of infection, while the softer notion of vulnerability was reserved for the maternal body, viewed as both the passive victim and the unwitting vessel of infection (Squire 1993:5–7).[34] Such characterizations of female culpability and vulnerability persist in reinforcing notions of safety in the heteronormative model of monogamous marriage and reproductive sex, belying the reality that for many women, married and unmarried, mothers or not, the greatest risk of exposure to HIV comes from their regular male partner(s) (Hirsch et al. 2009).[35] This pattern of HIV transmission is borne out by research in PNG, where findings from a nationwide sexual health study indicate that "housewives" are at greatest risk of becoming infected (Aeno 2005:5; see also Hammar 2007).[36]

The reductionist equation is evident in the media and popular representations of female gender in PNG, where "mothers" is the common referent for women. The maternal construction of gender also finds equivalence in nationalist and Christian discourses about women's domestic roles and responsibilities (Jolly 2002b:25; Jolly and Macintyre 1989:7). As noted previously, "gender" does not adequately represent the array of social relations in PNG that define male and female persons by age, rank, kinship, and reproductive status and that validate and give value to personhood. Of course, "mother" is not an inclusive term either. However, when the reductionist equation is not fully calculated, gender as a euphemism for "women" creates apprehension about an imported feminist agenda of liberation and empowerment. "Women" assumes an individuated autonomy unconnected to, and hence disruptive of, enduring relations of social reproduction, an assumption made especially apropos in the case of women who are perceived as either elitist or "wayward" (see Wardlow 2006). To complete the gender equation by reducing women to mothers makes the discourse of equal rights—and the talk about sex— more tenable in the PNG context where ideologies of male dominance and male sexual privilege persist.

The reductionist equation holds important consequences for how HIV risk is conceptualized. Pregnant women are the epidemiological indicator for estimating the prevalence of HIV infection in the general population, that is, the majority of people who are safely excluded from categories of people regarded as "high risk"—men who have sex with men and female sex workers. The idea that gender equals women equals mothers conveys a moralistic evaluation of those women perceived as deviating from the sedentary norm—women who do not marry or bear children, women who have multiple partners, women who exchange sex for material benefits, and women who keep pace with sexually active mobile men. The rhetorical emphasis on maternity negates embodied sexual desire and pleasure, the agency of young unmarried women, and the practice of nonreproductive sex, as well as differential needs for contraception and disease prevention throughout the life course. Once again, women are viewed either as victims and vessels (the "mothers") or promiscuous vectors (all others) in relation to HIV risk, a division that runs deep in the language of HIV prevention and feeds into the widespread misconception throughout PNG that "women" are responsible for the spread of the virus (see Butt and Eves, eds. 2008; Keck 2007:48). Countering these prevailing moral constructs often results in negating women's sexuality in the name of empowerment—the only strong woman is one who says no to (nonreproductive) sex (whether protected or not). It also undercuts recognition that for the majority of women, the likelihood of becoming infected with HIV is related to the sexual activity of their husband or intimate partner. Indeed, the portrayal of the HIV epidemic as feminized tends to reinforce perceptions that AIDS is a woman's problem—the problem affects only women or women are the source of the problem, a perception that in some areas in PNG parallels understandings of other sexually transmitted infections (Wardlow 2002).

The following statement, made at the 2004 PNG National Consensus Workshop on HIV/AIDS, reveals how gender bias becomes embedded in risk analysis of HIV: "If village girls are right into multiple sex practices, this will increase the exposure of rural communities to HIV/AIDS."[37] The statement suggests that as HIV manifests in rural areas, "village girls" has become the new category of epidemiological risk. Men generally do not perceive their sexual activity, imbued with notions of masculine prowess involving mobility and cash (Jenkins 2007:44, 47), as the pathway for viral transmission in the same way as what they perceive to be uncontrolled female sexuality. Commentaries by outsiders also influence biased gender representations of HIV transmission within the country. The following description of the PNG epidemic by a UNAIDS official was quoted in the media: "When women have multiple sex partners the epidemic really gallops, and that's what is happening in Papua New Guinea" (Corder 2005). The characterization of an epidemic out of control because of women's sexuality underscores the power of language in influencing perceptions of HIV risk and prevention and reinforcing the gendered dimensions of stigma and blame.

Gendered Agency, Social Reproduction, and HIV Prevention

The modes through which gendered representations of HIV risk are communicated influence how people engage with and personalize the information they receive. In many rural communities throughout PNG, information about HIV is linked to maternal and child health services, with health workers mandated to include HIV awareness in health promotion talks during antenatal and family planning clinics and immunization patrols. This has been the case in the Trobriands, where the VBA program also provides an important channel of communication. The integration of HIV and sexual health services within the primary health-care system is vital for responding to the global pandemic, and is especially important in contexts like PNG where the service delivery network is a main link to rural and remote communities, provided that facilities are open and functioning.

However, a consequence of relying on maternal and child health services as a key modality for HIV awareness is the subtraction of men and fathers, not only from the gender equation but from the defined "target audience" for receiving information. Elizabeth, a young Trobriand mother who participated in a group discussion with members of the Catholic Women's Fellowship, candidly expressed her concern that HIV awareness activities do not adequately reach men.

> I don't think the boys and men have much information about AIDS. This
> health education usually comes to the women whereas our men and boys are

having full freedom in the village without understanding all this health education. Like today, you came to talk to the women, to have them contribute to what you are doing, but only the women get this awareness from the VBAs, the health workers, or people like you. But for our boys and men, their interest, you know, trying luck with girls, it is very hard to get them to listen. [Taped group discussion, 29 July 2003]

The public health fixation on the mother-child dyad has "progressively extruded [men] from the processes of fertility and family planning" (Jolly 2002b:23). This extrusion is apparent in HIV communication as well. The portrayal of the HIV epidemic as feminized not only reinforces perceptions that HIV is a woman's problem, but it does not support men in taking an active role in the process of knowing about HIV prevention and taking responsibility for putting knowledge into practice. The extrusion also places further responsibility for the epidemic on women as the carriers and custodians of information and as the negotiators of condom use. The focus on the maternal body as the gendered site for HIV interventions necessarily involves questions of masculinity, particularly the role of men as fathers and members of families, the influence they have over fertility choices and HIV prevention, and how virility meshes with the values of fertility and expressions of female sexuality.

Trobriand women *do* mediate HIV information from their gendered subject positions as mothers and wives—and as future mothers and wives—and many women express a preference for community conversations that involve mixed gender and age groups. Women's desire for knowledge and clarification about HIV transmission and prevention reflects their concerns about marital trust, fidelity, and the health of their children (see Hirsch et al. 2009). In community discussions with groups of women, and in some discussions involving male participants as well, the question of the husband's fidelity during pregnancy and lactation invariably came to the fore in relation to the ABC prevention message, where abstinence was interpreted with specific reference to pregnancy and birthing practices. Many women recounted for me a Trobriand saying that encapsulates the entwined issues of abstinence and fidelity. "There is a saying in the Trobriands that we hear from our mothers. 'Avetuta basuma gala ulomwala agumwaguta. Avetuta bavalululu gala ulomwala agumwaguta.' When I am expecting a baby, my husband is not mine only. When I am giving birth, my husband is not mine only" (Taped group discussion, 30 June 2003).

Female sexual agency channels productively into pregnancy and lactation, taking an unambiguous social form in maternity. Male sexual agency channels into paternal support and nurture, a social form that also appears through purposeful action; however, men retain the sexual mobility and autonomy of youth, albeit discreetly. There is an uneasy balance between women's stated desire to practice abstinence to ensure the healthy development of their breastfeeding babies and the expected role of men to provide paternal support and nurture. Offsetting the balance is the common knowledge that men are likely to be sexually active outside of the marital relationship, generally with younger women who are not pregnant or lactating. A husband's sexual infidelity is perceived as potentially compromising the health of the mother and baby, and it is regarded as a contributing factor in childbirth complications and cases of maternal and infant mortality, particularly if the identity of the man's secret partner(s) becomes known to his wife. However, the demonstration of sustained material support from the father's *dala* is the greater measure of fidelity for ensuring the well-being of the mother and child. The father's ongoing provision of resources (*and* his sexual discretion) endows protective agency, further ensured by the mother's intentional disregard of her husband's sexual autonomy. The mother fully focuses on her baby and does not allow *uliweli*, or sexual jealousy, to distract her. The ambivalence shared by many women concerning the potential for husbands to be sexually active with other women during the period of pregnancy and lactation often finds expression in humor, as evident in the reference to nappies (baby diapers) in the following statement by a married woman, aged mid-thirties.

> It could be very hard to deliver the baby if the husband is going around with other women. But he still has the freedom secretly. But insofar as we can do anything about it, he can certainly do whatever he wants. One good thing about a pregnant lady and a lady after giving birth, one good thing is that the mother who is looking after the baby doesn't care about the husband going around; she knows but she won't care. The wife, if she finds out who the other lady is, then she will fight, but if she doesn't know who this lady is, she won't care. As long as the husband is helping the mother. The man will say, "I'll go look for nappies." Yes, like, two, three months looking for nappies! [Taped group discussion, 30 June 2003]

The following excerpt from a group discussion, involving thirty women participants of various ages and reproductive experiences, captures the mixture of acquiescence and frustration in how women view the disparity between male sexual infidelity and the sedentary discipline of maternal abstinence.

> Men are not to be trusted when we are having babies. Once we are breastfeeding, they leave us. Some are honest, they stay with their wives. Some are not honest. That's part of the advice from our mothers. When we are pregnant, the mothers give us advice. And they mention this to us. When you are pregnant, that's it. When you are free, OK, he is your husband and you are his wife. When you are pregnant, he is your friend's husband. That's part of the advice that our mothers gave us. And it is in us, true. So when we are pregnant—[*Another woman picks up the sentence and continues.*]—when we are pregnant and we go to our parents, we have to sacrifice. We *have* to sacrifice. Baby inside, at the same time, the father is another woman's husband. But we deal with it, until we stop breastfeeding or until we leave our parents and go back to our own home with our husbands again. [Taped group discussion, 29 July 2003]

Some women say they choose to *kalova*, or wean, their baby early, or resume sleeping with their husband while still breastfeeding, so he will not look for other sexual partners. However, because abstinence is a traditional form of birth spacing, they are concerned about getting pregnant again before their baby has reached its second year, which is also the period of birth spacing encouraged by the VBAs and health workers. Women recognize the benefits of modern contraceptive methods for reducing the period of separation and abstinence after giving birth, but they are concerned about physical side effects, including the effects of chemical contraception on their breastfeeding babies. They are also concerned that a shortened period of separation would appear to others as irresponsible behavior, saying that people would be critical of them for not demonstrating respect for their baby's well-being, instead thinking only of their own pleasure. A breastfeeding mother should also not think or talk about her husband or appear to be preoccupied with his comings and goings. Lisepa Tony explains:

> Talking about the husband, for the breastfeeding mother, it is not on. If the husband goes out to play soccer, chew with his friends, and the wife calls to him to come back, people say *nanali*, she is calling for her husband too much. It is shameful for the woman. So if he leaves her to go out, and she is looking after the baby, that's OK, let him go. *Nanali* is thinking too much about the husband. As soon as you do that, people immediately think that you are thinking about having sex with your husband. It is shameful, you should be thinking of the baby only. [Interview notes, 23 October 2003]

For many women, the timing of the return to their husband's village once their baby is weaned becomes the main cause of anxiety regarding the period of separation and abstinence. This transition requires the woman's family and *dala* relatives to mobilize food resources to reciprocate the paternal investment of support during pregnancy, childbirth, and lactation. Consequently, the timing involves collective decision making and often coincides with the yam harvest when food supplies are plentiful. Each time a woman moves back from her *dala* side to her husband's side, she must carry yams or bananas on her head and be escorted by her father and *dala* relatives. Women say it is shameful to arrive empty-handed in their in-laws' village; people would call her *nawokuva*, or empty-handed woman.

The other key issue that frequently surfaces as women mediate HIV information from their subject positions as mothers and wives is the transmission of HIV through breast milk. In particular, women are concerned about the susceptibility of their babies to HIV infection in relation to the valued practice of shared breastfeeding among women of the same *dala*.

> My aunt told us about this sickness, AIDS, and she said something about spreading the sickness through breastfeeding. So can you bring this advice to the ladies, if the mother gives the baby to her sister? Because here in the Trobriands, we have this sharing and caring in our hearts, some of us feed our sisters' babies. For example, my sister and our other sister and me, we had our babies at the same time and when one baby is crying for *nunu*, maybe it will go from my *nunu* to my sister's *nunu* to the other sister's *nunu*. That is exactly what we do here in the Trobriand Islands. [Female, aged mid-thirties, taped group discussion, 8 August 2003. Translated into English.]

The discussions and interviews held during my study revealed how HIV impinges on all aspects of social reproduction, confronting people with the imperative to reassess valued social practice. The following reconstructed dialogue reflects the issues that women articulate as mothers and wives in relation to their sexual and reproductive agency, and their implications for HIV prevention. The dialogue is an extract from a group discussion held in 2003, arranged through the United Church Women's Fellowship in one of the larger villages on Kiriwina, with a population of over five hundred. Held on the large shaded platform next to the church deacon's house, the discussion involved approximately thirty women, ten of whom had their breastfeeding babies with them. Some women sat on the platform with Ethel, Diana, and me, and some women arranged themselves on the ground in front of the platform. Women spoke in both Kiriwina and English, and Ethel and Diana provided translation during the taped discussion.

"The ward councillor was just telling me about your village, how many people live here, how many children are going to school," I begin. "He said you have a big population; that 'kids are pouring down like ripe mangoes.'"

The women smile and softly voice a confirmation, "*Mokwita*. True."

"I am interested in learning from you how you make decisions about having babies, when to have them, how many, and your views about family planning. I also want to talk about what you have heard and what you know about HIV and AIDS."

After a short, expectant pause, a young woman takes the lead in responding, speaking in English and projecting her voice loudly and confidently. "It is a good thing to have plenty of children, but maybe not so good. The elder mothers advise us to have more babies but now things are changing and the VBAs and clinic sisters are telling us different, we must take family planning."

I wait to see if she is going to continue or if someone else is going to speak. Then I ask, "Why is it a good thing, but maybe not, to have plenty of children?" Hearing myself, I suddenly realize how my question sounds very much like the "wrong question" to ask Trobriand women.

There is a momentary pause before an older woman quietly speaks in Kiriwina. "People who have plenty of children will have many things in the future; the boys will produce yams for the fathers and mothers. In the future when we are older, our children will return to help us. If we have plenty of kids, when someone dies, the *dala* can handle the burden of making *sagali*."

A young woman sitting on the ground stands up and says in English, "Some have heard the advice of the elder mothers; some have heard the advice of the VBAs. Things are changing; the environment is changing, so now we don't know which advice to listen to. We have a population problem. The soil is not good for growing plenty of yams. The trees are dying from too much cutting yam sticks. Things in the shops are going up in price. School fees are too high. We are not sure whether to have plenty of children or not." The woman finishes her statement with "*Agutoki*" (thank you) and sits down.

Another pause, and then a woman in her forties steps down from the platform and, striding away from the group, declares loudly, "*Makala*, because sex is *saina simwakaina* [very sweet]!" Everyone bursts out laughing. I quietly ask Diana if she is leaving because my question offended her, but Diana says no, she is just going off to prepare our food for after the discussion.

A pregnant woman in her mid-thirties, a mother of four young children, stands up and begins to address the group. Throughout her statement, she switches between English and Kiriwina, speaking clearly and confidently. The baby in her arms starts to fuss and another woman swiftly takes the little girl and carries her away. While the woman speaks, her small son wraps himself in her long full skirt and peers up intently at his mother.

"For family planning, it is also the case of not having steady supplies at the health center. This makes it hard for us to plan. For some women, it can also be the side effects, so they choose not to practice. For some, it's the balance between boys and girls. Keep on trying to have another boy or another girl to make a balance in the family. It is a combination of reasons: accident, custom, misunderstanding between partners, people's own choice to have big families. This HIV/AIDS awareness has been well-off, but people don't put it to practice. Because sex is so sweet, it is a careless pleasure. Customs and desires make it hard to practice safe sex. Single people have the right to have plenty of partners in order to find the right partner for marriage. Freedom is there for unmarried and married, especially on the man's side. People enjoy having the freedom and enjoy having the children, but through the 1990s and now in the 2000s, it has become a threat. HIV/AIDS is a challenge to our way of life so now people are trying to secure themselves from the habit of sex. Married men are trying to be stable. People are trying their best to be stable because they are fearful. We hear and fear the awareness talks but we don't know how to change our behavior. When we are short of sex, or when we are in need of it, then we forget. We must sit down and think of ourselves and our lives. Through education, we can come to live a good family life, a healthy life, a harmony life." Then in one graceful movement, the woman gathers the folds of her skirt, sits down cross-legged, and settles her young boy into her lap.

The women listen attentively and respond with nods and whispered words of agreement, "*Mokwita*. True." Then another woman adds, "There is a lot of awareness now but it is we the people ourselves deciding, how we choose to act on this information. We have the understanding but we still want a taste of the sweetness."

The pregnant woman stands up again and addresses me directly, "We want more awareness for the married men. This is the request, please, a recommendation for more awareness for men."[38]

The reflections represented here situate HIV holistically within the broader issues of social and environmental change, a direct reminder that HIV cannot be acted on in isolation from other concerns that affect people's lives and livelihoods. More specifically, the reflections productively demonstrate how sexual desires mesh with the broader pleasures of fecundity, bringing together the sweetness of sex with the sweetness of the physical care and nurture of babies and children. Through these representations of the values of social reproduction, I do not want to convey that pregnancy and childbirth are free from uncertain risk and danger for women and babies, or that all women embrace maternity with unequivocal expectation and enthusiasm (see Byford 1999; Mallett 2003). Nor is it my intention to endorse the essentialist gender equation by making a universalistic claim about the inherent value of female reproductive power while excluding the importance of male sexual and reproductive agency.[39] What I seek to illustrate is the relevance of the gendered constructs of maternity *and* paternity for situating knowledge in the relational person and for understanding mediations of HIV in relation to lived experience. These constructs hold meaning outside the moralistic binaries of vulnerability and culpability, of "mothers" and "others," of sex for reproduction as opposed to sex for pleasure. My intention has been to contextualize gendered agency in relation to the broader constructs of Trobriand sociality and social reproduction, and to bring to the fore the complementary domains of sexuality and fertility. I also stress a context of regeneration that transcends corporeal pleasures and pains and embodies the yearning of *Wosituma*, the celebrated ancestral wisdom of continuity and cohesion, which provides the opening frame.

Of course, most sexual activity is *non*reproductive, even when there is a strong cultural imperative for procreation (Jenkins 2004:4–5). My analytical intention, however, is to emphasize the social significance that sexual acts hold for the *potential* for reproduction, both actual and symbolic. The double bind of HIV communication for creating meaningful links between knowledge about HIV prevention and cultural knowledge lies within the domain of social reproduction. Approaches to HIV prevention that acknowledge the cultural values of fecundity and collective enterprise in social reproduction, as well as people's embodied capacities and potentials, will more effectively facilitate the process of knowing to support behavior change.

Controlling Fertility

Throughout the Pacific, constructs of fertility connected to ideals of fecundity, growth, and ancestral power also place a "persuasive stress on the *control* of human fertility" (Jolly 2001b:289). Sexual desire and the capacity and potential for reproduction are intimately tied to the concerns of fertility control. Despite *baloma* procreation ideology and the belief that pregnancy and viable fetal growth only results from sexual intercourse with one steady partner, Trobrianders acknowledge that women who have multiple sexual partners can and do conceive. The ability to control fertility is an integral aspect of exercising sexual and reproductive agency.

The desire to enjoy sex without worrying about unwanted pregnancy is a key concern for many women, both married and unmarried. In discussions and interviews, women candidly discussed the timing and prevention of pregnancy and described various methods they use for fertility control. But the concerns of fertility are not the sole purview of women (see Jolly 2001b:264). Men also voiced a vested interest in contraception and birth spacing, and young single men in particular stated that they worry about being named the father of a baby conceived in a casual relationship.

The regime of traditional fertility control in the Trobriands involves the knowledge and use of the leaves, roots, and bark of specific plants, referred to generically as herbs, prepared in various strengths and combinations for contraception, abortion, and permanent sterilization.[40] Herbs are also used to enhance fertility or restore ovulation after a period of contraceptive use. The plants are boiled to make a tea, which is then imbued with magical spells before drinking. Specialized knowledge about the plants, and the chants recited during preparation, are highly valued resources passed between close relatives, both male and female. Women usually obtain herbal methods from specialists within their own *dala*, but they may also seek the services of nonrelatives if the person is a well-known specialist.

Although infection and irreversible sterility are potential complications from the abortifacient dosage, women maintain that herbal infusions are very effective in terminating pregnancy and restoring menstrual flow. Knowing that herbal methods for pregnancy termination are both available and efficacious lends confidence to sexual agency. One village birth attendant explained, "Most young girls when they are out with boys they don't think about pregnancy. If they become pregnant they will *yopoi* [abort] with herbs. They don't worry really about it in the first place."[41] The actual use of herbal abortifacients is significant according to one older female specialist, who stated: "Young girls just go around, they get pregnant and then come to me asking for, you know, to get rid of [the conceptus], one or two months, it gets rid of it. Three months, it's a bit hard. Sometimes they get rid of it, sometimes they just carry on with pregnancy. So many young girls come I can't count. Even some married women come for that one." (Taped interview, 21 December 2000. Translated into English.)

A young woman's fertility management usually involves her *dala* relatives, particularly her mother's sisters or her maternal uncles, who provide her with the herbs and magical words to prevent conception or terminate an unwanted pregnancy. A young girl will often take herbal contraception at the behest of older relatives who are concerned that she not get pregnant while her mother is still having babies. Women say it is "big shame" to have another baby after becoming a grandmother. Women also report using herbal infusions when they have reached their preferred family size and do not want to have any more children, explaining that the herbs "shut their system down for good," an effect sometimes compared to tubal ligation. A young pregnant woman with a three-year-old daughter explained that her grandmother wanted her to take an herbal infusion to "block" her system after she previously had a stillbirth.

> When I had this [indicates stillbirth by holding belly], my grandmother, my mum's mum, came and she told me if she could, what, could make the village medicine for me to drink and block whatever system is in there. So she asked me and I said no, I want to have another baby before you do what you want. I'm wishing to have a baby boy and then I'll ask her to make that medicine for me to drink and then stop it. Stop everything. Rest for a while, give mum some support and assistance with the garden. [Taped interview, 19 December 2000]

Young girls and women also manage their fertility by observing their menstrual cycles and avoiding intercourse during ovulation. Girls refer to the weeks after ovulation and before menstruation as their "safe period" when they can engage in sexual activity without worrying about getting pregnant. Girls say they learn this form of contraception from their mothers and aunties, as well as from health workers and textbooks in the high-school library. Some women maintain that the ovulation method was used traditionally, while others say it was only recently introduced by Catholic laity.

Some women also use modern contraceptives, including the pill, injections, and condoms, which are available from the district health center. During annual visits to Kiriwina by specialist medical teams from Alotau Hospital, tubal ligation procedures are performed for women who request the method. Some women travel to Alotau to give birth at the provincial hospital so they can have a tubal ligation after delivery. Although family-planning services and contraceptives are meant to be available to all clients who request them, regardless of marital status, young girls remark that they do not feel confident going to the health center for contraceptives because service provision is implicitly focused on the needs of married mothers. "They say it is 'family planning' so it makes us young girls shy to go and ask," one young girl explained.[42]

A woman in her mid-fifties from a village on the north shore of Kiriwina reminisced about the time when she was a young wife in the early 1970s, when oral contraceptives first became available in the Trobriands, and she and her sisters and friends would put on freshly made *doba* and proudly walk the three hours to the clinic in Losuia to get their pills together. A review of the family-planning register at Losuia District Health Center suggests that women tend to go together in village groups to obtain contraceptives from the health center. Once registered, repeat supplies of pills and the quarterly Depo Provera injections are given to users during mobile maternal and child health (MCH) clinics. According to the register, injection is the method used by more than one-third of all "new acceptors" of contraception.[43] However, many women I talked to were ambivalent about taking Depo Provera, saying they fear the unknown long-term effects on their health and dislike the commonly reported side effect of sensitivity to cool temperatures, which they explain as an effect of the "cold" internal stasis produced by the drug when it "blocks" the regular flow of menstrual blood (see also Sobo 1993:62). When asked how this effect compares to traditional contraception, women qualified the difference by explaining that the intravenous injection produces a different internal state than that produced by drinking the hot herbal infusion.[44] One young woman told me she was thinking of getting a "DP" injection so she would get fat because she was too thin and looked just like a young girl even though she was a mother of three; however, she was reluctant to take it because of the cold sensation of blockage that others had warned her about. Women say they prefer the method because they do not have to worry about monthly periods or look after a packet of pills and remember to take one every day, and because it is given as a group during the MCH clinics.

I hold a vivid image of a group of women receiving their injections during a clinic visit to their village. About twenty-five mothers gathered at the church together with their babies—newborns to three-year-olds—and eased themselves up onto the raised communal platform, scooting and crawling under the low thatched roof until they were all comfortably seated. The MCH team—one nurse and two community health workers, all Trobriand women—arrived with the UNICEF-issued portable coolers filled with vaccinations, disposable syringes, and medicine. They proceeded to set up the makeshift clinic on the platform as the women shared betel nut and passed the babies from lap to lap, lavishing them with affection. The nurse called for the baby clinic books and the women passed them from one hand to another until they all reached her. She stacked them together and then began calling out the children's names one by one, weighed the babies on the hanging scale suspended from the roof beam, and then vaccinated them according to the schedule. Some of the mothers would quietly consult with the nurse about their child's health and get medication to treat a cough or fever. Halfway through the lengthy procedure one of the nurses pulled out a bundle of family-planning clinic cards from a worn canvas bag and began distributing vials of Depo Provera to about fifteen of the women who were due for a repeat injection. The small golden glass vials were lightly tossed from one woman to another across the crowded platform until they reached the right hands. On an unspoken cue, all the women began to gently shake their vials to "warm them up" before their names were called one by one to be injected. I was struck by the synchronicity of the movement and how it mimicked the fluttering motion of the *bisila* streamers in Trobriand dance. I mentioned this to the women I was sitting next to and they laughed at the comparison.

The women's collective presence and ensemble movement on the platform, replete with the busyness of babies, disrupted the views I held about Depo Provera as antithetical to the principles of reproductive rights and free choice. As the main contraceptive provided in many developing countries, the medicalized and efficient mass coverage of Depo Provera serves the interests of governments, international agencies, and service providers—the "population controllers" (Dixon-Mueller 1993)—but tends to elide the agency of the women whose bodies become "blocked." Maternity is used to recruit women as passive acceptors of contraception; they are given little or no information on potential side effects, and they have limited decision-making power and no access to comprehensive services and resources that ensure informed choice in relation to particular needs (Dixon-Mueller 1993; see also Basu 1997; Jolly and Ram, eds. 2001). Indelibly striking for me, however, was the shift in perspective from viewing the collective maternal body as the locus of coerced compliance to recognizing the sociality of service delivery and how the embodied practice of fertility control has an intersubjective dimension.

The provision of family-planning services in Papua New Guinea, while locally embedded in maternal and child health, is ideologically shaped by global paradigms concerning population issues and policies. There has been a major shift in these paradigms over the last two decades, from an emphasis on population control by means of contraceptive use to a focus on the enabling environments that support reproductive rights and responsibilities.[45] Contemporary shifts in addressing the issues of population and fertility control in PNG must also be seen in the deeper historical context, particularly in relation to the effects of depopulation during the colonial period in the late nineteenth and early twentieth centuries, primarily as a result of introduced pathogens (Bayliss-Smith 2006; Connelly 2007). Writing on the changing contours of fertility in the Pacific, Jolly argues that "the spectre of overpopulation in the Pacific present needs to be juxtaposed with the ghost of depopulation that haunts the recent past" (2001b:275). Concerns about depopulation in the Territory of Papua figured largely in colonial policy at the start of the twentieth century, and sexually transmitted diseases were seen as a particularly significant problem linked to declining birth rates in the Trobriands (Black 1957:233).[46]

In his critique of colonial sexual politics in the Massim, Adam Reed (1997:53–54, 66) argues that colonial administrators and missionaries alike viewed excessive sexual behavior as a key factor contributing to increased mortality and declining birth rates, and they specifically attributed depopulation to the perceived sexual and maternal irresponsibility of Massim women. Reed further notes that "a discursive explosion surrounding the subject of abortion and contraceptive practices epitomised this concern with feminine irresponsibility," and abortion was represented as "some kind of hidden explanation for the low birth rate" (66). The combined colonial and missionary strategy for addressing low fertility was to reform conjugality in the image of the European nuclear family and to encourage procreation within marriage by offering fiscal incentives to couples with at least four living children (56–57; see also Jolly 2001b:281). Missionaries sought to "refigure the female sexual body, containing its energies in a monogamous sexual practice" (Reed 1997:69).[47]

The "hidden explanation" for fertility control has been represented as a conundrum in the ethnographic literature on the Trobriands ever since Malinowski posited that Trobrianders do not recognize the physiological link between insemination and conception.[48] While Malinowski discounted the importance of traditional methods of fertility control, he pondered the seeming rarity of premarital pregnancy in the context of sexual freedom and speculated whether there was "any physiological law which makes conception less likely when women begin their sexual life young, lead it indefatigably, and mix their lovers freely" (1929:168). He later firmed up the hypothesis that "promiscuous intercourse, while it lasts, reduces the fertility of woman [*sic*]" (Malinowski 1974:60). In a commentary on Malinowski's postulation, Sidney Greenfield (1968:760) refers to both laboratory and social research that suggests an immunological basis for low fertility, wherein sperm-agglutinating antibodies produced by the female in reaction to semen from successive sexual partners prevents conception or successful implantation of the fertilized ovum. Biomedical research has advanced immunological theory in recent years, and current evidence from clinical studies on the female immune response to semen suggests that unprotected sex with multiple partners may in fact prevent the uterine conditions for successful embryo implantation and placental development in some women (see Robertson 2007). Indeed, it might be argued that the Trobriand model of procreation, with its emphasis on sustained sexual relations with only one partner, incorporates a method of fertility control that corresponds with immunological knowledge on the viability of conception.

In summary, I return to the opening vignette of this chapter and the woman's assertion about embodied capacity, which offers insight into the way gender as a cultural construct manifests in the capabilities of bodies and minds through an array of subject positions and social interactions. In the Trobriands, sexual and reproductive agency is a relational expression of volition, ideally involving mutual reciprocity of consensual pleasure and the projected desires of fecundity. In direct contrast, assertions of agency and empowerment in HIV discourse are framed individualistically and in the negative—"Just say no!" to (unprotected) sex. Such a proposition, based on the assumption of nonreproductive heterosex and extolling abstinence over protected sex, is antithetical to the inclusive assertion, "Because we can!" To be effective within contexts where the cultural imperative for social reproduction involves complementary constructions of sexuality and fertility, HIV communication must move beyond essentialist binaries and the individualist premise of behavior to engage with a diversity of meanings and intentions in sexual and reproductive agency.

CHAPTER 5

Youth Sexuality
Making Desires Known

Ulatile. That's boys looking for pretty girls and hardworking girls, that's what they have in mind. *Kapugula*, girls looking for handsome boys and hardworking boys, girls going out to other places, to other boys in other places.

—Amanda, aged twenty, 17 June 2003

Kapugula. Go out. Young girls, they go free. They get it from their grandmothers and mothers that they are free to go around.

—Village birth attendant, 18 December 2000

Ulatile, kapugula. Young ones go out at night to other villages. Because they are young, boys and girls are free to make their own choice, where they go out and how they attract each other and mix themselves up in a group. That's their freedom. Different girls from different villages, different boys from different villages. Some girls go to visit far distant relatives and that's where they pick their boyfriends. Just for the sake of visiting them, during *sagali*, stay for a while, find new boys. The boys will pick their ripe pawpaws [papaya].

—Middle-aged woman, 4 November 2003.
Translated into English.

The sexual exuberance that infuses the "Islands of Love" trope with such potency in the popular imagination is most powerfully evoked by the freedom that unmarried Trobriand youth enjoy in exploring and expressing their sexuality, unencumbered by repressive cultural ideology. The anticipated activation of sexual desire and agency during early pubescence locates Trobriand sexual culture in a unique place in relation to other parts of Papua New Guinea, and indeed many parts of the world, where social and religious norms commonly constrain or negate youth sexuality, particularly that of young females (Buchanan-Aruwafu 2007; Buchanan-Aruwafu and Maebiru 2008; Jenkins 1997, 2007; Keck 2007; Kelly et al. 2010). Perceptions of unrestrained and dangerous adolescent sexuality influence representations of HIV risk, evaluated in terms of early commencement of sexual activity, or "sexual debut,"[1] premarital sex, and unplanned pregnancies. These medicalized codifications of sexuality are important for reorienting HIV programs toward affirmation of young people's sexual desires and agency and their particular sexual health needs (Moore and Rosenthal 2006); however, the ways they have been mobilized in national HIV programs have served to define youth sexuality as a problem that requires correction (see Parikh 2005:128). Inadequate attention is given to contextualizing young people's desires in relation to cultural expectations and values regarding social reproduction (Setel 1999; Smith 2004), and to the ways youth sexuality reflects the ruptures and influences of social change and modernity, where assertions of newfound agency and expressions of love and romance are in tension with cultural norms and constrained by larger structural factors (Buchanan-Aruwafu and Maebiru 2008; Bucholtz 2002; Butt and Munro 2007; Parikh 2005; Wardlow 2006).

Trobriand sexual culture, and its celebrated value of the life stage of *kubukwabuya* in pursuing the endeavors of collective sociality, disrupts the representations of youth sexuality in HIV discourse. The sexual energy of *kubukwabuya*, or unmarried male and female youth, is visibly mobile in the social landscape, expressing productive capacity and reproductive potential by mapping out the broader social connections between people and places in overlapping networks of exchange. In this chapter, I further explore sexual desire as a "cultural production" (Tolman and Diamond 2001:36) by retracing the movement of *kubukwabuya* in their exercise of personal and collective sexual agency. I describe two distinct forms of cultural practice prominent in the sexual agency of young people. These are love magic and gift exchange. Sexual desires and intentions are realized through the use of *kwaiwaga*, or love magic, which secures the embodied desires of others and makes intimate relations visible in the larger social realm. *Buwala*, the gifts that young boys and men give their female sexual partners, signify the transactional dimension of sexual relations and the value of exchange in Trobriand society. I follow the gendered mobility of youth sexuality to its abrupt cessation in the transition to marriage and parenthood, but illustrate how this pathway is neither linear nor immutable, particularly for girls.

The Mobility of *Kubukwabuya* Desire

The Trobriand life stage of *kubukwabuya* embodies the autonomy to act on desire, to attract the desire of others, and to engage freely in sexual liaisons in the quest for a compatible marriage partner. The sexual freedom and mobility enjoyed by Trobriand youth are signified by the gendered terms *ulatile* and *kapugula*, the group activity of going out at night to look for *lubaila*, or sweethearts, ideally expanding the reach of desire beyond the familiarity of one's village peer group. Nothing quite exceeds the heightened sense of expectation and intrigue that embellishes young people's nocturnal mobility in the Trobriands. The night—particularly the moonlit night—belongs to the young. The witnessing presence of *tubukona*, the moon, swathes the night in soft light, creating an aura of safety and intimacy in the pursuit of desire.[2] On a clear night when the full moon casts enticing shadows and exudes a festive air, the movement of young people is especially energetic. Although I have never heard it stated explicitly, young people's nighttime activity is valued because it offers protection from the potential harm caused by malevolent *yoyowa*, or witches, who, along with disoriented and restless *kosi*, the ghosts of the recently deceased, also claim the hours of darkness.

Kubukwabuya sexual networks are intricately woven into the Trobriand social landscape, with the *valu*, or village, as the central axis. Young people typically commence their sexual activity in early puberty within the familiar social boundaries of their village *tubwa* cohort. Sexual networks then radiate outward based on traditional affiliations between villages as well as friendships established by preceding age groups. During a group interview with five men and young boys, an older man explained the protocol thus: "It's how villages go together and have an understanding. We have to be careful in making arrangements to show our respect, otherwise it's like stealing." A young boy then added, "Our thinking is this, if there is space in there for us, we can have it. If the space is covered up, no vacancies, then we will look elsewhere."[3]

This spatial conceptualization of sexual networks indicates a protocol of practice based on associations of place identity and relationality. Spatial rather than numerical accounts of sexual pairing were verified by several local interviewers engaged to administer the IMR baseline survey in the Trobriands in 2002 (see note 2, Chapter 2). The interviewers told me that standardized quantitative questions about individual sexual acts were not readily answered with a number on the survey form. When asked, "How many sexual partners did you have in the last month?" respondents tended to answer the question by recalling the names of their partners' villages and the locations where encounters took place. When numbers are used in relation to sexual acts, they typically refer to the equal pairing of respective group members during a planned outing rather than an individual tally of partners.

Young people report that casual sexual encounters generally take place in the bush, on secluded beaches, or at the old airstrip, where groups of boys and girls from different villages arrange to meet in the night and then pair off. The predominant pattern of *kubukwabuya* sexual networking involves a context where young people might have several concurrent partners whom they meet at different times, or where serial monogamy is practiced in the search for the right partner to marry. In describing the protocol of *ulatile* and *kapugula* activity, it is important to distinguish between "group sex," where sexual acts involve more than two partners at the same time, and group sexual networking, where young people pursue their liaisons together in a group with the intention of coupling with only one partner. Trobriand youth are quite clear about this distinction, explaining that they move as a peer group to look for individual partners.

> Young ones, they move in groups. They pass the messages where they are trying to go and meet. They write the names of how many girls or how many boys and that place for meeting. They would say, "Oh, we have ten girls, then plan for ten boys," and they would meet at a certain place and that's how they match people, you can have this one, you can have that one. But not even knowing the person, just the number given, and then the groups meet like that and spend the time there together. [Single female, aged nineteen, taped group discussion, 30 June 2003]

Young ones plan to go in groups, boys and girls. The girls will wait for a message or signal for when the boys will come in a group, and then they'll go and meet them where they agree, like in the bush or at the old airstrip, and from there it's one-one. Otherwise it is one-one from the start; just the boy and girl plan to meet up together and go to the boy's house. [Interview notes, 1 October 2003]

The negotiated pursuit of one's desires in relation to the desires of others is a key feature of *kubukwabuya* sociality. Solicitations and planned encounters evince the heteronormativity of sexual partnering, the homosociality within *tubwa* groups, and the collective agency of sexual desire. Arrangements to meet a desired partner for a private rendezvous, or to meet with a group from another village, are initiated primarily by the male suitors and typically involve preliminary negotiations. Younger siblings or cousins are often recruited as messengers to relay verbal requests, along with a few betel nuts to indicate intentions. "For us, the young girls, the boys come to us. It is embarrassing for girls to ask boys out. Mostly it is boys who try luck. They will send someone across with the message and maybe some *buwa* [betel nut]. If the boy tries and the girl says no he can always find someone else" (Interview notes, 1 October 2003).

In addition to verbal messages, notes and letters are also used to make intentions known and to broker arrangements in advance as a means to avoid the shame that comes with rejection. The style of written messages is exemplified in the following letter, which was shown to me by the group of young girls who received it. The girls told me that they did not respond because they were offended by the boys' exclusionary request, favoring schoolgirls over village girls, and there were not enough of them interested to make an equal match with the named boys.

[Name of boys' village]
Dear [name of village] Kubukwabuya Vivila,
Amakawani bwena wala kena? E pela yakamesa bogwa wala bwena. Gala goki avaka livalela taga yakamesa [name of boys' village] kubukwabuya tawau mainly [name of primary school] toginigini magimasi yokwami vivila ilemi [name of girls' village] beta kalubailasi. E magimasi Losuia Primary School toginigini e deli Kiriwina High School toginigini gala tosikivalu. Besa wala. Reply as soon as possible.
Igamesa yakamesa tawau,
[Names of six boys]

Dear Unmarried Girls from [name of village],
How are things for you, good only maybe? And for us, only good enough. No certainly, what we are saying but yes, our [name of boys' village] unmarried boys, mainly [name of primary school] schoolboys, we desire you girls from [name of girls' village] for friendship. Yes, that's so, and we want Losuia Primary School students and Kiriwina High School students, not those who stay in the village. That's all. Reply as soon as possible.
We, our names,
[Names of six boys]

Girls also make solicitations through letters, as explained in the following statement made during a group discussion with seven young women, aged seventeen to twenty-four years.

> It is like this, sometimes we write letters to other villages. So we will write, I can bring all of these girls, and tell their names one by one. And then we will wait for our boys to reply. And then the word will come by letter telling us where to go. So the village boys, who wrote the letter back to us, they come and wait, wait, where they told us to meet. So we go there, where we agreed to meet and then they will come and we, how will I say? We will share. They will choose, two by two, or pairs. The group leaders will choose which girl will go with which boy and so forth. You-you-you-you. [Single female, aged seventeen, taped group discussion, 4 July 2003]

Such arrangements can be thwarted if the numbers of willing male and female participants do not match up. The broader issue of gender asymmetry also poses a problem for villages with an unequal number of males and females in the *kubukwabuya* cohort. "More boys than girls in a village creates problems for boys. They have to look to other villages for their friendships."[4] In small village populations, a disproportionate sex ratio of live births in one generation can be quite marked.[5] People suggest that because young girls reach puberty earlier than boys and often partner with slightly older males once they become sexually active, the boys in their *tubwa* cohort get "left behind." They have to actively look for partners from different villages or wait until the younger *tubwa* cohort becomes sexually active. In villages where males far outnumber females, young boys feel disadvantaged and remark with dry humor that they are "wait-listed."

> We are the forfeit ones; we missed out because there are no more single girls in our village. So we keep our eyes open at *sagali*. We keep a watch to meet up with new girls that way. And we go to other places. We go by twos or more, we walk together, village boys. We ask girls where they are from. The oldest in our group is like the foreman, he does the asking. We can bring the girls back in our canoes. We always do things fair, equal numbers. If not equal, we will cancel the whole thing. And the girls must agree. Sometimes the girls from the other villages, their boys will catch up with them and then they have to cancel the whole thing. We have the problem that there are no girls in this village, but if their boys stop them, they have the right. So we have to cancel the plan. [Single male, aged twenty, taped group discussion, 15 October 2003]

The statement above illustrates the principles of equanimity, consensus, and collectivity that characterize the code of *kubukwabuya* behavior. Youth sexuality embraces the ethic of mutual desire and consent between partners. Young boys say that a boy must "study" a girl first to make sure she will agree to solicitations in order to avoid the shame of rejection and the homosocial shame among male peers that comes from coercing or "pulling" her against her will. The notion of shame not only ensures that casual sexual relationships are pursued discreetly and kept hidden from public view, but also upholds female sexual autonomy and protects against coercion.[6]

There is a custom where it would be shameful if the man tries to pull the girl. It would be a joke to all the boys. They would really laugh at him. So if the girl disagrees and walks away and he tries to pull her, and if there are other people around or she happens to tell all the guys, he will be really embarrassed because everyone would be making fun of him. [Single female, aged seventeen, taped group discussion, 9 January 2001. Translated into English.]

Once the boy tries luck on a girl, and if the girl doesn't like that fellow, she has to be very polite in answering him back. "Sorry, I don't think I am fit for you, I am not good enough, I don't look pretty enough," and all this. "Thank you for trying luck, but no thank you." We have to say it in a polite way that will make him understand and not feel shame because he will go back and think about the words we have just used and, "OK, this girl said it in a nice way," and he will accept it at that. But if a boy tries luck and you answer, "Look at yourself, you are really ugly, who would want to go with you?"—you know, these types of harsh words can make him grow angry and he will go back and think of other things to get revenge on the words that you have used. [Middle-aged woman, taped group discussion, 23 July 2003. Translated into English.]

While the prospect of shame associated with rejection mitigates coercion, it also holds gendered implications for sexual decision making, especially given the potential for retaliation by the spurned suitor. Because the responsibility for averting shame is largely carried by the female as the recipient of solicitations, a young girl's response to a boy who is "trying luck" may be diminished to passive submission rather than polite rejection. Her vulnerability to unwanted sexual advances is further increased by the possibility that he might retaliate with the use of love magic to *kivili nanola*, or "turn her mind," so that she loses her sexual autonomy and becomes sick with desire for him.

The protocol of *kubukwabuya* behavior also holds gendered implications in the management of sexual autonomy. The spatial boundaries of sexual networks are maintained by peer groups, with boys and girls from the same village keeping close watch on each other's movements (see Weiner 1976:171–72; 1988:68). *Uliweli*, or sexual jealousy, is considered an inappropriate expression of desire for unattached *kubukwabuya*. Perceived as the antithesis of freedom and mobility, it is the emotional preserve of married couples. Nonetheless, *kubukwabuya* demonstrate a strong group loyalty and are quick to criticize members of their village cohort who are seen to deviate too far from established patterns of networking. In this dimension of regulation the freedom enjoyed by young people takes on sharp gender divisions and a double standard, with boys generally more territorial and possessive about the movement of their female peers than the reverse, and with boys seeking more freedom of movement for themselves. Male privilege can be viewed in relation to the direction of movement in sexual networks, which mirrors the virilocal pattern of marriage where the woman moves to the man's residence. Young boys do not go to their girlfriends' hamlets or villages to meet with them; they arrange to meet them in a neutral location and then bring them back to their sleeping houses in their village. Young girls do not bring boys to their family home, not even their steady partners from the same village; their sexual mobility is directed outward.

Only girls can go to other villages, not boys. Boys will bring the girls to their village, to their house. Boys will agree to meet somewhere, maybe meet at the old airstrip. So all of us would meet up at the airstrip because that's where we chose. If our village boys find out, they are going to hit us. If it is boys from one village and another village, then they are going to fight, if they see us going or find out our plans. But if we [girls] just run away then the boys will fight each other. [Single female, aged sixteen, taped group discussion, 4 July 2003]

Gendered sexual mobility, particularly with regard to spatial boundaries and the frequency and distance of planned outings, can be the source of tension and intrigue for young people. Unendorsed group outings or secretive meetings embarked on by either boys or girls of the same village *tubwa* may precipitate a *yowai*, or fight, among themselves or with the implicated party from another village. The confrontation might be a planned ambush targeted at the outside group or it might ensue among members of the same village *tubwa* when the party held accountable returns home after an outing. Fights involving youths from different villages are typically restricted to the same sex, more often boys fighting boys in an expression of territorial pride. The potential for such fights to erupt is a perennial topic of intrigue, described with great fervor in the group discussions I held with young people. Physical confrontations over alleged waywardness and excessiveness in patterns of sexual networking are regarded by some young people as an acceptable punitive measure to restore respect for the village name. Yet young people also share the concerns of parents, church leaders, and village elders about the potential for contested outings and pairings to erupt into fights because such clashes can lead to negative repercussions for intervillage exchange relations and to the need to resolve festering conflict through the formalized exchange of yams. On the whole, the potential for disruptive conduct is moderated by considerable care and decorum in the pursuit and management of intervillage solicitations and relationships.

Young people's management of their sexual liaisons *within* the village requires even greater circumspection to avoid possible conflict and to ensure that amorous pursuits are carefully concealed from cross-sex siblings, who are often of the same *tubwa* group. The majority of steady relationships eventuate between young people from the same or neighboring villages, in contrast to the transient relationships pursued beyond the social sphere of one's *valu*. "Inside the village, everyone just has one steady friend on our mothers' advice. Only one friend. Otherwise, if you get two friends, they are going to fight. So steady partners mostly come from your own village. But you can't stop young ones. It might be four, three friends in the same village" (Female, aged eighteen, taped group discussion, 4 July 2003).

Fighting might erupt if a steady relationship is threatened by concurrent partnering. Usually in such cases, boys will fight each other to appeal to the girl's attentions, and girls will fight each other to assert their claim over the attentions of the boy. In some instances, a boy might "punish" his steady girlfriend for having a concurrent partner by striking her legs with a stick or metal chain. Such an assault is generally viewed as justifiable in a long-term relationship, symbolizing diminished *kapugula* mobility and intimating marriage by "folding the legs" of the woman. A young girl has customary recourse against such treatment and may seek retaliatory support from her *dala* kinsmen or choose to assert her autonomy by ending the relationship altogether. It is considered unacceptable for a girl to fight her boyfriend if she discovers him with another partner. Her retaliation is to fight the other girl or reject him outright.

The protocol of reciprocated desire and consent between partners and the judicious management of sexual networks help to mitigate the possibility of coercion and conflict. However, the most efficacious deterrent of physical confrontation and indeed the greatest restraint on the autonomy of personal will, is *kwaiwaga*, or love magic, used by both males and females. Fighting is inconsequential compared to the direct potency of *kwaiwaga* as both the cause and effect of one's actions, a potency that cannot easily be displaced by recourse to fighting or physical assault.

Sexuality and the Power of *Kwaiwaga*

It was Wednesday morning and the church building was enlivened with the presence of over fifty women and about thirty small children and babies sitting on mats on the linoleum-covered concrete floor. Dressed in homemade blue skirts and white blouses, the women were assembled in their uniforms for the weekly women's fellowship meeting, which on this day was followed by a group discussion on sexuality, reproduction, and HIV awareness for my research project. Our relaxed, free-flowing dialogue turned to *kapugula* and young girls' freedom of choice in making friendships with boys. An older woman spoke up above the others, directing her explanation to me. "If a boy loves, say this young girl here," and she playfully put her arm around a younger woman sitting next to her, "and if the boy really loves her but she refuses, he will not give up. He will try another way. That's where other business comes in."

"Other business comes in," I echoed, intimating that I knew what she was referring to. "Can you tell me about this other business?"

Immediately an unequivocal response was voiced by all in unison— "*Kwaiwaga!*" Peals of laughter followed. Some older children widened their eyes with excitement upon hearing the word and the laughter it ignited.

"*Kwaiwaga, that's* the other business!" another woman reiterated with emphasis. The laughter subsided and she continued to explain. "He will try another way. He will put the *kwaiwaga* in *buwa*, or whatever, sometimes in the lime pot, sometimes the mustard. He will use close relatives to offer you the betel nut. Once he makes *kwaiwaga* like this and you accept the betel nut, it won't take long. The boy won't come and get you; you will run to the boy's house! Even your relatives go and try to pull you back, they won't succeed because your mind has already been locked up in the boy's house![7]

Every group discussion held during the course of my research invariably turned to narratives about love magic. An endless source of intrigue, participants would eagerly launch into lively and impassioned explanations of *kwaiwaga*. To talk about sex is to talk about *kwaiwaga*, a cultural construct so potent that it ultimately defines and explains the embodied experience of sexual desire, seduction, consummation, and the surrender of autonomy to fidelity.[8]

Young people's sexual agency is mediated most directly at the interpersonal level by an individual's capacity to arouse desire in another person through the use of *kwaiwaga*, by *isivila nanola*, or "turning the mind." *Kwaiwaga* powerfully demonstrates the relational effects of personal agency, how one person's intentions and desires are simultaneously projected and reflected in the actions of another. Allaying the potential for rejection and shame, *kwaiwaga* provides the source of confidence for pursuing desired outcomes. The consummate ability to attract and persuade a potential sexual partner is consistently attributed to the use of *kwaiwaga*. The decisive use of *kwaiwaga* facilitates the passage to marriage by delimiting sexual mobility and promoting fidelity in a recognized partnership.[9] Although a young girl's rejection of a boy's sexual advances reflects negatively on his personal qualities, it ultimately indicates his lack of knowledge and competence in using love magic.

Kwaiwaga takes effect through a consumable substance such as betel nut or tobacco, or any substance or object that comes in contact with the intended recipient, such as the aromatic smell of coconut oil, "traps" along the road where love magic is strategically placed in the pathway of the desired one, or a love letter. Imbued with magical potency through ritual preparation by boiling special herbs in coconut oil and then reciting a specific chant and naming the intended recipient while chewing ginger, the medium carries the spell and causes it to enter the mind of the recipient.

Related to love magic is *kaimwasila*, or attraction magic, also made from herbs and coconut oil, which is used on the body to make it appear beautiful and arouse desire in others. *Kaimwasila* also refers to magic used in exchange transactions and public endeavors to enhance one's persuasion and charisma as a *kula* partner or a leader. I was told that there is no magic to keep unwanted suitors away in the first place, only a special form of magic, *kabisilova*, to break off an existing relationship or to cause someone to become estranged from their partner (see also Malinowski 1929:319). Personal vigilance is required to resist the power of *kwaiwaga*. An older village birth attendant explained, "When I was young walking on the road I didn't look upon the boys, I put my head down and was able to escape from *kwaiwaga*. I watched carefully; my mind was strong."[10]

Highly valued and guarded, the techniques of love magic are a distinct form of *dala* knowledge passed between close relatives. Magic can also be accessed from specialist practitioners for a negotiated payment, usually clay pots or cash. A well-known *toyuvisa* (literally, "one who untangles"), or specialist healer, explained to me the use and effects of love magic.

> In our culture when, let's say, man or woman, unmarried ones, doesn't find the right mate or when mates go astray, we have to help them. *Kaimwasila*, attraction magic. *Kwaiwaga*, love magic, very powerful. People have their own sources of *kwaiwaga* but they still come to me for this one. For making *kwaiwaga*, you cook herbs with coconut oil; you have *meguva*, or chanted magic, for different things or different strengths. It is a combination of the spell, chewed ginger and spit, and the sweet smelling plant combined. A young girl will have no chance of refusing because she is controlled by *kwaiwaga*.

There's the freedom but there's this other thing that pulls your mind. The effect of *kwaiwaga* can last one or two months, say like ginger traps along the road, but other doses will take you for life, you are locked for life. The overdose can be damaging, people will act like puppets or children with no mind of their own. [Interview notes, 16 October 2003]

Males are not the only purveyors and practitioners of *kwaiwaga* and other forms of *meguva*, or chanted magic. Rebecca, a married mother of four children, is an acknowledged and reputable specialist who inherited her knowledge of *meguva* from her maternal grandmother. She explained to me, "My grandmother loved me so much because I was the *bubu* who loved her best. That is why she gave this to me. It passes with the love. No love to pass it with, then the person will just rip it up, burn it, not pass it to the *bubus*. It will just die with that person."[11] Rebecca showed me the small address book she uses to record *kwaiwaga* chants. Frayed and stained with age, the book also is used to record her children's birth dates and as a clinic book for visits to the health center. In addition to ten different *kwaiwaga* chants, the book also contains several chants for *kaimwasila* and *kabisilova*, as well as spells for performance enhancement for athletes and students, protective magic against witchcraft and sorcery, spells for fertility control, remedies for ailments, and garden magic.

I asked Rebecca to tell me about one of the *kaimwasila* chants, *kala doba*, used on a new fiber skirt to enable the wearer to attract the boy of her desire. She explained, "Girls don't have to go looking for boys; they can attract boys to them with *kala doba*. Boys will come like biting mosquitoes! The girl can take her pick, have her choice, or she can say the boy's name in the chant and only he will come. It is shameful for a girl to go looking for a boy, it means you can't attract. But if you have strong magic, you don't need to look for him, he will come to you."

Rebecca then gave me permission to transcribe the English translation of *kala doba*, which poetically evokes the gendered aesthetics of mobility and desire.

Kala Doba
Bitatai [movement of body in doba]
Attract in front, side to side
Attract in back, up and down
Attract at side, where the skirt opens to show thigh and hip
Look like the chief's wife
Look like the chief's niece
Beautiful looking
Different people will be attracted from all directions, all walks
If you try luck
[Boy's name] will come to you
Short skirt will attract him
Pull his face down into your skirt.
(Name the parts of the skirt and repeat chant.)
(Name the shell decorations and repeat chant.)
(Name the breasts and repeat chant.)
Nupisi [budding breasts]

Nupiyakwa [breasts that stand up firm and tight or breasts filled
with milk]

Nutaiya [fallen breasts, whether dry or lactating]

The *kala doba* chant illustrates the power of female erotic appeal to transcend
the search for love, transforming "luck" into consummate effect by pulling the desired other toward the wearer of the skirt. Rebecca told me that most of her clients
for *kwaiwaga* are young boys whereas girls and women mainly use attraction magic
like *kala doba*. Consistent with the directionality of sexual pursuit, where boys
and men are the main initiators of liaisons, *kwaiwaga* is primarily perceived as a
male resource in the art of persuasion and seduction. However, many people agree
that the *kwaiwaga* used by females is far more potent than that used by males.
This perhaps reflects the gendered application of *kwaiwaga*; women say they use
it primarily for securing a partner's fidelity in steady relationships and marriage, a
feat perceived as requiring strong magic. In this sense, fidelity profoundly reflects
the transformative capacity of agency; the ultimate acquiescence to loss of sexual
autonomy and mobility is the effect of another person's action.

A frequently voiced concern is that the use of *kwaiwaga* is proliferating and
therefore the potential for misuse and "overdoses" has increased. The *toyuvisa* told
me that he is reluctant to provide *kwaiwaga* because of its overuse. Another common concern is that married men misuse *kwaiwaga* to gain the affection of single
girls. As one young woman explained, "We feel safe when we are with single men.
When we go out with married men, we feel frightened, scared if someone is looking at the back of us; scared that he will use *kwaiwaga* to spoil our minds. This is
how young girls end up marrying their friend's husband, through *kwaiwaga*."[12]

Coupled with these concerns is the view that women's increased use of
kwaiwaga reflects the relaxation of customary practice under the influence of modernity, which emboldens the exercise of autonomy and control. In this sense, the
repertoire of love magic represents a strategy for mediating social change, including new vulnerabilities brought by HIV (see Jenkins 2007:29–30). The shifting
perspectives on the uses and effects of love magic, and the sense of empowerment
engendered by its use, are apparent in the following excerpt from a discussion with
twelve adult women.

> **Patricia:** The ladies use it if their husbands are not trustworthy. To hold
> them back.
>
> **Janet:** It used to be only for boys to use on girls. But nowadays, everyone!
>
> **Patricia:** People used to say it is a shameful thing for a girl to use this *kwaiwaga*.
> And now—why are the ladies wearing boys' trousers, why is that?
>
> **Janet:** Now life is changing, ladies are wearing men's clothes so why not we use
> *kwaiwaga*, too? So that is westernized.
>
> *So you think the use of kwaiwaga is westernized?*
>
> **Janet:** Yes, it could be westernized, yes.
>
> *And does it work when the ladies use it?*
>
> **All:** Yes! It works!
>
> *Can you describe how it works?*

Mary: I'll describe. OK. [Big reaction from the other women, who begin to tease her.] No, I want to contribute.

Priscilla: She wants to contribute.

Helen: Let her speak.

Mary: OK. Once a lady gives *kwaiwaga* to a man, OK, she will be like, she has the freedom to go anywhere, leaving the man. Once this *kwaiwaga* works, the man has to cry for the lady. And during the night the man has to go and sleep in the lady's house. That's really bad! Before, not like that. Nowadays, because ladies do *kwaiwaga*, the man will run from his house to the lady's house.

Rebecca: This *kwaiwaga*, I use it too. I use it! I know! I work this thing. OK, suppose the man goes to another lady, OK, I use this magic and the man will just stay with me. Before only the boys and men knew how to use this. But now, girls and women also use it to hold the man. We cannot trick you. All of us use this one.

OK, so it is a way to keep your husband at home. That's a smart thing!

Rebecca: Oh, Kathy! Honestly, we use this one. We use it to keep the husband faithful to the wife.

Priscilla: That's the one!

And does it work?

Rebecca: It works! When we make this magic, oh please, the man will cry for the woman.

Janet: You have to use it the correct way. If the husband is too much going around, bringing diseases to the wife, then *kwaiwaga* is the way to help the lady keep him from going out, so he will stay and look after his family and his kids. [Taped group discussion, 29 July 2003]

As a cultural resource, *kwaiwaga* epitomizes the intersubjective qualities of social relations and how agency registers its effects through a process of exchange between different actors. The value of exchange in *kubukwabuya* sexuality, and Trobriand sociality more broadly, is further manifested in another kind of transaction that elicits and confirms desire between sexual partners and indicates the viability of a relationship—that of *buwala*, the obligatory gifts that young boys and men give their sexual partners after lovemaking.

Buwala and the Transaction of Desire

Men have the desire to give *buwala*; women have the desire to accept *buwala*. [Female, aged fifty, taped group discussion, 30 June 2003]

An integral aspect of sexual etiquette, *buwala* is regarded as a respectful gesture that symbolizes mutual pleasure between two consensual partners. While suggestive of gender asymmetry in sexual exchange, as a material affirmation of desire *buwala* serves to legitimate the intentions of a male suitor and validate the sexual act as a reciprocal transaction between two people. Moreover, the intimacy of *buwala* transactions situates the couple within the broader field of social relations, providing the means to communicate intentions, demonstrate viability, and assert marital preferences to relatives. A young boy draws on his social network for assistance in acquiring the gifts he gives, and in turn a young girl redistributes the gifts she receives to her relatives. *Buwala* is described as "the way to work out a relationship," that is, it is the means by which the seriousness of a relationship is revealed to others.[13] *Buwala* not only communicates the suitor's intentions to pursue a steady relationship but is the medium through which a girl indicates to her relatives whom she prefers as a steady partner. By redistributing her *buwala* gifts, she effectively seeks familial endorsement of the relationship.

> *Buwala* has two signs: Parents can see what the girl gets from her partner, what he is able to provide. Also, it is a signal that he is serious, there is something under it; he is thinking to marry. [Male, aged twenty, taped group discussion, 15 October 2003]

> *Buwala* is like the value of the boy; it's a measure of what he can give. If a boy has no *buwala* to give, he will ask his friends and relatives to help him. It is a must for them to help. It's a sharing thing for one another, a tradition to assist each other out with something for *buwala*. It's a credit for the boy to give something to his partner. The girl will not ask for it, will not complain for it. [Female, aged twenty-two, taped group discussion, 30 June 2003]

Sexual partners do not negotiate *buwala* transactions prior to coupling, nor do they enter into any discussion about it. *Buwala* transactions are polite, discreet, and always take place after a sexual encounter.

> The boy will prepare things. *Katubaiasa* [to prepare]. After, he will say, "I prepared this for you." If the girl is with him in his house, he would put it there for her to take when she leaves. That's if she is from the same village and she goes home before sunrise. Of a different village, he must walk her to her village and on the way he will give her *buwala* as they say goodbye. Or sometimes, *kabweli* [apology]. Suppose he had nothing to give, he would give his apology and say he will make up for it later. Or if it is not enough, something small, he will say, "I will give you something better next time." It is up to her, if she wants to continue the relationship. Yes, *buwala* is a must. If the agreement between the two is closer to marriage then they won't worry so much about *buwala* each time they get together. [Male, aged fifty, taped group discussion, 10 October 2003]

A range of items are used for *buwala*, including betel nut, tobacco, pieces of fabric, T-shirts, tortoise shell earrings, small knives, lime containers, and cash. But not only tangible items are used; young boys will also pass on highly guarded "treasures" such as magical chants. Imparting valued cultural knowledge in lieu of giving material items for *buwala* underscores the imperative of exchange in sexual relations.

> Sometimes if they don't have anything then the boys will give the ladies charms that would help them in their daily work, like growing sweet potatoes. Things they have, treasured things to pass to the ladies, like garden magic. They know the girl would need that, so they give them. That is when they don't have anything else to give, so they give their last treasures. [Male, aged eighteen, taped group discussion, 10 October 2003]

Boys typically acquire items to use for *buwala* from their *dala* relatives—aunties, grandmothers, uncles, older brothers (but not cross-sex siblings)—as well as from their father's brothers and sisters. Although parents are not generally approached for such items, fathers and mothers do make contributions if requested. An older woman told me that when her son would ask her, "Mum, can you give me K5 for my smoke and betel nut?" she would know that he intended to use it for *buwala*. Several young boys explained that some fathers take a direct interest in their sons' affairs by helping with *buwala* and advising on which girls to go out with. In effect, the contributions made to a young boy by his relatives are the equity he requires to be sexually active and demonstrate his potential as a future husband and in-law. The accrual of contributions forms part of a composite of familial and *dala* obligations that radiate outward to other exchange relations when the boy marries. In this sense, *buwalu* transactions set the basis for the subsequent exchanges between in-laws that seal the marriage bond. As a partnership becomes steady and the intention to marry is communicated, there is no longer the shared expectation to give and receive *buwala* every time the couple spends the night together. The cessation of *buwala* transactions signals the move to the more pronounced exchange patterns between in-laws once marriage takes place.

Similar in importance to upholding the ethic of mutual consent in sexual relations, *buwala* transactions are compelled by the moral concern to avoid the shame of contravention, dishonoring one's name and place identity. Like the transaction of desire itself, shame works both ways: a young boy would feel shame for not giving *buwala* and a young girl would feel shame in not receiving it. The imperative for gift giving and redistribution, and the shame in not doing so, was reiterated time and again during group discussions and interviews with both males and females, emphasizing the fundamental importance of *buwala* in the protocol of *kubukwabuya* sexual activity. The following explanations of *buwala* typify the gendered perspectives expressed during discussions, while hinting at the differential values of male and female sexuality. The first statement was made by a fifty-year-old divorced woman with four grown children.

> When the ladies *kapugula*, they meet the boys, and when they come back, the ladies must come back with *buwala*. It would be bad if they didn't, because those boys who went to the girls, those girls would come back to their village and one girl would say, "Oh, I came back with nothing." And then the groups of boys would hear the stories and they would turn to their friend and say, "Oh, you did nothing for that girl. Next time you will stay because you are spoiling the group's name, because you didn't give her anything." With a group of boys, every boy should give something. Because it is a group he must, or his friends will hear the stories and they will argue. And the girls who come back with plenty, they would say to the empty-handed one, "Oh, your man is not wealthy," or something like this. This is our traditional way of *kapugula*. In fact, if I go out with a man, he must, he *must*, it is a must that he gives me *buwala*. It is a must. So, if he won't, it will be the end of him.

How would it be the end of him?

Because what I bring, *buwagu* [*buwa-*, root word; *-gu*, first person possessive], I must give it to my family, my uncle. They would expect that I bring something from the man I go with. We give it to our aunties, our uncles—our mothers' brothers—or our mothers' uncles. If they agree with the friendship and they know the man I am going out with and his family, they would be happy and agree. If not, they will not accept him, they won't agree. They will try and stop me from seeing him. When the girl doesn't receive *buwala* people would say, "She was used for nothing." Women have a right to receive something from men. Otherwise, friends will be judging. If nothing from the boy then I won't agree for a next time and he will feel big shame. Girls outside of the boy's village must receive *buwala*; otherwise the boy's village will get a bad name. [Taped group discussion, 30 June 2003]

Similarly, the following explanation was given during a group discussion with five male participants ranging in age from early twenties to late fifties.

Young man: If no *buwala*, it would be a shameful thing because the man's friends would say, "Oh, you brought the lady [to your house], you slept with the lady and you did not give her anything."

How would his friends know?
The girl herself would tell her friends: "Be aware, don't go with him because he didn't give me anything." The word spreads. Men know they have to have something in stock before they go searching for girls.

Older man: *Buwala* is pride. In this manner, where you go with a lady and have sex with her in the night and in the morning she goes out and you give *buwala*, it signifies that you are having a close tie with each other and whenever you go back to her and ask her for another time to have sex with her then it will be possible because she will say yes. If you have sex with her in the night and you don't give her *buwala*, then it will stop the friendship. . . . Because the lady will go back and this thing you give her she will give it to her aunties and mommy and they'll, you know, "This is a very good thing that you will still go to that same person again if he comes to you." But if I don't give her very much presents, then that's it, the end of it. You see?

How do young people learn about buwala, that it is a must?
It is passed through the older ones . . . and as it is the rule, as you come up and start having sex, so when you bring a girlfriend to your house and sleep with her all the night, you must give her something. Or even the lady will go back if you don't give her anything, then her girlfriends will ask, "What did that person do when they slept with you? Did they give you anything?" It would be a shameful thing for her because she wanted sex, slept with her boy over there, then when she came home—*wokuva*, empty-handed. It is an insult. [Taped group discussion, 10 October 2003]

The above explanations suggest the importance of gender group affiliation and the influence of peers in upholding the ethical code of *buwala* exchange. The constellation of pride, respect, shame, and insult is persistently used to describe the significance of *buwala* transactions in legitimizing sexual relations. The image of arriving home empty-handed speaks of the larger cultural emphasis on the value of exchange in the Trobriands.

Because *buwala* often includes the exchange of *buwa*, or betel nut, it is tempting to interpret the word as deriving from *buwa*. However, Trobrianders make a clear distinction between the two words and do not draw a linguistic analogy.[14] In speech, the root word *buwa* is modified by the pronominal suffix of nearest possession, which designates relational terms and parts of the person that are inalienable (Lawton 1993). The unpossessed noun is conveyed by using the third person singular suffix, *-la*. It is significant that the pronominal suffix of nearest possession is used rather than the pronouns used to designate transactional and alienable possession. As Malinowski points out, this pronominal use "expresses an extremely close relation between the gift and both the giver and the receiver: in other words, that the gift is an essential part of the transaction" (1929:269).

Although the distinction between *buwa* and *buwala* is clear, the ubiquitous sharing of betel nut as the core expression of Trobriand sociality invites an association between the two words that underscores the value of exchange and distribution signified by *buwala* transactions. Stopping to chat along the road habitually entails an exchange of betel nut and the sharing of lime and mustard. Older women often respond to young girls' requests for betel nut with an allusion to the ready supply of betel nut that young girls are able to obtain through their *kapugula* mobility.

Trobrianders do not characterize *buwala* in terms of *mapula*, meaning price or payment, or as the material means for males to acquire sexual favors from females. Although young boys assert that they would not go out looking for girls if they had nothing to give, this reflects their concern about pride and respect rather than implying that sexual activity bears an economic cost. However, people do speak about *buwala* in terms of an equivalence of exchange, that is, in terms of replacing one thing for another, which suggests the interchangeable value of sex and goods as equivalent resources. Because *buwala* is given by males and received by females, it may seem logical to impute that females reciprocate the use of their bodies as a service for male sexual pleasure. Such an interpretation of *buwala* is suggested by Malinowski, who states, "This custom implies that sexual intercourse, even where there is mutual attachment, is a service rendered by the female to the male" (1929:268–69). While Malinowski discusses the "commercial" aspect of the transaction, he is quick to emphasize that *buwala* should not be misconstrued as prostitution (270). Yet representing *buwala* as a form of payment for female sexual services in a context of mutual consent and affection poses an unsettling contravention of Western constructs of prostitution and transactional sex, which involve the "implicit moral and analytical categories" that separate "real love," which is given freely, from monetary or material exchange (Swidler and Watkins 2006:2; see also Wardlow 2004; Zatz 1997).

The concept of transactional sex, defined as the exchange of sex for material benefits that typically involves multiple concurrent partners, has gained considerable mileage over recent years in analyses of factors that contribute to HIV transmission. The practice is generally construed as a problem that requires prevention to minimize the risk of HIV infection. Most analyses make a conceptual distinction between transactional sex and prostitution, identifying the interpersonal aspects of the former as significantly different from the economic terms of commercialized sex work. In particular, the concept of transactional sex carries assumptions about age and economic asymmetries associated with gendered power relations, construed in terms of "greater wealth of the male partner and a need or desire for monetary resources by the female partner" (Luke and Kurz 2002:6). Furthermore, the analysis contends that although female sexual agency is exercised to "extract" money and gifts from older male partners, power disparities delimit the ability of females to negotiate safe sex practices (6). Critiquing the dominant analytical narrative of transactional sex, Ann Swidler and Susan Cotts Watkins state, "The image of transactional sex as a desperate expedient of impoverished women seems to explain women's reliance on multiple partners in a way that Western analysts find comprehensible" (2006:2). Furthermore, they contend that the concept's emphasis on the "exploitation of poor, vulnerable women by wealthier, more powerful men" is based on the presumption of coercion to explain and justify women's participation in what is perceived as a deviation from idealized and normative patterns of sexual behavior (Swidler and Watkins 2006:n3, 28; Tawfika and Watkins 2007).

The practice of *buwala* based on mutual consent does not easily conform to the standard definition of transactional sex as the exchange of sex for money or material support, or of the gendered power asymmetries and coercion associated with such exchange. Nor does it offer a direct comparison to the ritualized practices of bride-price pervasive throughout PNG, which are increasingly becoming commodified (Jenkins 2007; Wardlow 2006). However, because *buwala* links sex with material transactions, the practice is particularly susceptible to monetary transformation and the emergent economic disparities associated with the cash economy. While the erotic appeal of money has been seamlessly incorporated into *buwala* without affecting the relational value of sexuality, there is now evidence that the terms of exchange are shifting in response to the influx of cash into the sexual economy (cf. Jenkins 2007; Nash 1981; Valeri 1994). This is especially the case in intergenerational partnering, where sex between adult men and young girls increasingly holds an expectation for cash payments, offered by men *prior* to coupling as the way to gain the female partner's consent. In this way, money is shifting the power dynamics between *men* of different age groups more significantly than it is reinforcing asymmetries between male and female agency. "Married men try luck by mentioning cash, especially if they go out to other villages. Young girls don't expect single boys to give them money." (Taped group discussion, 19 August 2003. Translated into English.)

One woman explained, "Cash is something we all desire and benefit from, so if it is offered it is hard for some to refuse."[15] A humorous expression used by some young girls to indicate their desire for cash is *Bapwaieki batagwala*, or "I'll be smoking and agreeing," meaning that the girl will be thinking of all the consumer goods she will be able to purchase if she accepts cash for sex.[16] The power of cash to arouse desire and truncate the protocol of "trying luck" also has the ability to supersede the seductive power of *kwaiwaga*, as typified by the following observation from a male perspective, "Magic is losing out to money. There's no need for *kwaiwaga* if you have cash to give."[17] Yet cash transactions are also talked about in terms of generosity and help, consistent with Trobriand notions of patronage, reciprocity, and obligatory support. "Because nowadays with cash already here, the man should really try to help the girl, maybe with K10, K20."[18] Viewed in this light, *buwala* offers an established cultural form and moral framework to accommodate new needs and desires engendered by money.

While the practice of *buwala* can be viewed as a particular cultural form of transactional sex, it is important not to distort the cultural meaning of *buwala* by a narrow frame of analysis that merely transposes Western concepts without interpretive depth. To appreciate the transactional nature of Trobriand sexuality represented by *buwala*, it is helpful to rehearse anthropological understandings of Melanesian concepts of value, which recognize that measures of comparison and equivalence are distinct from valuations in a capitalist economy precisely because of the social relations that obtain through gift exchange (Gregory 1982; Strathern 1988). The value of an exchange object reflects personal and collective agency in relation to its source of origin and is "constructed in the identity of a thing or person with various sets of social relations in which it is embedded, and its simultaneous detachability from them" (Strathern 1987:286). More than being a material measure of a girl's sexual worth and a boy's sexual interest, *buwala* represents mutual consent and pleasure, future fertility, and the interconnected social relations that shape *kubukwabuya* sexuality. Whether construed as reciprocal gift exchange or commoditized payment, *buwala* creates value through relational ties. And like other exchange items, cash also assumes relational value and is not transacted as an alienable commodity. *Buwala* is a particular manifestation of the generalized exchange and materiality of all social relations. Furthermore, it is fundamentally redistributive, underscoring how intimate transactions are embedded in a much larger field of exchange relations.

Nanola and the Agency of Desire

To further contextualize the embodied practice and transactional dimensions of youth sexuality in relation to the broader concerns of social reproduction, it is helpful to look more closely at how the notion of agency is conceptualized in the Trobriand social world. Autonomy is central to understanding the embodiment of social relations and, more specifically, how autonomous assertions and acts are ultimately, and paradoxically, expressions of situated relationality. The autonomous self is not the imagined atomistic individual of Western society, but is actively constructed in relation to social others, revealing the situational and relational core of personhood in the Trobriands and how the self takes form within the dynamics of exchange (Weiner 1976:219; see also Strathern 1988:89–90; Maclean 1994:667–68).

Nanola, the Trobriand word for "mind," encompasses by definition the principle of personal agency and autonomy, the "locus of an individual's thoughts, desires, and intentions" (Weiner 1983:692), and it reflects the measure of equity among all social actors regardless of rank and status.[19] Trobrianders do not outwardly speculate about the thoughts and desires of others, believing that "each person's mind is inviolate" (Weiner 1988:70), "protected and bounded from the intentions of others" (Weiner 1983:692, 695). From early childhood, Trobriand socialization allows considerable breadth for the exercise of personal autonomy in acting on volition and refusing to act on the requests of others (Malinowski 1929:45; Weiner 1976:136). "We don't know his/her mind" is a common disclaimer regarding the acts of others, thus preserving personal autonomy while absolving collective responsibility for individual acts.

Trobrianders are careful not to impute rationale or judgment onto another's action because doing so is likely to implicate them in chains of cause and effect. Counterbalancing the contrived concealment of individual intent are the strategies people engage to influence, seduce, and turn the minds of others by altering their thoughts, feelings, and actions. The dance of autonomy involves reciprocity between the desires of the self and the desires of others. In important ways, the effect of agency is the displacement—or eclipse, to use Strathern's term (1988:155, 219)—of autonomous acts, which tend to be viewed as the consequence of the persuasive power of others (see also Battaglia 1997). The use of magic wields tremendous power in enabling a person to exert her or his will over others, to guard against the unwanted desires of others, and, indeed, to affect the capacity to act in response to the desires of others (Weiner 1983).

Agency, thus, is "essentially a transformative capacity" (Demian 2006:151), which registers cause and effect in a social field comprised of multiple viewpoints. By acting with others in mind, the minds of others are turned back on the self or oriented toward a different viewpoint (Strathern (1988:272–73). The transformative capacity of the hidden mind demonstrates effect through relationality—"the mind is made visible in the context of multiple social relations with others" (Strathern 1988:164). On a fundamental level, *kumila* and *dala* encompass the autonomy of constituent members, such that the viability and capacity of the group is reflective of its component parts. In this dialectic of relatedness autonomy is socially constrained even as it is inviolable. Perhaps the autonomous mind is unknowable because of what is at stake—the impinging of one person's actions on others and, hence, the larger social consequences of such actions carried by the collective body. In this regard, it is socially important to preserve ambiguity about intentions until the decisive moment when action is made apparent through a potent event, whether a large-scale mortuary feast or a mutually arranged sexual liaison.

Assertions and transformations of relational personhood are made known to others in various ways but most visibly through acts of labor—the specific productive activities that make gendered agency appear in the social realm. In *The Gender of the Gift*, Strathern describes how labor is a "sphere of agency" oriented to social others (1988:156), which "produces or makes visible a relationship" (164). As discussed in Chapter 4, the value of labor in the Trobriand exchange economy is measured by its performative effects. Subsistence productivity is primarily self-determined in response to multiple social expectations and obligations.[20] Each person sets his or her own objectives and pace within specific forms of labor, which are essentially but not exclusively defined by gender. A person's *paisewa*, or labor, is directed toward activating and making visible valued social relationships—whether by cultivating yam gardens, producing *doba*, weaning and feeding an adopted baby,

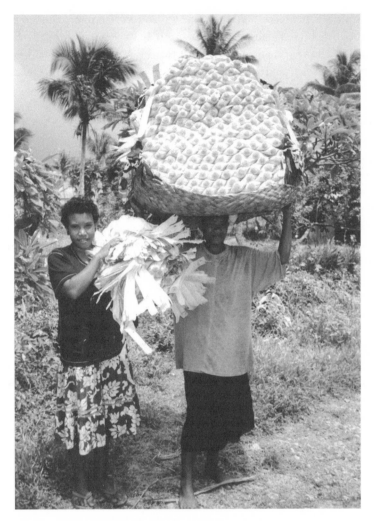

FIGURE 5.1. • Young girls carrying *doba* and *sepwana* from a *sagali*,
December 2000

caring for the sick and elderly, mourning for the deceased, or attending to the daily
chores of shared domesticity. Concurrently, labor is indicative of the very relationships that activate it in the first instance (see Demian 2000:94, 107).

In the Trobriands, work as an aesthetic sphere of agency often takes a mobile
and visible form in the action of "carrying" the investments and products of labor.
Gogebila means to carry on the head, which is almost exclusively a female form.
Katakewa means to carry on the shoulder or on a pole, which is a predominantly
male form.[21] Intent and purpose are set into motion by physically carrying objects
of exchange that represent social connections and, hence, social obligations and
responsibility. To move without visible intent from one defined social space to another—between dwellings, villages, and islands—or to arrive empty-handed as a
visitor is antithetical to the aesthetics of work and can be cause for social shame.
Carrying objects of exchange is an entrusted form of labor, a demonstration of

"working hard" that is as visually communicative as it is tangibly productive. From a young age, Trobriand children learn the value of carrying objects between people and households to signify reciprocity and social connectedness.

Yet *kubukwabuya* are also free to walk in full public view without carrying objects of productive labor or objects of exchange, especially when walking together in a *tubwa* group. Indeed, nothing quite exemplifies the freedom of youth so much as a leisurely stride unencumbered by the weight of a carried object. The shell necklaces, armbands, and earrings that adorn youthful bodies are symbols of the investments others make in their physical and social development, imbuing the carrier with the power of persuasion and seduction by enhancing their beauty and desirability. Young people proudly "carry" these adornments on their bodies, but the effect is one of display, not encumbrance. However, through the purposive action of carrying the objects of productive labor—firewood, water, fish, garden produce, *doba*, yam sticks, house timber—and acting with others in mind, young people freely demonstrate their potential to work hard and be fit for the productive roles of adulthood.

Moving toward Marriage

As a measure of the productive and relational value of sexuality, *buwala* demonstrates how exchange is used to communicate personal and group capacity through young people's sexual agency. The transactional dimension of *kubukwabuya* sexuality underscores the wider importance of mobility and circulation in the aesthetics of social exchange. In her ethnography of the Massim island of Sabarl, Debbora Battaglia focuses on the movement of exchange objects and their symbolic potency, observing that circulation is "kinetic 'evidence'" of relational pathways (1990:135). Following this insight, I suggest that *kubukwabuya* mobility, as the collective orientation of personal agency, registers kinetic evidence of social relations in much the same way as the circulation of objects of exchange, including *buwala* transactions. The consummate effect of the quest of sexually mobile young people as they move toward marriage is to make visible personal and group viability, building on established alliances between families, clans, and villages while exploring potential connections for future regeneration. Young people's embodied mobility is their contribution to collective productivity and social cohesion. In effect, it is their work.

A common remark made during discussions and conversations was that sex is regarded as a "play thing," an enjoyable, recreational pursuit that is not taken too seriously until the relationship becomes serious. Although sexual activity is often referred to as *mwasawa*, or game, which implies a competitive spirit, it is also euphemized with knowing humor as *paisewa*, or work. While this analogy is undoubtedly common in many cultural contexts (see, for example, Setel 1999:165), the comparison here is purposeful, underscoring the value of productive labor and the vitality of youth. "Hardworking" and "good-looking" are the commensurate qualities both males and females seek in their sexual partners and in their search for a compatible partner to marry. Parents advise their sons to "work hard in the garden so the girls will come to you." Young people talk of "studying" their friends to identify who would make a hardworking spouse. Many young people, both male and female, say they prefer to look for partners from further afield because the motivation to demonstrate one's capacity for hard work is bolstered by the prospect of expanding exchange relations and achieving recognition beyond their own village.

The quest to secure a steady partner is the undercurrent of *kubukwabuya* mobility. A monogamous relationship becomes visible to others when the young couple's autonomous mobility ceases, thereby activating the social obligations required for its legitimation. The timing of this transition and the choice of partner is largely the prerogative of young people themselves. Sometimes parents set demands or restrictions about who their offspring should marry, usually by intervening after the couple communicates their intentions. While the advice of parents and relatives is listened to, young people have the final say in the decision. An older woman explained, "Sometimes young people will agree to the decision of the parents, but mostly they will marry the one they truly love." [22]

Several people I interviewed mentioned how the path to marriage was a circular journey; after having a succession of relationships, they arrived back at the beginning and married their "true partner," the person with whom they first became sexually active. When I asked if the history of multiple partnering affected marital harmony, I was told that couples should not bring to the marriage any jealousy or hard feelings about previous relationships because every young person enjoys sexual freedom and autonomy. The caveat, however, is that a couple should never call to mind or openly mention their previous relationships to each other or to others; in effect, an artifice of marriage is the feigned erasure of one's *kubukwabuya* sexual history from memory. However, people concede that former partners often hold affectionate memories of each other and may fleetingly express their mutual fondness with a subtle exchange of betel nut when they happen to encounter each other along the road, at the market, or at a *sagali*. A commonly expressed observation, which indicates the gendered terrain of sexual competition and possessiveness, is that men "feel shame" when they see their wife's former boyfriends or encounter them on the road, whereas women "feel like champions" in front of their husband's former girlfriends.

Autonomy in marital decisions allows considerable flexibility for de facto and trial partnerships as well as mutability of marital status. *Vaipaka*, or divorce (literally, "marriage-break"), is fairly common in the Trobriands, and marriages might dissolve after a trial period if the couple finds they are not compatible. *Kwaiwaga* is often perceived as the underlying cause of such break ups. Such circumstances can cause friction between families and clans, and sometimes require an appropriate exchange of yams and other items to satisfactorily reach a recognized annulment.

The *bukumatula*, or "bachelor house" as Malinowski called it, symbolically synthesizes the Trobriand ideals of industrious masculinity, youth sexuality, and the passage to adulthood and marriage (1929:53). During early adolescence, a young boy establishes spatial autonomy by moving into his own *bukumatula*, which he constructs next to his parent's house or the household where he was a resident. The timing of this event is self-determined but often reflects other familial dynamics that prompt reconfiguration of shared domestic space, especially if a boy's younger sister has recently entered into the *kapugula* life stage. The paramount concern to keep cross-sex siblings' amorous pursuits separate and confidential from one another relates to the potency of love magic and the *sovasova* incest taboo (described in Chapter 6), which share a common mythological origin (see Malinowski 1929:456–59). The anxiety over the possibility that a sister will accidentally come into physical contact with her brother's love magic is a core reason for sibling segregation. At this important transformative stage in a young boy's life, he will also commence his active engagement in formalized exchange relations by making a yam-exchange garden for a man who has been directly involved in his upbringing (Weiner 1976:146). By building a *bukumatula* and engaging in yam cultivation for exchange, the young boy publicly demonstrates his economic viability as a future husband and in-law in the productive transition to adulthood.

Although I seldom heard these dwellings referred to as *bukumatula*, when I used the term people would concur with me. The most commonly used term is *bwala kubukwabuya*, meaning house of an unmarried youth. I do not know if this is a contemporary expression or if it has a long history of usage.[23] The gender-neutral age category as a modifier is noteworthy, as only young unmarried men build and reside in these houses, while *kubukwabuya* girls continue to live with their parents or other adult relatives and do not directly engage in house construction except to help plait the roof and wall thatching used for family or communal dwellings. *Bwala kubukwabuya* are often transformed into family *bwala* when a young man and his steady partner establish residence as a married couple.

The *bukumatula* is also the sanctioned private space where young people engage in sexual relations before marriage (Malinowski 1929:53; Weiner 1976:169). The dwelling offers a different kind of intimacy for nighttime liaisons than the other locations where groups of young boys and girls rendezvous, often signifying the seriousness of a steady relationship. Under the veil of darkness, a young boy will meet his girlfriend at a prearranged location and then bring her back to his dwelling for the night. And then before the break of dawn, the young girl will discreetly leave the house and return to her family dwelling, taking care that no one sees her, especially her boyfriend's sisters. If she is from a different village, her boyfriend will escort her to the road or path leading to her village, where she will quietly slip back into her family dwelling before dawn. If she arrives back after sunrise, a young girl will be mindful not to attract attention to her tardiness. She might casually assume a domestic task or join the early morning activity at the tide pools and wells, where younger girls are busy washing cooking pots and collecting water. If a girl does not leave the *bukumatula* before dawn, she will stay quietly in the house all day, unseen, until she can make a stealthy exit when night falls again.

Like young boys, girls exercise considerable freedom in determining their labor contributions and cannot be forced to work against their will. *Kapugula* girls apply their productive labor to domestic tasks that involve washing and cleaning, as well as caring for younger siblings. They also learn from their mothers and aunts the craft of *doba* and mat plaiting, and the intricacies of *sagali* preparation and participation. Young girls' labor takes its most public form in the work of carrying exchange objects between households and villages. The productive mobility of young girls is regarded as complementary to their youthful beauty and sexuality, with an analogy drawn to work that enhances cleanliness.

Kapugula shouldn't be cooking, just go chop firewood, collect greens from the bush, peel the yams and wash them, help to wash dirty saucepans, but not cooking on the fire. We come to high school, learn home economics, and it is a problem for the young girls, they feel strange. Cooking is like making them dirty, the smoke, the charcoal. It occupies their time in the house when they should be going out, enjoying themselves. Washing clothes and pots at the pool, these are clean jobs. They keep their bodies clean at the same time as they are working. *Vivila kapugula* should be clean. [Interview notes, 6 November 2003]

The value of labor, and its correlation to sexuality, is also underscored by the strict protocol of youth coupling that prohibits the sharing and eating of food in each other's presence. Like the cooking of food, which is the work of married women and mothers, the consumption of food is also perceived as the antithesis of *kubukwabuya* sexuality. A girl does not eat when she spends the night in her boyfriend's *bukumatula*, even if she does not make it home before dawn and remains in the house all day. Girls explain that they would feel extreme shame to eat in front of their boyfriends or to accept food from them because it would make them appear hungry, which would be perceived as greediness and undisciplined insatiability. They also say that eating would show a lack of respect for the young man's capacity to grow yams as a potential in-law and would be tantamount to insulting his family, as though they were already responsible for feeding her as a new wife. They further explain that to eat food in the boy's house is shameful because it would imply that his mother is already cooking for her even though they are not married. This constellation of reasons for shame relates to the value of affinal exchange relationships and the obligation of a married man to provide food for his children (cf. Young 1986). The prohibition on prenuptial food consumption directly endorses the act of matrimony (discussed in Chapter 4), which takes place when a young couple shares a meal of yams together for the first time. It also reflects the situation of early matrimony, when a young bride goes to live with her in-laws but does not cook until the mother-in-law prepares for her a new *kailagila*, the cooking hearth made with three stones, a symbolic event that further marks the transition to being a married woman.

The passage from being single to being married is often seamless and subtle, made visible initially through the inconspicuous transactions between two families and the simple meal eaten together. Yet at times the transition has a profound effect. One of the most dramatic acts of *kubukwabuya* autonomy and volition occurs when a young girl immobilizes herself in her boyfriend's house. In her refusal to leave, or to let her relatives *biu*, or "pull" her, she also refuses to eat. Such determination compels her relatives to honor her decision to become married to him (see Malinowski 1929:74).

One morning in January 2001, I was visiting a friend in the small dwelling that her husband had recently built for his growing family, shortly after another inconspicuous event in the life of the village—the birth of a baby. It was just a few hours after Cecilia had given birth to her fifth child. She was sitting up on the mattress admiring her newborn and stroking his face when she motioned with her eyes for me to peer out the tiny window cut in the thatched wall. "Look over there, the newlyweds!" she said with amusement. The window framed a lively, jovial gathering of about ten people across the hamlet yard at the *bukumatula* built by Tim, aged twenty-seven, the adopted younger brother of Cecilia's husband.

Tim was just a toddler when his *kadam*, or maternal uncle, adopted him after his mother died. Originally from a distant village on the far northwestern side of Kiriwina, he was determined to marry a girl from the same place to reinforce his paternal ties. His older brothers in the village arranged for him to meet Mary, eight years his junior. Tim built a *bukumatula* and began courting Mary.

Peering out the window at the gathering, I spotted the young smiling bride wearing a brand new grass skirt, freshly cut at the knees. I then recalled how late one moonless night a few weeks earlier, there was an urgent knock on my mother-in-law's closed front door and voices called out, asking if we had seen Mary. Her parents were on a resolute search for their wayward daughter, having walked the three hours from their village, and were now going door to door in our village, a small flashlight lighting their way. They suspected that she might be with Tim but didn't find the couple in his *bukumatula*. Mary had been staying inside Tim's house for several days and her parents had come to *bibiusi*, literally pull her out of the house. They didn't approve of the relationship and they wanted to take her back home. But the equally determined couple was well hidden, and if someone knew their whereabouts they didn't reveal it, for Mary's parents went home without their daughter. A few days later it was fait accompli. Mary had stubbornly stayed inside Tim's house, refusing to leave, and to demonstrate her resolve and soften her parents' objection, she did not eat. Word got back to her parents that she had made up her mind and nothing could change it. So they arranged for *katuvila*, the series of marriage transactions between the two families, and arrived at the hamlet that morning with a small entourage of relatives carrying several baskets of uncooked yams and platters of cooked food for Tim's adoptive parents. Tim's mother tied a new grass skirt around Mary's hips and draped a piece of bright red material over her shoulders. Tim's father presented Mary's father with a shell necklace. And Tim and Mary sat on the small veranda of the *bukumatula* and ate yams together.

Later that afternoon I saw Mary at the water tap, nonchalantly filling several pots with water. She was glowing radiantly but became demure when I congratulated her. Several days later she energetically joined in a rambunctious game of *randasi* (from English, meaning "around us") with a crew of children outside my mother-in-law's house, and she slammed the ball with gusto when teammates yelled out, "*Katuvila!*" (literally, to turn something back in the direction it comes from; the word is used in the game to signal to the striking player to hit the ball backward). Mary had become a fully visible resident of the village, and although now married, no longer *kubukwabuya*, she still participated in the impromptu games of young people.

Bidubadu and the Plenitude of Desire

Balancing the competing priorities and goals of *kubukwabuya* mobility and multiple partners with the quest to find the right partner in the path toward marriage is often talked about in terms of disciplining the boundaries of desire. Young girls especially say they try and "limit" themselves in their sexual pursuits. A twenty-year-old single girl, who characterizes herself as "already old," spoke of her mother's advice about relationships and setting limits in the pursuit of desire.

> I have the freedom. I walk around but my mother keeps telling me that I can walk around but I must also have the time to help her in the garden and house-work. My mother is saying, don't walk a lot, otherwise you'll get pregnant on the way and then you'll bring a single child back to the house and you would have to learn to look after that child. So when I walk around I must limit myself. My mother said I must stick to one partner and learn from that man whether he is the right one for my future husband because I am already old. If I have a steady friend that's the time I can really learn if, who, the man, the boyfriend is. But if I keep jumping to the next I won't know who that person really is. [Taped group discussion, 13 January 2001]

The word *bidubadu*, or plenty, is commonly used to describe the level of sexual activity among young people, evoking the plenitude of *kubukwabuya* freedom and mobility. The euphemistic phrase *bidibadu mitasi* (plenty eyes, third person plural), expresses the collective abundance of *kubukwabuya* desire as well as the ability to attract multiple partners. I first became aware of the colloquial use of *bidubadu* in a conversation with six young girls, aged between twelve and fourteen years, during the World AIDS Day parade on 1 December 2000. Led by the district health center ambulance, with siren blaring, health workers paraded up and down the two main roads in Losuia, carrying handmade signs on butcher paper with cursory messages about risk and prevention. Written in English, the messages included the following:

> Are you at risk of AIDS?
> Decide now to:
> • Have sex with one faithful partner
> • Use a condom when having sex
>
> AIDS is a killer. To prevent a killer:
> • Use condom when you want sex
> • Have one faithful partner

I asked the group of girls I was standing with to tell me about the messages. After whispered discussion between them in Kiriwina, one girl stated in English, "Us young girls must stick with one boy." I asked, "Is it the same for boys? Stick with one girl?" The immediate response was "Yes." Then one girl said, "There might be one or two," and someone else picked up the sentence and said, "or three or four," and then two girls laughed and said, "*Bidubadu*. Plenty!" I then asked, "So a young girl or boy might have plenty of partners before marriage?" The response was immediate and unanimous: "*Mokwita!* True! *Bidubadu!*"

A short time later, I once again encountered the word during a discussion with seven unmarried girls, aged between sixteen and twenty-two.[24] My question about how many boyfriends they would have before making plans for marriage was met with whispers and giggles until they all answered in unison, "*Bidubadu.*"

"*Bidubadu?*" I echoed, and they all burst out laughing. "Is that what you said?"

"Yes!" they answered with suppressed amusement.

"I hear that word a lot, I tell you!" I said jovially, and they laughed some more and whispered in Kiriwina language.

Diana, who was facilitating the discussion, said, "They say you're joking and everyone is laughing."

"But I do hear that word a lot. And I don't know what it means. I know it means 'plenty' but what does plenty mean? How many is plenty?"

"Let's say it is a plural," Diana offered after a pause.

"As many as . . . ?" I pressed.

Mari answered forthright. "As you can. Until our life stops."

"Would it mean three?" I asked, pushing for a number.

Diana said, "No, three is not that much."

Mari then suggested, "*Bidubadu* is ten, twenty."

"And you said, 'Until our life stops.' What do you mean by that?" I asked.

"Until we are getting satisfied."

"Until you are satisfied," I repeated.

"Yes."

"And what happens when you are satisfied?"

"When we are satisfied, that's the time we choose the right partner."

"So how many until you are satisfied?"

The girls broke out in laughter again, finding my persistence amusing, and Jenna playfully scolded, "Upwards twenty. Don't ask!"

Bidubadu indicates how young people's search for the "right partner" typically entails an extended period of multiple partnering and casual sexual encounters before the transition to adulthood—"We have a lot of time to enjoy ourselves before marriage."[25] Importantly, while the notion connotes the freedom and plenitude young people enjoy during the period of *kubukwabuya*, it does not convey a sense of promiscuity or indiscriminate excess. Young people represent their sexual freedom as a process of decision making that involves careful discernment and studied selection, not careless abandon.

The transformative shift into reproductive forms of adult sociality is achieved through childbearing, marriage, and the establishment of affinal exchange relations. As expressed by the idiom "until our life stops," this critical point of social repositioning in the Trobriand regenerative cycle is associated with the consummation of youthful desire and the cessation of sexual autonomy and mobility. The abruptness of the transition between youth and adulthood is captured in a statement by another young girl, who declared, "If I stop, that's the end of me."[26] However, the extended life stage of *kubukwabuya*—of sexual exploration and experimentation, of being attractive and pursuing desire, of testing out potential partners in an expanding social field—is ultimately directed toward assuming the relational status of mothers, fathers, wives, husbands, and in-laws.

The transition between exercising sexual freedom, which is hidden from public recognition to retain autonomy from formal exchange obligations, and finding the right partner to settle down with, which carries public acknowledgment when families and clans become linked by the relationship, holds tensions in terms of its timing and disclosure. The timing is especially problematic for young girls because, unlike boys, the longer they retain their *kubukwabuya* status, the more likely they are to be seen as undesirable marriage partners. In this sense, maternity becomes an important objective for a young girl, whether or not it leads to marriage. By becoming a mother, a young girl transforms her sexual agency into a reproductive achievement that carries her into a new life stage. However, the potential reversal of this transition allows sexual autonomy and *kubukwabuya* mobility to be reactivated if desired.

The temporal shifts of relational subjectivity and the power of the autonomous mind are made clear in the self-account of a twenty-year-old mother who, acting on her decision not to stay married to her baby son's father, told me: "My mind is strong; I am still a young girl if I want." Such an assertion speaks of willed transformations rather than a teleological life course. Her decision to leave her husband reflects the mutability of marriage in the Trobriand context when a young couple find they are not compatible after a trial period. The weaning and adoption of the baby son by her big sister, who was herself infertile, made possible the young mother's decision to *vaipaka*, or divorce, and reclaim the social status of a young girl (see also Demian 2006:147). Her purposive choice to reposition herself as a young girl in relation to others, and no longer to appear as a wife and mother, is testament to the exercise of personal autonomy in the expression of sexual and reproductive agency. Her reclaimed single status was demonstrated by appropriate gendered forms of productive labor—moving back into her widowed father's household to care for her small sisters and elderly grandmother. The visible acts that redefined her social status in the eyes of others allowed her to reenter the realm of *kubukwabuya* where, paradoxically, she had to take care to *katupwana*, or hide, her amorous pursuits. The young mother's assertion of reclaimed *kubukwabuya* status reiterates the theme that sexuality is as productive as fertility in forming and transforming social relations.

Single Mothers and "Fatherless" Children

The fluid transformations of maternal and marital identities reflect the temporal variation of desire and circumstance within and between life stages. Reclaiming single status and *kapugula* mobility might happen as the way to resolve an untenable relationship, as in the case of the twenty-year-old mother whose older sister adopted her baby. A single mother who has never married also resumes the status of a young girl when reclaiming *kapugula* mobility once her baby is weaned. In such circumstances, maternity is not denied or concealed by the young woman's reactivated mobility; it simply no longer assumes a dominant form. In fact, a single woman's maternity can effectively elevate her desirability as a potential wife by affirming her reproductive viability and, by inference, the viability of her *dala*. A single mother is sometimes said to be "out of circuit," a colloquial phrase in English that refers to an unmarried woman's period of abstinence during pregnancy and breastfeeding. But a single mother is able to reclaim *kapugula* status after her baby is weaned, or even before she stops breastfeeding if she is willing to risk the potential vulnerability that such action is believed to place on the health of the baby and accepts the possibility that people may judge her character negatively.[27]

Amanda was a twenty-year-old single mother of a seven-month-old girl when I interviewed her in 2003. She became pregnant several months after graduating from Kiriwina High School. In reflecting on her maternity, Amanda spoke of the assuredness of customary support that single mothers can rely on, the ethos of maternal abstinence, and the anticipation of resuming *kapugula* status after breastfeeding.[28]

> Our customs are like this. When you are five months pregnant, if you are married and staying with your husband, then you have to return to your own parents and wait to give birth. If I ask my parents, the husband can come and stay with us while I'm pregnant, but we won't stay with them, at the boy's parent's, that's not good. So if I had been married, I would come home at five months, but then [*laughs*], as I was single, I was already here! Ladies feel that this custom is like a way of preventing a problem with the pregnancy. It's a way of avoiding problems because the babies are still growing, they are still small, so it is good to concentrate on them. For me, I'll just stay with my parents. I'll just stay and look after my baby until when I decide I can go and look for someone. Somebody I want, who is man enough to look after myself and my child.

> *Will it be a problem if he knows you already have a baby?*
> Yes, some men think of this. Some do. But some men want to get married and settle down. But I'm just thinking that when my daughter is adopted and when I try to find a friend, maybe he will love me and care for my daughter. My parents will adopt her. As I am living with my adopted parents, she will go to live with my real parents. I'll stop feeding her, but I can still carry her, I'll go to the garden—I can go out! [*laughs*] If I go out now and go around and look for boys, old ladies will talk about me, say that I'm still breastfeeding and I'm looking for boys. Our customs are like this. Even though we are young and not married, but when we are still breastfeeding, we are not allowed to go around and look for boys.

Amanda's story also reveals that the transformative capacity of reproductive agency does not necessarily make a young girl appear as a mother in her relationship to others. Amanda explained that her father did not approve of marriage to the baby's father and continued to treat her like a small girl even though she had already given birth. She spoke with regret that she had not yet fulfilled her father's expectations that she would find a job as a result of her education, highlighting how early maternity at times becomes problematic in relation to the imagined future.

> But as for marriage, my father does not want this small girl's father. He told him to go back to his place. Because when I was expecting, he [the boyfriend] does not want to come to me. But when I gave birth, he thought to himself, this small girl looks exactly like me so then he wanted us. But my father told him, no, he does not want me to go with him. My father tells me that I must look for a job, and he gets worried that he has wasted all the money on my schooling, yes, after all he has done for me. He wants me to focus my eyes and see and look for a job so I can help my small sisters and brothers with their schooling.

Even though I gave birth already, he is still treating me like I am small, like I am still a schoolgirl. I am a woman with a baby, my own baby. I don't have to be treated like small kids. . . . I enjoy looking after my daughter. And everybody in the village, like young girls, old women and men, they all like carrying my daughter. So I feel happy and just like a woman who is in the house. And because the father's aunties are here in this village, when he comes to see them, they carry this small girl to him, to the father. My daughter's *bubus* [father's aunties], they love her, they always bring her something, and they carry her at church, they carry her to their friends, they will always want to carry her.

So your daughter will know who her father is?
Yes, she will know. And he sends money, clothes, when his uncles come around, so he still thinks about this little girl.

Amanda confidently asserts her maternal status even though her father continues to treat her like a small child. Her story speaks of the personal pleasure of caring for babies, as well as the pleasures of collective nurture and the importance of paternal care and recognition through material support.

Changing Patterns and Constructions of Premarital Pregnancy

Identity transformations between life stages also invite consideration of the broader transitions of social change and the dynamic factors that influence such change. As discussed in previous chapters, the conundrum of cultural continuity and change is often raised during community conversations about HIV and sexuality in the Trobriands. The benchmark question invariably posed is whether or not young people today are becoming sexually active at an age earlier than that of previous generations, which in turn raises the proxy indicator of whether or not there are now more premarital pregnancies than before. While the degree of change remains contentious, Trobrianders say that it is relatively common for young girls to have their first pregnancy before marriage *tutabaisa* (nowadays).[29] Indeed, pregnancy and childbirth often precipitate a marriage agreement. Pregnancy can even be a strategy to gain parental approval for marriage, as one village birth attendant explains, "If a girl wants her boyfriend but her parents don't approve, she will get pregnant so she can marry her boyfriend."[30] However, as Amanda's story suggests, this strategy is not always reliable. People also speak of situations where a woman chooses to remain single after becoming pregnant, sometimes acting on the advice of her relatives. Other observations suggest that more women are choosing to remain single during early motherhood and are having children fathered by different men. Related to this pattern is the expressed concern that single mothers with several children may have difficulty finding a partner willing to marry them.

Young unmarried mothers explain their maternity with various euphemisms, such as, "somehow I found myself this way," "somehow the baby found me," "I missed my step," "the burden the man gave me," or "the problem I made for myself." While such self-reflections suggest that premarital pregnancy creates a predicament of displaced agency and encumbrance, there is no social stigma attached to being a single mother. A young girl can act with the assurance that if she does becomes pregnant, her maternity will be accommodated by her family and *dala* relatives whether or not the pregnancy leads to a temporary or permanent partnership with the child's father. Furthermore, she can be assured that her family and *dala* relatives will lovingly care for her child.[31] The customary practice for a pregnant woman to reside in her natal household in preparation for the delivery of her baby and throughout the duration of breastfeeding provides young single mothers with the same familial and domestic support as married women. Because of the residential arrangement, single mothers do not face uncertainties about where support will come from, nor is their domestic situation different from that of married women who are pregnant and lactating. If paternity is known and acknowledged, the father and his female relatives often take an avid interest in the child even if marriage to the mother never eventuates, as Amanda's story demonstrates.

There is general consensus, however, that it is hard to carry the "burden" of parenting without a husband. Yet some young women say that single life is preferable to marriage. In one discussion session held after a women's fellowship meeting, a young woman with a baby and a toddler sat quietly behind the main group of participants, actively listening to the other women. She spoke up for the first time when the topic turned to premarital pregnancy. She said, "Some of us single mothers don't want to get married. Our family ties are strong. Our relatives will always provide care to raise the children, so why should we bother with marriage?" I asked her if she was single and she said she was divorced; her husband had left her for a younger girl. I asked if she planned on getting married again and she categorically answered, "*Ga!*" (No!). Then I asked if she would still want to enjoy herself in a relationship without getting married, and she said that because she is still breastfeeding she is not interested in making friends but maybe later she will look for someone.[32]

Diana offers the following perspective on the contemporary situation of premarital pregnancy:

> Let's say that unwed mothers are a new trend but we don't really take it as a problem. Women can survive without a husband. Parents will always welcome their daughter's children. Mothers want their daughters to have children. The problem comes during the MCH clinic, when the nursing sisters ask for the baby's father's name. Then it is shame because the mother cannot answer. It is like the mother saying to her child, your father is this man, but he did not want us. Shame also comes if a mother is still having babies when her daughters start having babies. [Interview notes, 29 September 2003]

The perceived changes to patterns of premarital pregnancy can be traced to some extent in the ethnographic literature. Malinowski (1929:166–72) speculated on the apparent rarity of "fatherless children" in a context of premarital sexual freedom with seemingly little or no use of contraceptives. He also stressed a purported aversion among Trobrianders for bearing children out of wedlock (1929:167). Weiner's observations (1976, 1988) suggest that premarital pregnancy was not uncommon during the 1970s. She argues that because female reproductive agency is accorded high value in the matrilineal kinship system, Trobrianders regard premarital pregnancy as neither anomalous nor reprehensible. Asserting that the Trobriand procreation ideology of *baloma* impregnation is "used as a protection for the innate sexual power of women" (1976:193), Weiner uncritically applies the "virgin birth" model as evidence that this strategic "disguise" upholds female sexual freedom while exonerating potential shame if pregnancy does not led to marriage (223). However, as with Malinowski, Weiner's main emphasis is not premarital pregnancy per se but the consequences of the lack of paternal nurture if marriage does not follow the birth of the baby. Weiner refers to the Trobriand word *gudukubukwabuya* as a pejorative that means "fatherless child" (1976:127; 1988:61).[33] She recounts an inflamed incident of "hard words" when the insult was used to cause shame in retaliation for a perceived misdeed. By contrast, I was told by several research participants that the word *gudukubukwabuya* does not normally carry a pejorative meaning but is simply used to refer to a child born when the mother was single.

Trobrianders offer various explanations about the perceived increase in premarital pregnancy by referring to historical processes. There is some recognition that the improvement of overall health status, resulting from better nutrition, childhood immunization, and the availability of antibiotics to treat infectious disease, has accelerated the process of puberty and has increased fertility (see Jenkins 2007:35–36; see also Worthman 1998).[34] Other explanations suggest that, with the availability of modern contraception, traditional methods of fertility control are not practiced as widely as before and yet young unmarried girls are not able to readily access contraceptives from the health centers. The most frequent explanation is that premarital pregnancy is more common nowadays because young people's sexual activity has increased because of new desires and the trappings of modernization and the cash economy. In one group discussion, when the topic turned to the age of first sexual activity, an older woman explained that, compared to her time of youth, nowadays girls become sexually active at a younger age because they are sexually stimulated by the modern way of living. When I asked her to describe the modern way of living, she replied, "You know, wearing *dimdim* [white people] style clothes. Before we only wore grass skirts." The woman then lifted up her blouse and held her breasts while continuing her explanation. "Before our breasts grew slowly because we didn't wear any clothes. Nowadays with clothes rubbing against the body the breasts grow faster so the girls get sexual feelings at a younger age." The older woman's demonstrative remark elicited much laughter and a chorus of *Mokwita!* (True!) and *Aiseki?* (Who knows?).[35]

The conjecture and debate about changing patterns of youth sexuality is influenced also by how the formal education system has created a uniform category of "adolescence," which involves specific social conformities and prospects that produce tensions in relation to the Trobriand values of *kubukwabuya* freedom, capacity, and potential (see Herdt and Leavitt, eds. 1998). Young people encounter these contradictions as they shape their social identities and sexual networks in relation to their educational status, affiliations, and parental expectations. For some, being a *toginigini*, or student, also holds a distinct appeal in terms of *kubukwabuya* desire, as illustrated in the letter recounted earlier in the chapter. Furthermore, as Amanda's story indicates, premarital pregnancy is specifically perceived as problematic for a "schoolgirl" as opposed to a "village girl," in that it impedes a promised trajectory of future opportunities for education and employment in the formal wage sector. The moral values encoded in this binary extend to young boys as well, although not in relation to paternity as much as in terms of how formal education represents a future in the labor market.

Identifying premarital pregnancy as a problem that reflects social change is largely prompted by the biomedical and public-health discourses that inform HIV communication, wherein "teenage pregnancy" is modeled as an epidemiological category of risk assumed to have negative outcomes.[36] My emphasis here is on the signification of the term as a social construction rather than on the reproductive health implications of early childbearing and unprotected sexual intercourse. Construing premarital pregnancy as a social problem occludes questions of agency and desire (Arney and Bergen 1984; Smith 2004). While the euphemism of a "missed step" used by some Trobriand single mothers to refer to their maternity does suggest an acknowledgment of mistiming and displaced agency, the cultural response to premarital pregnancy in the Trobriands is not constructed in terms of a mistake that produces a negative corollary.[37] The following statement by a middle-aged woman summarizes the views commonly expressed in group discussions and interviews, which indicate that premarital pregnancy is viewed not as a deviant or undesirable experience of sexual activity, but is accepted as a possible and sometimes deliberate effect of *kubukwabuya* agency and desire: "Pregnancy is important for many women. Women think, I am happy to have babies for the clan. Many unmarried girls have three or four children without having a husband and they have ways to look after them. The families will help out. Some girls don't mind, they'll just go and go until baby comes." (Taped group discussion, 31 October 2003. Translated into English.)

HIV communication that employs the categorical assumption that premarital pregnancy is a social problem that requires intervention is likely to produce alienating effects in contexts like the Trobriands, where the issue has more to do with questions of capacity and desire related to the value of social reproduction. Approaching the interconnected sexual and reproductive health needs and concerns of sexually active youth as socially problematic does not recognize the legitimate agency of youth sexuality and young people's rights to information, services, and support (see Ingham and Aggleton 2006).

Representing Agency and Desire

In her monograph, *The Trobrianders of Papua New Guinea*, Annette Weiner begins the chapter entitled "Youth and Sexuality" with a section headed "Waiting and Watching," which describes the period of *kubukwabuya* as working toward the attainment of adulthood, measured by the exercise of personal autonomy and the ability to influence and control the agency of others (1988:65–66). Weiner (1988:66) elaborates her argument as follows:

> With young people, the strategies for influencing others are sharply developed during adolescence. For them, however, the means of persuasion are not with yams and other kinds of material wealth because these are controlled by adults. Instead, adolescents learn to deal with the wills and plans of others

through their own sexuality. Their abilities to negotiate their sexual desires and seductive intentions are backed by their youthful physical and social beauty, made even more potent with love and beauty magic. Clothes, decorations, even the flowers and herbs thrust into armbands and hair heighten the aura of seduction. For young people, intention is written on their bodies, in their walk, and in their eyes. The shell decorations that are worn point to a young person's social status, and the flowers and the coconut oil enhanced with magic spells. . . . "Make somebody want you."

Often in books housed in academic library collections the reader encounters musings in the margins of the pages, penciled in by a previous reader. In one particular copy of Weiner's monograph at the Menzies Library at the Australian National University, there are numerous penciled comments, one of which caught my eye for its comparative observation. In the space underneath the paragraph cited above is written, "Same as us." While the "us" of this reflexive observation is not clear, it can be assumed that the inclusive pronoun is of Western persuasion. The universalist sentiment immediately calls into question the propensity for ethnographic accounts to inscribe exoticism in the "other" when the practice described appears axiomatic in purpose and intent. The penciled comment gives me pause when writing my own account of Trobriand youth and sexuality. My hesitation relates directly to how perceptions of adolescent sexuality, like "culture," take on negative values in relation to HIV risk, framed in terms of promiscuity and undisciplined desire and agency. I do not want my ethnographic representation of the Trobriands to feed into the penchant for exoticism and bounded notions of cultural diffence, nor do I want it to be used as evidence for moralistic evaluations that judge sexual desire to be responsible for the HIV epidemic.

The affinity revealed in the "same as us" comment resonates with the words of many Trobrianders who unreservedly describe the sexual freedom and exploration of youth as "the natural feeling," wherein "natural" implies a universality of human experience, albeit one based on a decidedly normative heterosexuality. Yet most Trobrianders are acutely aware of the particularity of their cultural ideology, especially in relation to other cultures in PNG, and they are mindful of how encounters with hegemonic models of meaning pose tensions for evaluating and reconciling difference. Trobriand moral and aesthetic constructions of sexuality and, in particular, the embodied experience of young people's sexual agency and desire contrast sharply with the narratives produced in the discourse on HIV risk behavior. Such disjuncture between models of meaning creates ethical and practical challenges for mediating and acting on information about HIV prevention. HIV communication that builds on a foundation of respect for both the commonality and diversity of human sexual desire and experience—and young people's capacity to act—has greater potential for reducing vulnerability and risk.

CHAPTER 6

Converging Meanings

> This kind of sexual behavior [having multiple partners] is part of our custom so it is not really surprising to us about AIDS, because maybe we already know this disease through *sovasova*. Because we have the clan system and we follow it in our sexual behavior and if we don't follow it we get sick. So maybe people from other places don't understand about the clan system and they have too much mixing of the same kind and that is how this virus has spread and made so many people sick. But here we know this sickness and we have treatment. We can control the spread.
>
> —Benjamin, aged mid-thirties, 4 November 2003

The Trobriand phenomenon of *sovasova*, or chronic illness that manifests from the breach of clan exogamy when members of the same matrilineal clan have sexual relations, exemplifies how disease etiologies and effects are socially constructed and constituted. As a form of cultural knowledge that links sexuality and disease, *sovasova* directly influences comprehension of HIV and AIDS in persuasive yet problematic ways. The topic of *sovasova* emerged unprompted in nearly every discussion during my research, demonstrating how an established model of meaning provides an interpretive framework for making sense of new phenomena. The consistent association Trobrianders draw between *sovasova* and AIDS reflects a logical attempt to resolve uncertainty about the presence of HIV in the Trobriands and to temper the seemingly paradoxical representation of AIDS as a new disease of sexual risk that has no immediate symptoms and no available treatment or cure. Such a construct is antithetical to the traditional model of medicine and contradicts popular notions of modern biomedicine as well, commonly perceived as having a diagnostic regimen of drug treatment for almost every named disease. However, as the statement above suggests, knowledge of *sovasova* empowers confidence in the local ability to treat symptomatic illnesses and to control the spread of HIV.

Sovasova and the Problem of Sameness

Sovasova occurs from sexual intercourse when the same blood or same clan recognizes itself. The same blood cannot mix properly, it is neutralized, and so germs can grow inside the people who are affected. Sexual fluids carry clan "signatures," maybe a bit like DNA. If two people with the same clan blood have sex, the sexual fluids do not mix and germs are able to grow. [Provincial disease control officer, 9 April 2003]

When same clan has sex, *sovasova* is passed through blood or genes; in English you might say chromosomes. Because they are the same clan the blood cannot mix, so sickness will result. Sickness forms inside like a tumor or thickness. There is no direction either way, it just gets stuck and doesn't move. [Traditional healer, 16 October 2003]

Maybe there is no sickness there but as we believe, that sickness passes between same clan, from one to another through sexual fluid, it passes both ways. [Ethel Jacob, 23 September 2003]

Sovasova[1] refers both to the exogamous proscription against intraclan sexual relations and marriage between cross-sex siblings and to the ethnophysiological ailment that results from the breach of this incest taboo. Descriptions and explanations of *sovasova* follow a consistent schema but vary according to people's knowledge, experience, and ability to draw analogies with other knowledge systems, particularly biomedicine, as evidenced in the statements above. All descriptions emphasize the problem of the "sameness of substance" (as discussed in Chapter 4; see Malinowski 1929:422); sexual intercourse between members of the same clan fails to be socially and physically productive because the "signature" sexual fluids of the clan are unable to promote the reciprocal flow and mixing of difference. *Sovasova* etiology is concerned with two levels of causality—the origin or underlying cause, and the immediate cause that commences the pathological process (see Foster 1976:778; Ingstad 1990:32). Fundamental to the underlying cause of *sovasova* is the breach of exogamy, which threatens social order and the basis for social reproduction through established patterns of exchange between different clans. The immediate cause of *sovasova* is sexual intercourse between two people of the same clan. As a cultural scheme, *sovasova* "links sickness to moral concerns and social relations" (Farmer 1990:23). The dual meaning of *sovasova* illustrates how "individual pathologies are homologous with social pathologies" (Sobo 1993:54).

Theories on the universality of incest taboos often suggest that such proscriptions generate exchange between different social groups (Lévi-Strauss 1969; Meigs and Barlow 2002). The Trobriand phenomenon of *sovasova* highlights the relationality of sexual practice, which ensures the potential for regeneration through the corporeal mixing of clan difference and reinforces important social ties and exchange relations. The Trobriand homology between social and physical flow and good health is consistent with other models of disease etiology present in societies that place a high value on reciprocal exchange as the basis for creating social networks and collective health (see Sobo 1993:54; Taylor 1988:1348).

The "neutralization" of sameness caused by violating the *sovasova* taboo results in internal congestion or stagnation, providing the ideal conditions for the growth of *minumauna*, or *maunauwela*, described as germs or wormlike parasites that produce debilitating effects in the host. The illness of *sovasova* is associated with a spectrum of discernible signs and symptoms, including severe stomach pain, abdominal swelling, "dusty" skin, pallor, boils, joint inflammation, wasting, and malaise. *Sovasova* is experienced as a chronic and recurring ailment that becomes more pronounced with age. Explanations suggest that while the breach produces effects in both sexual partners, the degree of illness may be more severe in one partner than in the other, depending on their general state of health prior to the breach. There is disagreement as to whether *sovasova* diminishes reproductive capacity and the viability of offspring born to parents of the same clan, with some people holding that such babies are born sickly and die prematurely.

Sovasova is treatable with a combined regimen of botanical and magical remedies, called *kelawodila* (literally, "trees of the forest"), which purge the *minumauna* out of the body and restore healthy bodily flow. The specialized knowledge of treatment is highly valued, safeguarded within lineages, and obtained from *dala* members or *toyuvisa*, the specialist healers. Regarded as highly effective, treatment dosages and courses vary according to the severity of the breach, whether a casual liaison or a long-term relationship.

In practice, while the rule of exogamy between *dala* is strictly adhered to, the rule between members of the same *kumila* is flexible and is often breached in casual sexual encounters and occasionally breached through marriage (Malinowski 1929:432; Weiner 1988:74). Because of the availability of treatment, people regard the breach of *kumila* exogamy as a safe possibility even if socially undesirable. People are willing to breach the taboo for casual relations, believing that illness only becomes a chronic problem in steady and long-term relationships or marriage. The perception of risk is related to the extent of the breach, tempered by the flexibility of the proscription and the professed efficacy of treatment, as suggested by the following explanation: "If they keep on going to that person for quite a number of times then that's where *sovasova* comes in. If only one night, then it doesn't come in as a risk. People won't really worry about *sovasova* if it is only one night."[2] Some people speak of using the treatment like a "morning-after" prophylactic to prevent the onset of illness resulting from causal one-off encounters between fellow clan members.

In his various accounts of *sovasova*, Malinowski treated with particular relish the willingness of people to breach the taboo as evidence of the "complex currents and undercurrents which form the true course of tribal life" (1929:433).[3] Noting that the supreme taboo falls away with the gradual classificatory extension of the brother-sister relationship, Malinowski imputed that the breach is regarded in various degrees as "daring and dangerous, but not abominable" (443–44); "a desirable and interesting form of erotic experience" (430); "a thing both smart and desirable, owing to the piquant difficulties in carrying it out" (1953:96); "and a spicy, not very repressed prohibition" (97). Malinowski observed, with a distinctly masculinist tinge, "The moral shame of such incidents is in reality small, and as with many other rules of official morality, he who breaks it is a smart fellow" (1953:99). He further acknowledged that the botanical and magical treatment for *sovasova* is "absolutely efficacious" (99), "well-nigh universally known and is used very freely" (1929:431).

While the willingness to engage in sexual relations with a fellow clan member is disputed, the most powerful reason given for the willful breach of *sovasova* is love. The source of desire for someone of the same clan is attributed to *kwaiwaga*, reflecting the mythic origin of the incest taboo, which tells of a brother and sister who die in each other's arms after coupling on the beach, overcome by the power of love magic (see Chapter 5, note 8; see also Malinowski 1929:456–59). There is also a popular narrative that speaks not of an ancient but a modern love unencumbered by the use of *kwaiwaga*, where people's strong feelings of love empower them to reject the taboo of *sovasova*, if not the ethnophysiological consequence of illness. As the *toyuvisa* explained to me, "In the past, *sovasova* was very taboo but in present times people don't care. The mentality about *sovasova* is changing because of love. People are accepting that they can have this sickness if they really love each other."[4]

Because *sovasova* illness is the inevitable outcome of violating the incest taboo, prevention is relatively straightforward to negotiate by disclosing clan identity to a potential sexual partner and choosing not to engage in sexual relations if both parties are of the same clan. People do not construct the risk of *sovasova* in terms of taking a chance with an unknown outcome. The following excerpt from an interview with Meg, a married woman in her early forties, indicates the protocol involved in negotiating sexual encounters to avoid partnering with someone of the same clan.

> My mother gave me advice about *sovasova* in grade five. I heard people talking about it and was scared of it. It is a continuous sickness unless we have strong medicine. I have seen people suffering. I saw it with my eyes; OK, it is true. It is only through carelessness, that's how they get involved with this sickness, *sovasova*. We ask, *"Avaka kumila yokwa?* What clan are you?" "Oh, sorry, my brother!" if he is same clan. And we go our separate ways.
>
> *And do you feel shame if he is your brother?*
> No, not if we don't know each other, say if we are from different villages. But mostly, young people take care who they go with. They send messages, use messengers to plan the meetings, so they know before who is the right partner for them. [Interview notes, 11 October 2003]

Meg's declaration, "I saw it with my eyes; OK, it is true" underscores the palpability of symptomatic evidence in establishing the "truth" of disease etiology. As a cultural model that links sexuality with disease, *sovasova* explains the causality of a spectrum of physical ailments while dissociating such effects from other causal agents of suffering, in particular the malevolence of witchcraft and sorcery. To this extent, there is broad and irrefutable consensus that *yoyowa* (witchcraft) and *bwagau* or *bogau* (sorcery) do not factor in the cause or consequence of *sovasova*.[5] However, while the etiological explanation for *sovasova* lies within the sexual agency of willful transgressors, people acknowledge that those affected by the illness are more vulnerable to the exploits of witches and sorcerers. A traditional healer explains, "*Sovasova* is like STI between same clan, but sometimes the symptoms can be caused by *bwagau*. People become open to sorcery if they are already sick from something else."[6]

Although *sovasova* is described by the idiom "STI between same clan," people maintain a cognitive distinction between *sovasova* and *pokesa*, the generic term derived from the English word "pox" and used for a range of sexually transmitted infections, including syphilis, gonorrhea, and genital ulcers. More generally, *pokesa* refers to any ulcerous sore on the body. Underscoring the distinction between the two disease phenomena is the belief that, unlike *sovasova*, sorcery and witchcraft can be a cause of *pokesa* and other STIs, even though the association between sexual practice and *pokesa* symptoms is acknowledged. People also attribute *pokesa* etiology to the breach of prohibitions placed on betel nut and coconut trees by their owners to prevent pilfering and early harvest.

> *Pokesa* is different from *sovasova*, it is a sore on the outside. People usually go to the health center for *pokesa*. They recognize it as a disease they can get medicine for. [Middle-aged male, taped group discussion, 26 June 2003]

> *Pokesa* is different. We know it is gonorrhea. Some people use magic to make people get this one. Because we have certain people in the village having this magic, so we must look around for someone who can cure it. If we go to the hospital, OK, they can help, tablets can help. But most of the time our people, old people, have certain herbs for it.

> *How do people explain why they are sick with* pokesa?
> Some they say people made *bwagau*, they got their underpants or whatever to make magic on it. When they see us hanging our pants or skirts or whatever on the line, OK, in the nighttime they see that nobody is watching, they go and get it out and they do something on it, put magic on it. Then we'll be staying there and not long we'll feel something paining, then it turns up that we are sore, the sore comes up, so we have this from magic. [Taped interview, 14 January 2001]

"A Mixture of Ideas":
Historical Interplay of Disease Etiologies

The etiological distinction drawn between *sovasova* and *pokesa*, the incorporation of the disease spectrum of "pox" into an extant etiological framework of supernatural powers, and the use of both traditional and Western medicines for treatment illustrate the historical interplay between different models of meaning. Indeed, the generic naming of the word *pokesa* after the English "pox" resulted from the epidemic waves of foreign pathogens—particularly syphilis and gonorrhea—that swept over the Trobriands during the late nineteenth and early twentieth centuries, and the medical interventions that followed. The new word represented a range of new disease symptoms associated with the arrival of *dimdim* foreigners. The "Islands of Love" mystique of a primitive sexuality was an illusory contrast to the realities of the effects of introduced sexually transmitted diseases (STDs) in the early colonial period (Hughes 1997:235; Connelly 2007).

Concern about the demise of the population, which numbered approximately ten thousand people in 1905, prompted colonial officials to embark on a mission to eradicate the "baneful diseases" of syphilis and gonorrhea (Black 1957:233–34; Hughes 1997:234; Spencer 1999:75). Colonial medical interventions were dogmatic and confrontational, engendering dread rather than confidence in the new system of diagnostic and treatment procedures based on biomedical models of disease etiology (Maddocks 1975:29; see also Denoon 1989 and Perez Hattori 2004). Much depended on the qualities of particular doctors in gaining the trust and acceptance of villagers, such as the "tact and perseverance" of Raynor Bellamy in the Trobriands, who was able to allay "native prejudice against European medicine" (Black 1957:194). Upon taking up his appointment in 1905 as general medical officer and assistant resident magistrate in the Trobriands, Bellamy was put in charge of the newly built "lock" hospital, so called because of the legal power to confine infected patients granted by a regulation made by the Native Regulation Board in 1904. His initial approach was punitive, rounding up and incarcerating infected patients until they were either cured or dead (Young 2004:386). According to Bellamy, Trobrianders had no prior knowledge of how venereal infections were spread, and his patients were "incredulous" when he instructed them on the mode of transmission (Black 1957:234). Apart from the fear and indignity of being lined up and examined, Bellamy noted that people resisted hospitalization because it removed them from their relatives and economic livelihood (Black 1957:234; cf. Perez Hattori 2004). Reports suggest that Bellamy quickly gained the confidence of Trobrianders "beyond his most sanguine expectations" and that people began to come voluntarily for treatment, although Bellamy noted that women were less willing to do so (Black 1957:234).[7] In 1906, Bellamy estimated that about 10 percent of the population, including children, showed symptoms of STDs, and in 1908, he commenced a program of systematic examination and treatment of every man, woman, and child (Black 1957:234). Bellamy's regimented approach, which involved punishment of absconders, is credited for reducing the incidence of STDs from 5.22 percent in 1908 to 1.37 percent in 1915 (Black 1957:234), and by 1926, Bellamy reported that the percentage of infection was below 1 percent and no longer had an effect on birth and death rates (Bellamy 1990:300).[8]

Medical interventions to control the spread of STDs in the Trobriands continued to be carried out by successive colonial authorities. In 1939, a venereal survey of fifty-four hundred persons was conducted by Dr. Ford, who reported no difficulty in gathering people for examinations, a feat he credited to the effectiveness of Bellamy's years of service. Indeed, Ford remarked that "the occasion was accepted as a gala event" (Black 1957:236). (There could be an unintended pun in Ford's description, as *gala* means "no" in Kiriwina language.) My research questions did not prompt any personal or collective memories about such events, apart from the occasional humorous recounting of a scenario where people ran into the bush when they heard that the medical patrol was coming to their village. By contrast, nowadays the blaring siren of the health center's ambulance making the rounds on immunization patrols (the supply of gasoline and vaccinations permitting) is met with squeals of delight by young children. In whatever ways Trobrianders collectively responded to the colonial patrols that involved populationwide examinations in search of diseased genitals, the effects of these historical interactions have been absorbed into current understandings of disease etiology and approaches to treatment. As Jenny Hughes points out, the interventionist approach to STDs in colonial PNG, which involved the corralling of patients for examination and incarceration in lock hospitals, sets a precedent for attitudes in the era of AIDS, particularly the popular sentiment in PNG that the only way to control the spread of HIV is to lock up those who are positive (1997:244).

Sitting in the STI testing laboratory at Losuia District Health Center in October 2003, I search for a residual presence of a bygone era but find only the predictable air of resignation that seems to hang over many rural health centers in Papua New Guinea. The facility's chronic lack of maintenance and refurbishment produces the sediment of neglect, betraying the genealogy of clinical medical practice in the Trobriands, particularly the recent past in the 1960s and 1970s, when the center thrived as a surgical hospital under the directorship of a medical doctor.[9] People continue to refer to the health center as the *ospeta*, or hospital, as though it were still the bastion of colonial and missionary presence or held the promise of development under the newly independent nation state. But expectations have diminished along with the standards of health services, which were decentralized under state reforms in the mid-1990s, and the disintegrating infrastructure, plagued by constant disruptions to the supply of water and electricity because, yet again, the pipes are broken or the generator has run out of gasoline. The disheveled state and scattered contents of the room where I sit accentuates the paucity of available supplies and equipment. The layers of grime and mold on the walls and shelves suggest an acquiescence to neglect that says something about local capacity and function as much as the effects of tropical humidity. But the general disarray goes far beyond localized laxity; it speaks strongly of the indifference and marginalization not only from provincial and national levels but from the global centers of power that condemn out-of-the-way places to mediocrity, even failure (see Mallett 2003).

I clear aside a space at the table to review the clinic register book that the laboratory technician gives to me after I obtained permission from the district health manager. Clement Moseturi, from Tukwaukwa village, has worked at the health center for many years since his initial student training in allied health sciences. Although his official position is lab technician, he assumes multiple roles as ward orderly, STI clinician, and health promotion officer. He tells me that for the last several years he has looked after communicable diseases and has been on the nursing roster in the center's two wards because of the number of patients and the chronic shortage of personnel. In particular, the number of patients admitted for tuberculosis over the last few years has put pressure on existing resources. The TB ward currently has three patients, a young woman in her early twenties, and a mother and her infant baby. There have been twelve TB cases so far this year, with a total of eighty-five TB patients admitted since 2000.[10]

Clement is adept at drawing posters. One of his posters on the wall in the TB ward shows a bone-thin patient with an outstretched hand ready to receive the daily dose of drug therapy. The handwritten text, in English and Kiriwina, describes the elements of DOTS, the directly observed therapy short-course strategy for TB treatment. When I was here in 2000, his hand-drawn AIDS awareness poster was taped on the exterior wall of the outpatient clinic, depicting various situations in the Trobriands identified as potential sites of HIV transmission (see Chapter 7). Today he is busily working on one of several posters he has started; this one is about the risk of HIV transmission during *Milamala*. As Clement draws, I begin to copy data from the STI register. I ask him to explain the record book and what it reveals about the STI situation in the Trobriands.

> We do STI testing—gonorrhea, syphilis. For donovanosis we send the smears to Alotau. We don't do HIV testing, there's no facility due to power problems. There are a great number of people suffering with gonorrhea. We do contact tracing and bring patients in for review. We supply the patient with contact cards to give to their partners. However many they need, we give them, but it is not effective. We need to physically follow up, go out to the villages, talk to the people directly and not expect them to come to us. There is embarrassment and shame to come here with the card. In many cases, people say their contact was a "market spin," they met on the road, or the partner is from far away, so it is hard to follow up. No names are exchanged between the partners, maybe only place names, so the person can tell us only this village or that village. With our system it is impossible to determine patterns in STI prevalence. We have to assume that every village, every area has STI problem. You'll see from the book that villages close to town and the guest lodge are the most commonly infected areas, especially on the female side. But maybe it's just that they come to the clinic for treatment because they are close by. Men from outer areas are more mobile than women, so infection is taken back to the villages that way. We cannot specify which group, which village is most infected unless we take a survey. We presume HIV is already here. One positive case has been seen. It is already spreading but it is not yet known. People don't see it yet. [Interview notes, 23 October 2003]

The register book records a total of 122 diagnosed cases of STIs for the period from January 2000 through October 2003. As Clement notes, the data indicate a high rate of gonorrhea (88/122) as well as a high level of unmet need for services, particularly among females. The low number of registered females (12/122) reflects various factors, including the gender sensitivity of services, accessibility of services, the effectiveness of contact tracing, and the willingness to access services.

Clement's acknowledgment of the ineffective approach and reach of available clinical services and his mention of the need for a survey to map STI infection rates can be understood in relation both to the seeming historical efficacy of medical patrols in controlling STIs before the age of antibiotics and to the penchant for epidemiological surveillance in the age of AIDS. From a service-delivery point of view, his descriptive assessment of the STI situation raises uneasy questions about HIV voluntary counseling and testing and its integration with existing sexual and reproductive health services. Clement's remark that HIV is already spreading but not yet known because of its invisibility underscores the significance of symptoms in Trobriand constructions of disease. Moreover, it accentuates the clinical difference between diagnosing STIs that manifest in recognizable and visible symptoms and testing for evidence of the invisible virus.

The importance of symptoms for making sense of disease, the diagnostic comparisons between the symptoms of *sovasova* and other disease symptoms, and the interplay of different interpretive frameworks in Trobriand articulations of disease etiology are all illustrated in a statement by the health extension officer (HEO) at

Losuia District Health Center. Ridley Mwaisiga was responding to my question about his views on Trobrianders' perceptions of HIV and AIDS.

As for people's understanding of HIV/AIDS, you would know about *sovasova*, believed to be from a sexual relationship between same clan members. I have to bring this into my awareness talks because people have the question in their minds. When people reach old age or have some illness, they say the sickness is because they were with their own clan members, that's why they have those symptoms. Pain, weakness, weight loss. You could say it was just old age. On the health side, I regard it as UTI, PID presentation [urinary tract infection and pelvic inflammatory disease]. On clinical grounds, this is how I see the sickness of *sovasova*.

It's a traditional belief, that same clan and opposite sex, during the sex act, the release and exchange of fluids from both men and women during the penile ejaculation and female orgasm. Because the fluids exchanged are from the same clan members, that's why there is *sovasova*. . . . If a young person is sick they will take it as *sovasova*. For example, malaria symptoms, they will still consider it as *sovasova* if they know they have had sex with same clan. The idea is very vague. It is passed on from generation to generation. It is hard to explain anatomical composition of fluids in the body. There is no clinical documentation of this sickness. But for transmission, it is not like a disease going from one person to another, no, but it is about exchange, the mixture when the fluids come together. Absorption is taking place. The male absorbs the female, the female absorbs the male. To me personally, I can't explain here what happens between members of different clans. Let's say it is an exchange of difference. Mixing of difference. With *sovasova*, there is nothing different to exchange.

The man and woman manage *sovasova* in the traditional way. Other times, if the problem is so significant, the person cannot contain it with the traditional system so they run to the health center. They might see then that the symptoms can be treated with a mixture of ideas. It is a misconception with sexually transmitted infections and urinary tract infections. Some people come to realize that *sovasova* is really pelvic inflammatory disease and UTIs. Before when donovanosis and syphilis were very common, people were able to know the difference between gonorrhea and syphilis and *sovasova*. There is a distinct difference between ulcerated STIs and *sovasova*. People can recognize *pokesa*, or genital ulcers. But not all would come to the health center for treatment. It is the level of literacy. Some resort to the traditional methods. They take it as the normal thing. Not all sickness is treated. Some who have symptoms take it for granted and once the sore goes away they think the sickness is gone. [Interview notes, 10 December 2003]

The immediate reference that Ridley, the HEO, makes to the conundrum of *sovasova* in relation to HIV and AIDS indicates the conceptual association that people invariably make between the uniquely Trobriand phenomenon and the new and unknown sickness. Speaking as a health professional, the HEO was understandably concerned that his comments reflect a clinical interpretation of *sovasova*.

Yet the enduring cultural logic of *sovasova* is apparent in his explanation as well. His description of diagnosis and treatment and his comment that the symptoms of *sovasova* "can be treated with a mixture of ideas" is indicative of pluralistic understandings of illness and how the complementary application of different models of therapy assists in obtaining desired outcomes.

Commenting on medical pluralism with particular reference to Papua New Guinea, Shirley Lindenbaum states that the successful provision of culturally appropriate health services "is achieved not by manicuring Western medical categories to fit local conceptions, but by broadly appreciating indigenous definitions of the desirable paths to take in order to achieve control of destiny in illness and health" (1991:177). Indeed, it could be argued that the "mixture of ideas" reflects a conceptual preference for models of relationality and reciprocity in dealing with health and disease (see Street 2010), a preference that emanates from the core Trobriand cultural value of mutual difference in achieving collective well-being. Pluralistic and reciprocal approaches underscore the importance of HIV communication that acknowledges how divergent models of meaning interact and shape new understandings. The facilitation of dialogic mediations between preexisting models of disease and information about HIV and AIDS as new disease phenomena is critical for producing knowledge that will enable prevention (see Farmer 1990, 1994).

Converging Frameworks: *Sovasova* Compared with HIV and AIDS

People tend to think that HIV/AIDS is not necessarily a new problem but has been around for a long time, just called something else, *sovasova*. [Provincial disease control officer, 9 April 2003]

Some people say we already have the cure for the disease HIV/AIDS because it has been here a long time; we already have this sickness *sovasova*. [Ethel Jacob, 20 June 2003]

We were told that some Trobriand people, who live in Alotau and Port Moresby, who have the *sovasova* treatment, have given it to people who are sick with AIDS. For that, I don't believe it, that it would work. Because I know that AIDS has a different virus and *sovasova* has a different *maunauwela* [germs]. [United Church pastor, 13 November 2003]

Cecil Helman observes that throughout the world, "AIDS has become the preeminent 'folk illness' of the modern age, absorbing, in each local context, a variety of indigenous images, metaphors and cultural themes" (1994:348). Documenting the emergence of a collective representation of AIDS in rural Haiti, Farmer illustrates how the "'adoption' of a new illness category into an older interpretive framework" provides "organizing principles" and "preexisting meaning structures" for people's shifting understandings and experience of the new disorder as the HIV epidemic develops in a particular setting (1990:20, 22). Although the broad comparisons that Trobrianders draw between *sovasova* and representations of HIV and AIDS pose contradictions and create tensions, the preexisting interpretive framework has significant influence on mediations of new information (cf. Ingstad 1990). Trobrianders comprehend HIV infection and prevention in relation to their cultural model of sexual disorder and the valued capacity of sexuality and sexual networks for maintaining relations of difference.

Representations of both *sovasova* and HIV are conceptually associated with behavior that deviates from normative moral and sexual codes. However, there is evident dissonance in the values of sexuality represented by the two models of disease etiology. The organizing principles in the *sovasova* paradigm, which link disease to unproductive sex between partners of cosmological and corporeal sameness, do not readily accommodate representations of HIV as caused by sexual promiscuity and infidelity. Furthermore, the extended period of multiple partnering that defines *kubukwabuya* sexuality is valued as life-affirming social practice, the antithesis of disease and death associated with HIV.

There are dissimilarities as well between the models of *sovasova* and AIDS etiology in the conceptualization of disease transmission and, hence, disease prevention. The violation of the sexual taboo does not *spread* infection from one body to another in an asymmetrical direction; rather, disease is generated between two bodies with the same clan substance as the result of the nonabsorptive exchange of sexual fluids. Preventing *sovasova* is as straightforward as declaring clan identity, unless people are overcome by the power of *kwaiwaga* or desire. Most awareness information about HIV infection is constructed around the notion of transmission from one body to another, so that infection is generally conceptualized as a singular event involving a unidirectional source of infection. The language of HIV epidemiology further reinforces this notion of unidirectional transmission from purported sources of infection in the construction of moralistic categories of risk, such as "sex workers" and "men who have sex with men," which inscribe "otherness" rather than sameness. Additionally, communication about HIV transmission and prevention invariably raises questions about the invisibility of HIV before the effects of infection become apparent in a human host and how confirmation of HIV antibody status is not possible without blood testing. The time lapse between cause and effect does not easily support a conceptual link between sexual practice and HIV infection, nor does it readily compel immediate action to minimize and prevent potential transmission. Indeed, it is this invisible aspect of the viral complex that solicits the inscription of epidemiological categories of "risk." While *sovasova* etiology also involves a hiatus between sexual activity and the presentation of symptoms, the question of prevention is not obscured, nor troubled, by the invisibility of the causal agent.

Information about the use of condoms as the barrier means of protection against HIV transmission, especially as protective of the male bodies on which they are placed, also tends to reinforce perceptions that the source of viral infection is contained within bodies marked by epidemiological categories of risk, in particular, female bodies (Hammar 2007; Wardlow 2006). The question of whether condom use can prevent the effects of *sovasova* between bodies belonging to the same clan poses a particular conundrum, as reciprocal flow and mixture of sexual fluids is desirable, unlike the admixture of sameness that results in diseased stagnation. Because condoms as a contraceptive method are already associated with unproductive sexual contact, counteracting the desired mixing of difference, the proposition that condoms might work as a barrier method for *sovasova* seems redundant and counterintuitive to many people.[11]

A further point of dissonance between the two models of disease etiology lies in the problematic question of HIV treatment, which is also counterintuitive to Trobrianders' way of dealing with illness. The information people receive about HIV and AIDS consistently carries the misleading message of "no treatment, no cure," which instills fear and dread of the "killer disease," with the tacit intention of motivating prevention through behavior change. The representation of HIV and AIDS as having no treatment or cure creates a moral conundrum when existing HIV drug therapy cannot be provided or accessed, compounding the uncertainty about the presence of HIV infection and its potential transmission between sexually active bodies, and creating fear and ambivalence among Trobrianders (see Chapter 2). Yet the preexisting interpretive framework helps mitigate fear of the unknown through reference to a known phenomenon and the cultural resources for alleviating symptoms and managing sickness. The following statement made during a group discussion with women of mixed ages and marital status reflects how the *sovasova* framework provides a pivotal point of reference for alleviating fear of the unknown.

> The reason why we are afraid of AIDS is that we do not have any experience with it. We wonder what a person with AIDS feels like, looks like. We have no experience with the symptoms. It is hard to know because we can't tell who would have the sickness. We know people get the sickness but we don't know the symptoms because of the time it takes. Talking about fear, it is the same for *sovasova*, how we feel about AIDS is the same as *sovasova*. But with *sovasova* we have the treatment so we are not so afraid. We haven't tried *sovasova* treatment to see if it could work for HIV/AIDS because we don't know who might be sick with the virus. If someone we know has AIDS, then we could try the treatment to see if it works. [Middle-aged male, taped group discussion, 19 August 2003. Translated into English.]

The issue of treatment is perhaps the most important area of concern in Trobriand mediations of AIDS. Although asymptomatic HIV infection is difficult for people to imagine, representations of "full-blown AIDS" are immediately associated with the debilitating effects of *sovasova*: weight loss, pallor, malaise, and chronic illness. Consequently, there is a commonly shared perception that knowledge of *sovasova* treatment holds the potential means to mitigate, if not resolve, the effects of AIDS. People speak with confidence about the efficacy of known herbal and magical treatments to manage *sovasova*, and they speculate with varying degrees of confidence about the potential to treat the new sickness. "Some people feel that AIDS might be the same as *sovasova*. So they say we can use the same treatment for curing AIDS, this is what we feel, because we don't have any treatment for AIDS. I think, because AIDS, the symptoms are, well, slight difference from symptoms of *sovasova*. But I think if we use this medicine for *sovasova* to treat one of the AIDS carriers, I think it will help them" (Female, aged fifty, taped group discussion, 6 June 2003).

The concerns of prevention and treatment also overlap with the importance of sexually transmitted infections as cofactors in HIV transmission. Given the Trobriands' history of medical interventions for sexually transmitted diseases, perhaps it is perplexing why the cultural model of *pokesa* is not readily brought to bear on HIV, especially as the new epidemic represents the latest wave in a long history of infectious pathogens that come from beyond the horizon. I suggest that the causal and physiological distinctions made between *sovasova* and *pokesa* transect the moralistic renderings of AIDS as a novel, deadly disease caused by transgressive sexual behavior, which has no immediate visible manifestations and no cure. Similar to representations of HIV and AIDS, *sovasova* is an internalized chronic ailment with no immediate cure and aligned with a heavy moralistic narrative, whereas *pokesa* refers to the visible signs and symptoms of genital infections, which can be treated and healed. While *pokesa* is generally accepted as a possible consequence of sexual activity, it is not regarded as symptomatic of deviant sexual practice. The cause of *pokesa* is most often explained as the discontent of malevolent agents of witchcraft and sorcery. And yet, as the HEO explained, regardless of etiology, *pokesa* symptomatology is recognizably visible and often taken for granted "as the normal thing," a view that undoubtedly affects treatment decisions.

Importance of Cultural Models for HIV Prevention

Because of what we believe about *sovasova* it happens that way. [United Church pastor, 13 November 2003]

The Trobriand phenomenon of *sovasova* illustrates how the cultural construction of illness is symbolic of moral issues, social identity, and social relations (Pelto and Pelto 1997:150; Craddock 2000:154). Furthermore, *sovasova* demonstrates the *dynamic* quality of cultural models and the ambiguities and inconsistencies that are inherent in all interpretive frameworks (Lewis 1993:212). The fluidity of explanation about a culturally specific illness like *sovasova* suggests that mediations of a new disease complex like HIV and AIDS are also likely to produce pluralistic interpretations. Nonetheless, as a persuasive paradigm for social and sexual relations in Trobriand society, *sovasova* provides an important preexisting interpretive framework for integrating new information. This, of course, raises the broader question of the utility of diverse cultural models of sexuality and disease in HIV communication, and the consequences of converging interpretations for the prevention and management of HIV infection.

I suggest several areas of consideration regarding the convergence of models of *sovasova* and HIV and AIDS and regarding the significance they hold for communication about HIV prevention and management in the Trobriand context. Firstly, because most information about HIV infection is constructed around the notion of transmission from one body to another, HIV is commonly viewed as deriving from a single event and a unidirectional source of infection. This has implications for the extent to which the moral discourse surrounding the epidemic in PNG and elsewhere is negatively preoccupied with identifying and blaming the perceived source of infection (Hammar 2007; Butt and Eves, eds. 2008). The etiological model of *sovasova* is significant for its emphasis on the interaction *between* bodies and the recurring effect that *every* act of intercourse has on the course of the ailment. *Sovasova* is generated between two people of the same clan; it is not transmitted from one person to another. This feature of the model might contribute to a clarified understanding in the Trobriands of the importance of cross-infection and reinfection *between* bodies in the disease progression of HIV. Knowledge of this dimension of HIV transmission is important—especially in a context like PNG with a generalized epidemic, limited testing and condom use, and limited availability of treatment—not only for transforming sexual practice but also for potentially shifting negative attitudes toward categories of people perceived as responsible for spreading the virus.

Secondly, *sovasova* raises the fraught issues of fear, stigma, and blame surrounding HIV and AIDS, which have largely defined the collective response to the epidemic throughout Papua New Guinea. I suggest that the cultural vocabulary provided by the *sovasova* paradigm enables Trobrianders to discuss collectively the subject of HIV and AIDS with a confidence that alleviates negative and harmful reactions. While *sovasova* is a socially undesirable condition that carries a measure of shame, the breach of taboo does not produce reactions of discrimination or reproach. Because the breach represents the antithesis of productive social relations, and as such is an illogical and unproductive strategy, Trobrianders primarily regard *sovasova* violation as a matter of imprudent choice and conduct. Transgressors bear the consequences of chronic ill health and perhaps incur some mild gossip, but they have recourse to available treatment and the community does not ostracize them. Importantly, the power of love, both mythic and modern, can be appealed to rhetorically to legitimate relations of sameness. It remains to be seen whether the moral framework of *sovasova* might positively influence the tone of response in the Trobriands to people affected by HIV and AIDS, or whether a discourse of blame attributed to witchcraft and sorcery will be invoked. Nonetheless, the capacity to discuss candidly the interrelated topics of sexuality and disease opens channels for potentially engendering a measured and compassionate response to the challenges of the HIV epidemic. The mitigation of fear lessens the prospect that discrimination, stigma, and blame will define the response to HIV and AIDS as further direct experience with the epidemic shapes people's collective understandings.

Treatment is a critical area of consideration, especially given the resource constraints for an effective clinical response to HIV in the Trobriands. The beliefs and practice associated with the etiology of *sovasova* and its treatment have direct consequences for the way Trobrianders mediate information about HIV prevention and for decision making regarding treatment options for HIV-related illness. The potential for traditional treatments to provide efficacious symptomatic treatment bears serious consideration when antiretroviral therapies for HIV infection are not currently available at Losuia District Health Center. Of course, this proposition raises ethical concerns about the use of alternative treatments for the management of HIV-related illness, as well as the larger structural disparities and global inequities of resource distribution that have tremendous bearing on the capacities of governments, communities, and people to effectively respond to the HIV epidemic (Farmer 1999; Reid 2004). Furthermore, regardless of whether herbal treatments for *sovasova* are pharmacologically efficacious from a biomedical point of view, if AIDS is conceptualized as similar to or the same as *sovasova*, the confidence about the capacity to deal with HIV infection through traditional methods of *sovasova* treatment may undermine HIV prevention efforts and encourage complacency about the potential impact of the epidemic.

Although people are quite clear that witchcraft and sorcery do not factor in the etiology of *sovasova*, it is uncertain whether Trobrianders will attribute AIDS to witchcraft as more people confront the experience of living with the debilitating effects of HIV infection (Haley 2010; Hammar 2007). As is the case throughout much of Papua New Guinea, witchcraft and sorcery are powerful explanatory constructs in Trobriand cosmology that on some level, whether immediate or underlying, hold an etiological link to all illness, misfortune, and death. Indeed, either witchcraft or sorcery is perceived to be the root cause of disease and death in virtually all cases (Malinowski 1929:137, 192; Weiner 1988:39–41). And because terminal illness represents the loss of clan vitality, witchcraft and sorcery are the ultimate threat to maintaining the relations of social reproduction and social order. *Sovasova*, with its dual cause and consequence, represents the one exception in the Trobriand model, although there is acknowledgment that those who breach the proscription are more vulnerable to the exploits of witches and sorcerers. Of course, *sovasova* also threatens social and moral order by undermining the relations of difference that ensure clan vitality and social reproduction, but the cause of illness remains a question of internal agency, not attributed to an external malicious force. In this sense, *sovasova* stands outside the paradigm of witchcraft and sorcery and offers a particular salience for mediating HIV and AIDS. Yet it is also an unsettling bridge to the questions of symptoms and treatment, which become the focus for responding to the underlying cause of sickness.

The following statement by a traditional healer pinpoints the explanatory power of malevolent magic as the "reason underneath the sickness." The man's reference to Africa suggests a perceived correlation of context in the global geography of AIDS between HIV prevalence and places where the fundamental cause is attributed to supernatural powers.

> Every sickness should have a treatment and every sickness should have a cause. People want to know what causes sickness. For HIV, in our terms, our understanding, the belief from custom, from our parents, it will be seen to be caused by *bwagau*, not by sexual activity. For example, like malaria. We know the parasite comes from the anopheles mosquito but how does the malaria get into the mosquito? Who put the malaria into the mosquito? We think that the spell of *bwagau* or *yoyowa* put the sickness in there. The mosquito is just the carrier. So there is always a reason underneath the sickness. For AIDS, the thinking will be the same. The natives of Africa, some of them have very strong *bwagau* there. AIDS does not just come out by itself, it is not automatic. It was put there in the first place by magic. [Interview notes, 20 October 2003]

In whatever ways the immediate cause of AIDS is understood in terms of viral transmission, the explanation above links AIDS etiology to the core moral concern of magic and the ongoing struggle against malicious intent (see Ashforth 2002:129).

When the cause of illness and death is understood in moral terms and attributed to the malicious actions of others, treatment and healing assume paramount importance in the struggle to protect and restore social balance. Fundamental to this process is the need to identify the social source of illness and make it visible.

Treating the Reason underneath Sickness

As the explanation by the traditional healer indicates, whatever the immediate cause of life-threatening illness might be, at a fundamental level the bodily experience of disease is understood in Trobriand terms as a manifestation of social and moral disorder caused by malevolent magic. Symptoms are evidence of the underlying disorder, but the restoration of bodily and social well-being requires more than merely symptomatic treatment; it requires treating the reason underneath sickness by making it visible through an evaluative process that employs magic, prayer, herbal medicines, and clinical treatments in various combinations to achieve remedial effect (cf. Lindenbaum 1979; Lepowsky 1990). The etiological explanation that physical suffering has a magical source shifts focus away from the sick person as independently responsible for the cause and management of the condition, and promotes the mobilization of social resources to defuse the effects of illness and restore equilibrium, not only in the patient's body but in the social body (Weiner 1976:86; see also Scheper-Hughes and Lock 1987:7, 15).

In the Trobriand paradigm, *yoyowa* and *bwagau* provide the generic reason underneath the sickness, but the particular circumstances that might explain the motivation for malicious action are not necessarily speculated about nor pursued in the process of healing. Neither does the response to illness necessarily involve any form of retribution toward the identified source of suffering. While reprisal is likely to be carried out with a counteraction of magic in due course, it rarely involves immediate and physical confrontation. The politics of conflict that may be linked to an episode of illness are responded to in a different social arena from that of healing. The focus of healing is on revealing and naming the source of suffering, not explicating intent or engaging in retribution.

Naming the Source: A Story of Healing

Members of the women's church fellowship gathered at the home of Susan's parents on Sunday evening to show support for the thirty-two-year-old mother of five, who had been seriously ill for more than two weeks and was just beginning to show signs of recovery. Washed and dressed in fresh clothes, Susan sat cross-legged in the doorway of the house, her husband at her side holding their nine-month-old baby daughter. An older daughter sat behind them along with Susan's older sister. Next to Susan was a large bouquet of frangipani, hibiscus, and bougainvillea flowers. The women arrived with pots of cooked food and placed them in front of her on the veranda. Susan was still frail from her debilitating illness and although she appeared restful, she exuded a sense of sorrow and loss. As the large group of women quietly settled into place on the lawn and veranda, a profound vulnerability and uncertainty seemed to hang over everyone. Was this summoning of support a turning point to invigorate the promise of full recovery? Or were the efforts of healing still locked in a struggle with the malevolence that might pull Susan under once again?

The *toyuvisa* and his young apprentice son were also in attendance, sitting on plastic chairs next to Susan's father by the cookhouse. Several men from the village had arrived as well and sat together in a group, most of them carrying young children and babies. But the gathering was foremost an expression of solidarity among the women of the village. Sitting across from Susan on the veranda, the fellowship president led a devotion with an opening statement, speaking quietly about how everyone was praying for Susan and wishing her a speedy recovery, and how the community had to stand together to provide support in a time of need. The deacon's wife led the first hymn and read passages from the Bible. Sitting on the veranda with the women, I was touched by the solemn demeanor of the gathering and the collective outpouring of love and concern. I thought about the intimacy of village life and how these women have known each other all of their lives and continually bear witness to each other's minor and monumental struggles and delights.

Susan's mother then stood up on the front step leading to the veranda, a position that put her comfortably in the center of the gathering where she was able to address all in attendance. She spoke in a confident but soft tone, recounting the hardships her family had faced over the last two years—several illnesses, the death of her sister, and now Susan's ordeal. She apologized for not yet making *lubwau* for those who supported them with food and assistance during their previous trials, explaining that she had been working very hard preparing for her sister's *sagali*. She appealed to the community to give the family time to prepare *lubwau* properly. When she finished, everyone clapped the village signature clap—two, then three, then one final clap. We then went forward one by one to kiss Susan and shake hands with her husband before we departed. Susan wept silently, gratitude in her eyes. Her husband looked refreshed, having shaved and changed into clean church clothes, and he smiled broadly but with a restrained dignity, clearly appreciative of the communal expression of support.

Twelve nights earlier, at the height of *Milamala*, the harvest season when the spirits of the deceased arrive from Tuma to move among the living, the *baloma* of Susan's recently deceased father-in-law visited her while she was sleeping. He communicated three messages to the family, one about his son's yam-exchange garden for the coming year, another about the planned cementing of his gravesite, and the third about the welfare of his elderly mother. Susan awoke from the dream with a high fever and had difficulty breathing. Her husband carried her on his back to the health center just after midnight to seek medical treatment. She was given an injection for malaria and was put on a course of antibiotics. In the morning, news of the spirit's visitation traveled swiftly throughout the village.

That afternoon, I happened to meet Susan with her husband and several of their children on the main road by the trade stores. She looked weak and pale and was wearing a jacket because she felt cold. She told me that she was discharged from *ospeta* because the ward was officially closed due to the chronic water problem. The water tank at the health center was dry and the pipe leading from the main district tank was broken. When I asked her how she felt about going home before her course of treatment was finished, she responded with an air of resignation, "Nothing I can do about it. How can I stay there without water?" In order to complete her treatment, she had to return to the health center every six hours to get injections. As we walked back to the village together, Susan described her symptoms: high fever, chills, and chest pains. I asked what she thought the sickness was (not what the health center diagnosis was) and she said it was probably malaria. In fact, such is the endemic nature of malaria in the Trobriands that it has become a generic term for any illness that involves high fever and headache. This is reflected in clinical treatment as well, where chloroquine is overused as a standard drug therapy for a range of symptoms. The word "quinine" is used colloquially to represent any drug therapy, including antibiotics. Later in the day, I learned that Susan had been feeling unwell on and off for several weeks with a bronchial infection and had been spending most of her time in the house making mats for the upcoming *sagali* for her mother's deceased sister. Susan never mentioned her dream to me and I never asked.

Two days later Susan took a turn for the worse, her fever and pain stronger than before. She had not slept or eaten since taking ill and she was withdrawn and uncommunicative, often appearing catatonic. These symptoms made her sickness assume significance in the daily life of the village, in contrast to milder illnesses or ailments that people deal with privately within their immediate household or hamlet. Everyone was concerned about Susan's prognosis, and there were many quiet conversations about her condition, the reason underneath her illness, and ways of dealing with it. The consensus circulating in the village was that the visit by her father-in-law's spirit made her vulnerable to the exploits of witches. This was clearly the work of a well-known *yoyowa*, and although no name was uttered the inference was explicit.

In the early evening, Susan's husband carried her over to one of his clan member's house for specialist treatment. She sat cross-legged inside the entrance of the small thatched dwelling, rocking back and forth, eyes glazed and staring straight ahead. Her husband looked exhausted and anxious but was fully attentive to her condition. He had been staying by her side at all times, not sleeping either, and he had not shaved or changed clothes since the ordeal began. The male clan member brewed a dark herbal tea in a large pot on the cooking fire while his wife stoked the flame. The man was well known for this particular remedy, which he learned from his father, one of the first Trobriand Methodist missionaries. Susan was given some of the tea to drink and then it was sponged on her body with special leaves while the man chanted protective magic.

Susan was escorted to the Sunday church service the next morning, freshly dressed in a white blouse and blue skirt, arriving with her husband, children, and parents. She looked weak but was smiling. Her attendance was a clear effort to assert a positive image to the community and to resume normality. People welcomed her warmly and special prayers were offered in the service. But there had been little improvement in her condition since washing in the herbal medicine. Her sleepless night had been filled with terrifying hallucinations, and consequently she was carried to her parents' house in another hamlet where the family gathered in vigil. And then after church she took another turn, regressing into a possessed state that gripped her throughout the following night. She would angrily strike at her hallucinations, her body writhing and contorting in pain, and she made strange, guttural sounds and high-pitched screeches. She wrestled with whoever tried to restrain her and several times she attempted to run away from her parents' house.

For the next few days, ongoing accounts of her condition circulated in conversations around the village. That the herbal medicine was not able to exact the anticipated effect and cleanse Susan of her sickness was not an indictment on the specialist's knowledge or skills, but instead affirmed in people's minds the particularly powerful nature of the force at work in her body. Some people contended with straightforward confidence that Susan's continued high fever, cold sweats, and hallucinations were due to malaria, stating that the medication simply takes time to work. It is often like this, I was told. People get sick and go for treatment at the health center and expect an immediate improvement from medication, not realizing that medicine takes time to have an effect. Then they stop taking medicine before the course is finished and start treating for witchcraft or sorcery. Then they get worse and blame it on the effects of the medicine and they then resort solely to herbal treatments and magic. I was told that Susan had stopped going for the course of medication at the health center and that her father had commissioned the *toyuvisa* from a nearby village to treat her. Engaging the services of the *toyuvisa* indicated the elevated concern and urgency with which Susan's family viewed her condition. Such a decision requires a significant payment. *Toyuvisa* do not set the terms in advance but generally expect one or two clay pots and a cash payment of up to K50, depending on the length of engagement, plus a limitless supply of tobacco and betel nut during the course of treatment.

The *toyuvisa* did not proceed surreptitiously but conducted his business in full view of the community, walking confidently down the main road from his village to Susan's parents' home and back again, a canvas bag hanging authoritatively from his shoulder, his adolescent apprentice son following in step, carrying his betel-nut basket and lime pot. The engagement of the *toyuvisa* conveyed a public statement about familial agency; by enlisting the power of the healer, Susan's father communicated an offensive position against the supernatural forces that threatened his daughter's and his family's well-being. The community also assumed an offensive stance, augmenting the specialized intervention of the *toyuvisa* by gathering as a collective body on the ground outside the family's house at dusk on Wednesday evening in a demonstration of support and to offer prayers and cooked food for the family. The children played quietly, people shared betel nut and chewed, and several women in turn led whispered prayers and softly sung hymns. Cries of distress and anguish occasionally broke through the stillness from inside the house, and the crowd exchanged anxious expressions. By nightfall the gathering dispersed, and a single kerosene lantern glowed from inside the quiet dwelling.

Susan continued to fight demons for the rest of the week. Her head would roll and she would snarl at her husband and children and say hateful things to their faces. The children were frightened and began to stay away from her, sleeping at relatives' houses. Her husband was emotionally and physically exhausted but remained vigilant and determined. The *toyuvisa* worked steadily with Susan and the family to expel the *yoyowa* from her. He was "on call," making routine daily visits, attending to Susan at night, and instructing the family how to care for her, what food to feed her, and how to prepare it properly. His main healing practice was to help Susan visualize the source of her malady by summoning the *yoyowa* when Susan was in a dream state. When the name was finally drawn out after several attempts, vulnerability swept over the entire village as the news passed from one household to another. This was highly dangerous terrain; the revelation had to be contained. Christian prayer was appealed to in people's conversations and retellings: we don't want bad feelings, this is not good for the community, there is no point in calling names, let's just forget it, these are satanic powers, we need spiritual strength and prayer. Having successfully revealed the source of illness, the *toyuvisa* called for a combination of prayer and medical treatment to restore Susan's health.

A community health worker from the closed *ospeta* began attending to Susan to administer a course of malaria treatment and antibiotics and to put her on a saline drip. I talked to him outside the house when he arrived for an injection, which was given every eight hours, pulling the disposable syringe and medicine vial from his trouser pocket. He told me he had to work together with the *toyuvisa*, that it was a combined effort. He confirmed that Susan had malaria, but she was made weak and vulnerable to infection by *yoyowa*. "It is impossible to say which came first, but the *yoyowa* will always go for the weak ones. They use infections to their advantage." He also told me that he was happy to help out with the medicine. "It is not the people's fault that the health center is closed, so they shouldn't have to suffer because of it." Besides, he added, he was related to Susan's mother's father, part of the same *dala*, so there was no question but that he should help.

Several months later, I made a brief visit to the family household. It was the first time I had seen Susan since the women's fellowship gathering. I talked to her briefly from the doorway as she sat inside the darkened front room. Susan had not yet fully recovered from her ordeal. She remained weak and pale and had lost a significant amount of weight. But her prolonged illness was no longer the subject of conversation and focused attention; it had receded into the background of village life, settling into an invisible stasis, folded away into the interior space of her family's dwelling. She continued to live with her parents and had not yet resumed attendance at church or community gatherings. She did not attend her aunt's *sagali* that she had been making mats for when she fell ill. Nor did she attend the primary school graduation ceremony the previous week to watch her daughter perform the circle dance with her classmates. And because of her poor health, she had not resumed breastfeeding her baby. Then a few weeks later, I learned that Susan had shifted to her big sister's house. She had regained enough energy to start tending to the kitchen garden, she had also resumed breastfeeding, and her husband had traveled to Alotau to look for bolts of fabric to help prepare for her *lubwau*.

This narrative illustrates the power of witchcraft, which is perceived as the core reason for sickness, and how pluralistic responses to disease involve interactive and complementary methods of healing (Frankel and Lewis, eds. 1989). Underlying the centrality of medical pluralism in managing and treating disease, the situation presented in the story shows the synergistic interaction of biological, environmental, social, and structural factors in disease etiology, and indeed the direct interactions between different diseases themselves (cf. Singer and Clair 2003). Foremost, the story highlights how making sense of disease is fundamentally a social process, dependent on the strength of social relations for charting the desirable path toward the restoration of well-being. It is within this context of converging meanings, shaped by the dynamic interplay between colonial medicine, contemporary health services, Christianity, witchcraft, and traditional regimes for defining and responding to disease, that HIV assumes its presence in the Trobriands.

CHAPTER 7

Fitting Condoms on Culture

One day in June 2003, I noticed a familiar image on the exterior wall of a newly constructed *bukumatula*, built by a young unmarried man next to his parent's house, just across from the church in Orabesi village. The image that caught my attention was the "Show You Care" HIV awareness poster produced by the PNG National AIDS Council Secretariat in 2002 (see Figure 7.1). Aimed at sexually active young people, the poster represents youthful modernity and consensual heterosexuality in a photographic montage of a smiling young woman with a frangipani in her hair and two confident couples in fashionable attire. The text reinforces the ABC hierarchy of HIV prevention (Abstain, Be faithful, or use Condoms) that is the cornerstone of the national awareness campaign. It states: "There is no cure for AIDS and the best ways to protect yourself are not to have sex or be faithful to one partner who is also faithful to you. But if you decide to take the risk, you must use a condom *every time you have sex*." The message goes on to say, "Condoms should be seen as part of making love. They protect against unwanted pregnancies and sexually transmitted infections. And, in this way, they show your partner you care." The tagline message at the bottom of the poster states: "So remember. . . . If you're thinking about sex, think about condoms" (see NACS 2002). The poster implies that sexual activity, while deemed to be risky, involves a process of deliberation and decision making. Notably, the poster allows intimacy and consensual pleasure to be part of an idealized heterosexual experience, countering the widely held perception throughout PNG that condoms represent infidelity and distrust in sexual relationships.[1]

It is telling that this particular poster found its "target audience" in a Trobriand village, engaging the imagination of a sexually active young man. When I pointed out the poster to the woman I was walking with, she said, "Yes, some of our boys do think about these things. It is like a reminder to his friends." Sudi, the young man, later told me that he got the poster from the local health center. He said he liked it when he saw it and asked the nurse if he could have it, so she gave it to him on the promise that he would put it up where people could see it. He also told me that he gets condoms from the health center and sometimes uses them with his partners. By displaying the poster on his dwelling, Sudi enhanced the HIV prevention message with contextual signification. Juxtaposed thus, the poster on the *bukumatula* became a potent symbol of how Trobrianders' conceptual engagement with HIV is mediated by cultural knowledge and lived experience. Moreover, the

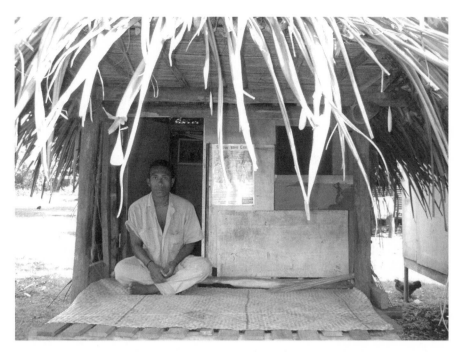

FIGURE 7.1. • Sudi with HIV awareness poster on his *bukumatula*, June 2003

signification poses the challenge of reconciling the perturbing relations between notions of "risk," HIV prevention, and the embodiment of cultural practice.

Landscapes of Risk

I heard a WHO statistic on the radio, coming up to World AIDS Day on December first. Every fourteen seconds a young person is infected with HIV somewhere in the world. So I am thinking, what is the Trobriand statistic? Every day? Every hour? How long will it take to wipe us out? People are scared when they hear about this disease, the death it brings, but fear does not stay with them when sex is on their minds. People put fear out of mind so they can still act free. Freedom is like a feather in Trobriand hair, our pride. It is young people's time to enjoy. So it is very hard to change our ways, very hard for us to think of fear when we are enjoying ourselves. But we need to break away from customs that put us at risk in this time of AIDS. [Linda, aged mid-forties, 08 November 2003]

"Risk" has become a central cultural construct in industrialized societies to signify not only the probability of an event but also how dangerous or negative its outcome might be, situating the individual agent in relation to an array of choices mediated by societal constraints (Petersen 1997). As a metaphor for danger, risk is increasingly "invoked to protect individuals against encroachments of others" (Douglas 1990:7), inviting a direct association with discourses of regulation and blame. The concept dominates biomedical and epidemiological models for predicting disease trends and managing and controlling health outcomes (Skolbekkan 1995). Risk is the pivotal concept on which HIV interventions are based, representing not only the threat of the pathogen but deviance from forms of sexual behavior regarded by the biomedical paradigm as normal and safe. HIV communication draws heavily on the language of risk to identify and describe modes of viral transmission and exposure and to buttress prevention messages. The moral deployment of risk in the language of HIV reinforces perceptions of "otherness," effectively constructing an impenetrable dichotomy between us and them, inside and outside, such that prevention options are estranged from cultural meanings and the embodied experience of sexuality (Herdt 1992; Lyttleton 2000). The notion has become so entrenched in HIV discourse that even deliberate reconfigurations of risk to guard against the language of stigma and blame—by moving beyond individual bodies and groups of bodies toward settings and social structures, and by introducing the notion of "vulnerability" as the passive counter to intentional agency—continue to draw bounded circles around practices deemed unsafe and deviant.[2]

Among Trobrianders, perceptions of HIV risk reflect these rhetorical configurations and are commonly expressed in terms of an external difference located beyond familiar boundaries. By contrast, notions of belonging and attachment to place provide a sense of resilience and immunity to the novel pathogen. The observation that "Trobriand Islanders feel safe and relaxed in their way of life; HIV is not an issue for them" captures the significance of cultural identity in people's orientations toward HIV risk.[3] Yet as the experience of the epidemic evolves at the national level and spirals out to encompass the diversity of local contexts, the language of HIV risk shifts the imagined boundaries of protection, increasingly implicating local settings and "cultural practices." As shown in Chapter 6, the mounting tensions between introduced risk, cultural risk, and cultural resistance in the time of AIDS reflect a deeper history of encounters with new disease phenomena able to penetrate place identity and borders of being.

As Linda's statement above conveys, the HIV pandemic is modeled statistically as a ticking time bomb, threatening even out-of-the way places with decimation and imposing dramatic rupture from the familiar as the only recourse. The HIV awareness messages reaching the Trobriands have shaped a local landscape of risk where the intermittent arrival of cargo, fishing, and tourist boats represents the main mode of potential transmission. The wharf at Losuia signifies the site of concentrated HIV risk—the local "hot spot" of infectivity.[4] Young girls and boys are warned by adults not to go to the wharf when the boats arrive and not to "involve themselves" with the crew and passengers but to restrict their sexual encounters to their own Trobriand peers. Similarly, the two guest lodges on Kiriwina signify potential exposure to HIV brought to the islands by foreigners and traveling politicians, public servants, and businessmen seeking local sexual hospitality in the "Islands of Love."

Jowell Topeula, a Trobriand man in his early forties involved in HIV peer education and community awareness theater, recounts how people typically respond to AIDS information and the ABC prevention message with amusement and dismissal, expressing a strong sense of place identity in opposition to the foreign and holding the view that such models of disease, risk, and death are incompatible with local knowledge and experience.

> Whenever we mention about wearing condoms, or sticking to one sexual partner, or not having sex, then everybody starts laughing. Because, you know, they tell us, this AIDS you are talking about, we know nothing about it, it doesn't come here. This AIDS is only for *dimdims*. We natives, we don't have this AIDS business. We only know that we stay around in our village and if *bwagau* comes then we die. We would never know if somebody dies because of AIDS. You see? The idea is that AIDS is just a foreign word or sickness, a *dimdim* sickness only. We Papua New Guineans, we Trobrianders, we don't have it. [Taped group discussion, 10 October 2003]

The denial of AIDS as evoked here does not suggest a disempowered position of defensiveness in the face of an escalating epidemic (see Campbell 2003:110, 192), but instead projects a confident, well-rehearsed cultural incompatibility with, and immunity to, the imported moral discourse of risk. Similar expressions of denial were described by Dorothy Ruguna, a widow in her mid-fifties who was one of the *asples* researchers with the benchmark national study on sexual and reproductive knowledge (NSRRT and Jenkins 1994; see Chapter 2). Dorothy has a long-term perspective on the evolving responses to HIV and AIDS in the Trobriands, having been sporadically involved in awareness work since 1994. During a group discussion in her village, she voiced cynicism about the effectiveness of awareness programs in promoting behavior change, characterizing people's attitudes as "don't care." In a follow-up interview, Dorothy reiterated her concern. Her account illustrates how the perceived boundaries of protection shift closer to home as the discursive presence of the epidemic settles into the local landscape.

> When health workers come to do AIDS awareness, people say we don't care about this one because we don't have it here in our village. We don't carry this AIDS virus. They say, our body is our own body, we control our own body. But I've already talked to them, you say it's your body but you will never know if you'll be carrying AIDS around, you might get it somewhere and then bring it back here. The community health worker talked to them about it, he put posters on the walls in the aid post. But people say we are free, we don't have this sickness here at home. They control their own bodies by having choice in what they do, who they go to, their partners. They have the freedom so they are not thinking about a sickness like AIDS. [Taped interview, 13 December 2003]

The confident dismissal of the possibility of acquiring or transmitting HIV suggests that the representation of risk linking multiple sexual partnering to viral exposure has little salience compared to people's empowered sense of freedom and choice in exercising their sexuality. As explored in Chapter 6, even the consequence of breaching the *sovasova* taboo, which *is* conceptualized as a sexually transmitted disease, is not perceived as risk in terms of taking a chance with an unknown outcome. And while *sovasova* does represent moral danger, it is concerned with the effect of *sameness* rather than *otherness*.

Dorothy's reflections on people's attitudes about HIV risk were interspersed throughout the interview with accounts of the use of love magic. When I asked whether the effects of *kwaiwaga* undermine people's ability to "control their own bodies," Dorothy explained that although people "can't help themselves because their mind is caught, they know what *kwaiwaga* is, not like the sickness of AIDS." As a medium for exercising control over the agency of others, *kwaiwaga* bolsters confidence in sexual pursuits while diminishing the uncertainty of the outcome. Similar to Jowell's account of how *bwagau* explains death, Dorothy's answer also indicates how the cultural knowledge of magic provides an interpretive framework for mitigating uncertainty (see Gammage 2006) and lends weight to the cognitive denial of AIDS.

Resistance to the notion that HIV can penetrate local boundaries also stems from the representations of risk that impute moral judgment on sexual behavior. Jowell spoke about the provincial HIV training workshop on peer education and community awareness theater that he attended in Alotau in 2000, and how he formed a local troupe of young people upon returning to the Trobriands. On World AIDS Day in 2001, the troupe performed a play based on a script from the workshop. The written synopsis of the play, called "Rasta Boy," tells of a young man out for a spin at the market who "automatically gets AIDS" from a *pamuk* (Tok Pisin for prostitute), then goes back to his village, infects his wife, and suddenly dies. The play's redemptive plot tells a parallel story of a young couple who go together to the health center to get tested for HIV before they get married.[5] Jowell recalled how the play was not well received by Trobriand audiences. He explained, "People did not agree with the *pamuk* character because we don't see this kind of thing happening here. Young people are free to go around. Sex is a free thing. For the messages, we have to come up with different ideas for the Trobriands."[6]

Aside from the gross misrepresentation of the disease progression of HIV, the play's stereotypical characterization of the prostitute as the vector of the virus, who seduces the hapless young man and then kills him, perpetuates the myth that female bodies are the source of HIV and undermines people's capacity to comprehend HIV risk in relation to social structure and sexual practice. In the Trobriands, as elsewhere, the representation of the *pamuk* character offends people's experiential understandings of sexual agency and sexual transactions, resulting in embarrassment, denial, and disengagement (see McPherson 2008). The use of community awareness theater to disseminate information about HIV and AIDS and to encourage local participation in the response to the epidemic has been supported widely throughout Papua New Guinea as an important medium of communication in contexts where literacy levels are low and access to television and radio is limited. However, the standard scripts and stock characterizations tend to reinforce rigid categories of risk settings and behaviors, playing to moralities and prejudices rather than empathic identification with real-life characters and situations.

Given that denial is a common response to HIV and AIDS in the Trobriands, it is not surprising that *katuigaki*, meaning a flippant disregard of warning, is the Kiriwina word most often suggested as best capturing the notion of risk, indicating as well how the imported construct communicates heavy moral undertones about individual behavior. I was told that health workers sometimes use the word in re-lation to family planning—scolding women who understand the importance of birth spacing but still have babies at close intervals. Under certain circumstances, blatant disregard of warnings can also signify admirable prowess and confidence, for instance when going out fishing in inclement weather. Additionally, the word *besobeso* (literally, "this way and that way"), alluding to a random carelessness or displaced action contrary to social conventions, is likened to the notion of risk. While both *katuigaki* and *besobeso* can signify sexual practice that does not con-form to the protocol of mutual consent and collective endeavor, the corollary of such action is not linked to the perilous exposure to disease, except in the case of *sovasova*. However, the dialogic transaction between constructions of HIV risk and Trobriand interpretations does not readily support an understanding of risk as the potential disease outcome of unprotected sexual activity. For young boys in particular, sexual risk represents the potential shame of rejection, not the danger of infection, thus explaining the importance of *kwaiwaga* in controlling for the desired outcome of sexual agency.

Yet the language of risk in HIV communication, heavily predicated on danger and otherness, does translate directly into fear. As Diana observed, "The preven-tion side of HIV risk is taken as a joke but the sickness side creates fear." Denial and humor appear as an impervious front to the underlying fear generated by HIV awareness. In fact, the manifestation of fear is where magic and people's percep-tions of HIV directly intersect. Probing for what constitutes *kokola*, or fear, I was told that fear of death from sorcery or witchcraft is foremost on people's minds. The fear of famine or of not having an adequate harvest also weighs heavily, be-ing the immediate concern of several villages on the northwest side of Kiriwina in 2003 because of localized drought. Some people mentioned the fear of wars in other countries, such as the war in Iraq and whether that war might reach the shores of PNG as did the battles of World War II, still vivid in the memories of elders. Undoubtedly due in part to the subject of my research, and thus the under-lying topic of our discussions, such reflections also included the fear of dying from AIDS "because there is no treatment or cure." However, the fear of AIDS is not constant like the vigilant fear of death from sorcery or witchcraft, but is suffused with ambivalence and uncertainty. For some, the obscurity of AIDS translates into a metaphor for juvenile discipline: "We just take the word AIDS as a threatening thing. If a small child gets into something they shouldn't—'Hey, you, don't touch that, you will get AIDS!' That's how people use the word now, as a threat or a scolding word. But mostly, we still don't understand why it is like this, so we just hear this word and get frightened" (Female, aged 50, taped group discussion, 30 June 2003).

People also contemplate whether fear might be transcended if they could only "see" AIDS or have the experience of caring for someone who is sick with AIDS. The capacity to care for the sick and dying and to overcome the underlying adver-sity that illness and death represent is an ongoing obligation, socially and cultur-ally assured. Such reflections indicate how the process of seeing and knowing holds the prospect for alleviating fear and countering the potential for stigma to grip the response to the epidemic.

During a discussion with members of a women's fellowship group, Florence spoke of the evolving responses to messages about HIV risk, the incompatibility of casting sex in terms of risk, and the ongoing struggle to reconcile fear and desire through behavior change.

> When the message about AIDS was first introduced here, people took it as a joke. They thought it can't be true. But then by repeating the message and talking with concern, the thoughts about AIDS have changed. Now everybody is concerned. Like before, Trobriand Islanders take sex as fun. Sex is not a risky thing. But nowadays it is no longer taken as fun because of what has now been introduced here, HIV/AIDS in the Trobriand Islands. It is very frightening. Before it was only the concern of the health workers, but these days, everybody is concerned. Before, young ones were like butterflies going from one hibiscus to another hibiscus. Nowadays they try to stick to one partner. But, I believe, talking honestly, speaking in the church, not forgetting that we are in the church doing the interviews and discussions, that not one person has one partner only. Everybody has more than one boyfriend or one girlfriend, until they find the right partner to get married to. And though there might be fear of AIDS, that can't stop people from having sex. They still take it as fun. [Taped group discussion, 22 July 2003]

"Steady with Custom"

As the language of HIV risk becomes assimilated through reiteration, including messages about the implied moral hazard of not taking risk seriously, perceptions of risk undergo change. As indicated by Linda's words in the epigraph to this chapter, Trobriand mediations of HIV and AIDS increasingly represent a struggle between fear and desire, between the risk of becoming infected with the deadly virus and the "freedom" to practice their culture.[7] Perceived boundaries of safety dissolve and the familiar landscape of culturally sanctioned sexual practice is reconfigured so that sex becomes synonymous with risk. As a village birth attendant asserts, "These days, with HIV already here, when young ones go for sex, they are going for risk. Sex is a risky thing."[8] Men say that male sexual infidelity during the period of pregnancy and lactation is "the biggest disease in Trobriand culture," echoing the concerns of women (see Chapter 4).[9] HIV prevention messages are inverted with irony, given new interpretations cognizant of cultural vulnerability (see Schoepf 1992; Setel 1999). Commenting on the ABC slogan, Clement observes with wry humor, "In the Trobs, 'steady' is sticking to our community lifestyle. Both boys and girls have multiple partners; we are steady with custom."[10]

For World AIDS Day in 2000, Clement made an AIDS awareness poster for display at the outpatient clinic at the district health center. Drawn in black marker on a large sheet of butcher paper, the poster depicted various situations in the Trobriands that Clement identified as conducive to HIV transmission. The message in Kiriwina language stated: "AIDS can come from all these activities from the hiding place: harvest festivities, when people gather for lovemaking, on the road, the place full of coconuts. AIDS has already come to our place. Use condoms each time you have sex male or female."[11]

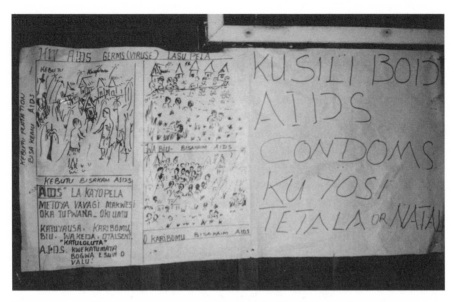

FIGURE 7.2. • HIV awareness poster at Losuia District Health Center, December 2000

The influence of culture on susceptibility to HIV is viewed more broadly as well, encompassing a way of living that values sociality and collectivity, as one policeman noted: "In the Trobs, people live close together, do things together. It's always togetherness here, group behavior. Whatever people do, it is in togetherness. The likely spread of this sickness will be because of the togetherness" (Interview notes, 22 July 2003).

Mediation of HIV risk also reflects the broader landscape of cultural continuity and social change, and the tensions between tradition and modernity, customary beliefs and Christianity. During a discussion about abstinence and faithfulness, Elizabeth spoke about the difficulty of acting on HIV prevention in the context of "a race between good and bad" practices.[12]

> From my point of view, these two things are racing each other, the good and the bad. Some customs are good, you see, and some new things are good. Some old things are bad and some new things are bad. So what I am saying, these two words, good and bad, are racing each other, and who will get ahead? Like before, divorces, or too many partners, the one man going from one lady to another and then back to the original one. But now it is because of the religion that people are being faithful. So the Christians won't let these traditional beliefs affect them. But the use of magic is coming up. Even our very religious couples are using it so they will have permanent partners and stick together. By using this magic you will be faithful. On the other hand, before the children had to grow and walk and run before another baby came, but now the baby is just sitting or crawling and another child is already on the way. What I am saying, these two things are racing each other, the good and the bad. Here in the Trobriands it is very hard to get these things to balance. [Taped group discussion, 29 July 2003]

The principal of Kiriwina High School also sees the problematic tension between tradition and modernity as contributing to the shifting landscape of risk in the Trobriands, specifically in how the "ways of the village life" detract from the value of formal education. He shared his views shortly after the grade 8 graduation ceremony.

> Retention continues to be a big problem for our students. They are tangled in sex and a "don't care" attitude. Yes, there are other factors like school fees that make it hard for some students to stay in school, but I am concerned about the ways of the village life. The nightlife in the village pulls them; they cannot help themselves. It is the culture. I know for a fact because I am a village man, too. I speak as a village man. The night activities are very strong on the youth and makes it so they don't really care about their education. [Interview notes, 19 December 2003]

As the discursive epidemic spreads, perceptions that HIV risk lies within "culture" and the landscape of the village have become more pronounced. Of all cultural practices, *milamala*, the yam harvest season, has come to epitomize the risk of HIV in the Trobriands. In recent years, harvest festivities have assumed a commercial dimension to attract tourists and generate local revenue. Promoted as a cultural event, the annual Milamala Festival is funded by provincial government grants and organized by local committees representing business interests, the district government, and host villages. During the festival period, the subject of HIV enters more frequently into conversations as people speculate on the heightened levels of sexual activity and the influx of visitors who come to the "Islands of Love" with sexual expectations. While I was walking with a group of friends on the crowded street by the wharf in Losuia during the 2003 inaugural Milamala Festival, all of us admiring the many young people who were dressed in traditional finery for dancing, a middle-aged woman spontaneously remarked to me, "While we are promoting our culture, we are promoting the spread of the AIDS virus."[13] This perceptive observation is not a mere indictment of the so-called risk of cultural practices. During the conversation that followed this remark, the broader context of risk was described: increased mobility involving tourists, visiting government officials, and public servants; cross-generational partnering of younger women with older men, whose longer sexual histories hold greater potential exposure to HIV and other sexually transmitted diseases; and the sudden influx of cash, which influences levels of transactional sexual activity. Yet "culture" as the embodied expression of place identity carries the burden of culpability for viral transmission.

In particular, perceptions of cultural risk focus on *karibom*, the all-night dance promenade in the central clearing of a host village when people of all ages walk in a slow, rhythmic pattern in counter-circles to the steady beat of drums. Considerable local mystique surrounds the subject of *karibom* and the ramifications it holds for sexual intrigue and abandon. Performed only during harvest festivities, *karibom* is described as "*mwasawa*, a game of enjoyment for everyone to participate in," men and women, married and unmarried; its inclusivity means that established relationships are temporarily suspended and "people don't let *uliweli* [sexual jealousy] get in the way."[14] *Karibom* can also take the form of *kayasa*, a competitive event sponsored by a chief or senior man of high rank to celebrate an abundant yam harvest. The liberty of the sponsor to set the terms of participation was raised as an issue by a number of people who I interviewed. I was told about several occasions in the recent past where the sponsor decreed to the participating village that any married person who complained or who chose not to take part would get "paid" with a pig or yams. Moral emphasis was placed on greed: the reluctance to participate implied that one is overly possessive or jealous of his or her spouse or steady partner, "too greedy to share," while payment for such behavior projected further greed on the recipient (and also obliged them to reciprocate the payment at a later date). The collective pressure at the village level to participate took precedence, while the shame of being recipient to the sponsor's largesse compelled everyone to take part regardless of their willingness.

Whether staged as a cultural showpiece for an audience of tourists, as a sponsored competition of obligatory participation, or simply as the spontaneous culmination of harvest festivities, people acknowledge that the event of *karibom* is ripe with sexual possibility *and* the risk of infection. Joseph, a young Trobriand man involved in HIV peer education, views the risk as inherent, explaining, "the sexual side of *karibom* is taking place in there, so you see, HIV and other STIs can go right through the dance and spread so quickly."[15] Yet participants in a group discussion described how HIV prevention is far from people's minds during *karibom*.

> In the *karibom* way, the drums will be beating and you go around in circles in opposite directions, boys and girls, and then join, like dancing, hugging, and holding hands, whatever. But for real sex, no, that's after, if it's agreed between two partners, whatever they do, they can go underneath the mango tree, or underneath the pawpaw tree, or in the house. But for the time of dancing, it's only a merry dance, a happy dance; people are not having sexual intercourse right there. Those who are aroused, they move out. But people are concentrating on enjoying themselves; no one is concentrating on condoms. Assuming they don't have condoms with them and they have sex with anybody there, then the disease might be spreading from anybody. So whatever we are arousing in our culture, there are two things here: people should think about HIV and think that this dance will lead to sex so we have to take precautions. But you see, we had the politicians there and they don't think about these things [HIV prevention]. [Male, aged forty, taped group discussion, 10 October 2003]

As indicated here, some people regarded the risk of *karibom* as an indictment on the failure of leaders and festival organizers to adequately address HIV prevention in the context of harvest festivities and to ensure the wide availability and distribution of condoms. The 2003 festival brochure encouraged visitors to "feel free to participate in all the activities and join in the fun" but prohibited the taking of photographs during *karibom*, deeming it to be "culturally sensitive" (Milne Bay Tourism Bureau 2003). The ban gave rise to speculation that it was actually a "cover-up" by the festival organizers, knowing that photos would provide evidence that programmed activities were "going against AIDS awareness." However, people also acknowledged that the local member of parliament briefly mentioned the HIV epidemic in his speech at the closing ceremony, appealing to young people in particular to "look after themselves" and "avoid the sickness."

Such appeals echo the moral doctrine of the church and the sentiments expressed from the pulpit by deacons and pastors, whose veiled references to the epidemic do not inflame fear or shame but encourage young people to "look after your bodies like good Christians" and "avoid the sickness by limiting your behavior." Rhetoric that personalizes the epidemic in terms of young people's individual and collective risk is becoming more common, with an emphasis on young people's own agency as well as their elders' agency in safeguarding their future. Raymond Kautawata, a village court magistrate, pinpoints how the celebrated freedom of *kubukwabuya* sexuality offers the opportunity for informed choice, as opposed to the suppression of knowledge, which delimits agency. "Our freedom lets us think twice about risk so we have to make the best choice. We have to give young people the best advice, stick to one partner or use condoms. Young people have to think carefully about HIV/AIDS because it's their life" (Interview notes, 24 September 2003).

Raymond's words reveal the sense of responsibility adults have for guiding young people in their decision making, suggesting the importance of intergenerational as well as peer participation in HIV communication. His words also indicate that thinking carefully about HIV risk involves more than personal discipline and restraint; it involves thinking about condoms as the means for protection and prevention.

Thinking about Condoms

U'ula condom pela baisa kokola AIDS.[16]
[The reason for condoms is because of the fear of AIDS.]

This statement was mentioned to me many times, like a well-rehearsed mantra, indicating the widespread awareness among Trobriand men and women about the use of condoms for preventing HIV transmission. When I asked people to recount the HIV awareness messages they were familiar with, it was common for people to invert the well-known ABC slogan and begin by identifying condoms ahead of abstinence and being faithful as the main prevention strategy. Although marital fidelity is a vigorously contested issue, particularly in relation to abstinence during pregnancy and lactation, conversations often would be reduced to fits of laughter as people contemplated the proposition of not having sex at all. Most Trobrianders do not perceive condoms to be at the bottom of a moral hierarchy of prevention. These views sharply contrast with the general tone of resistance toward condom use in PNG as reflected in the circulating discourses of media, churches, government officals, and health workers, which inscribe condoms with risk and disease and associate their use with promiscuity and infidelity (Hammar 2007:76–77, 2010; *National* 2010).[17] In the Trobriands, the response to awareness about condoms as an effective means of HIV protection and prevention has been positive and pragmatic (cf. Keck 2007; Wilde 2007). There is also growing evidence that condom use is transforming the landscape of risk and desire in the Trobriands, and observations like the following are common: "Before this sickness came, no one knew about condoms but now young ones are using this thing. We see condoms in the men's baskets. When we walk on the paths, we see used condoms on the ground" (Interview notes, 13 November 2003).

Traversing the islands by foot, I kept watch on the roadsides and bush tracks for evidence of condom use and came across plenty of empty wrappers and the occasional used condom. The reach of condoms throughout the islands and increased awareness about HIV risk are largely attributed to the village birth attendants program, which serves as the main condom distribution network in the Trobriands. The women volunteers obtain supplies of male condoms from the district health center and provide them free of charge in their villages, although they report that the supply is irregular and insufficient to meet potential demand. Some of the women volunteers also have a few female condoms provided as samples during a training workshop where they were instructed on how to insert them. Jane has been a village birth attendant since the program commenced in the early 1990s, long before HIV awareness and condom distribution became program activities. She told me that at first everyone laughed about condoms but now people, including the young girls, are coming forward. Martha, who also has been with the program from the beginning, says that as a village birth attendant she feels *tuvalua*, or free from shame, to speak about condoms. She tells the young boys that if they are shy to approach her for condoms they can go to her husband or son instead. She tells the girls that they should also carry condoms so if someone asks them for sex on the road and they agree, they already have their protection with them. When she gives community talks about HIV and condoms, she uses herself as an example to encourage others not to feel shame.[18]

The effectiveness of the VBA condom distribution program reflects the confidence engendered by working through established and trusted social and kinship networks within communities. As one young man asserted, "Condoms are becoming part of life and friends are reminding friends."[19] Local networks of support alleviate the shame that prevents young people in particular from accessing condoms from the health center. Moreover, health workers in the Trobriands are not averse to promoting and providing condoms, unlike health workers in other places throughout PNG (see Hammar 2007; Wardlow 2008; Wilde 2007). Ridley, the health extension officer, views the challenges of condoms primarily in terms of the difficulty of persuading people to accept condom use as part of sexual practice. "Condoms are the only effective measure to prevent HIV/AIDS in Trobriand Islands, as well as most STIs. Plus they can prevent unwanted pregnancy. So it works both ways, disease prevention and contraception. But it is very hard to get people to use condoms. They want skin to skin" (Interview notes, 10 December 2003).

As Ridley frankly notes, the general acceptance of condoms for preventing the spread of sexually transmitted infections *and* preventing pregnancy is difficult to reconcile with the valued aesthetics of *bilamapula*, the reciprocal movement between partners during sexual intercourse that results in orgasm and the ideal exchange and mixing of *momona*, or male and female sexual fluids. Some people contend that condoms are "wasteful things," turning potent sexual fluids into rubbish to be discarded. Men joke about how the awkwardness of putting on condoms during sexual arousal makes them abandon their intention to use them. They also explain their nonuse in terms of their partner's preference, saying that women and girls dislike the feeling of condoms inside them. Women, too, speak negatively about the effects of condoms on the pleasures of lovemaking. The following statement by a mature-aged woman beyond her reproductive years is a candid reminder that HIV prevention efforts must be attentive to the spectrum of human sexual desire and agency across the life course.

> People aren't serious about condoms because they stop the whole emotional feelings. For me, I've had experience with condoms. My partner asked to use the condom. He tried that one, used it when we had sexual intercourse. I said, OK, give it a try, but then I said, "Oh, I feel uncomfortable with this thing!" So he took it off and threw it out. It just doesn't agree with the system. Whenever I'm in the middle of sexual intercourse and the excitement, you know, the time when the mind is boiling, but the condom stops it, stops the feeling of orgasm. The condom is already in the way so it's not, it's not so exciting. Now you see, I don't like these condoms! Truly! [Female, aged fifty, taped group discussion, 30 June 2003]

Apart from questions of physical and emotional pleasure, the association between condoms and disease also inhibits people's willingness to adopt condom use. A young man explains, "People think that if you use condoms, or want your partner to use one, it means you are carrying a disease."[20] Such understandings tie in with the "othering" of disease and the persistent view that HIV risk exists beyond the spatial boundaries of familiarity. Young men report that because of the limited condom supply, they tend to save condoms for use when they have sex with someone from outside their immediate network of relationships. Comments from several village birth attendants confirmed this strategy. One VBA explained, "When the young boys here are getting other girls from other villages, they come and ask for condom. But with their own girlfriends from here, they don't."[21] Another VBA reported that she tells the young women of her village, "If you want to go around with other men from other villages, then you should use condoms as protection."[22] As discussed in Chapter 5, young people's preference for forming steady relationships with partners from their own village or villages nearby reflects the way sexual networks assume spatial dimensions that define both *tubwa* membership and established exchange networks within and between affiliate villages. Such affiliations add to the sense of resilience and protection against a disease associated with "others" from outside familiar spaces.

The perceived safety of familiar boundaries also conceals the problematic issues of trust and fidelity at the interpersonal level while reinforcing a moral binary between married and unmarried sexual partners. The ABC slogan implies that "sticking to one steady partner" is the panacea for avoiding the risk of HIV transmission, promoting a false sense of confidence in young people who engage in successive steady relationships in their search for the "right partner" to marry. Following the hierarchical logic of the ABC message, some people perceive condoms as undermining trust and fidelity between steady partners, as Marianne, a twenty-year-old single mother, explained: "Maybe if you make a steady boyfriend, I don't think there is any danger of getting AIDS. Those who have steady partners and they trust each other, then it is just not right for them to use condom. But there are those whom you don't know, like maybe you are together for the first time, then you use these ones. But it's embarrassing to ask the man to use condoms" (Taped group discussion, 30 June 2003).

Embarrassment also pervades the reluctance of women and girls to obtain condoms from the health center and VBAs. They contend that because "condoms are a man's problem" and are "fit for the man's body," made to wear on the penis, men should be responsible for getting them and using them. At the same time, many women and girls indicate curiosity about female condoms and express an interest in trying them. Some young boys report that their female partners will remind them to use condoms and will even have one ready for them to use during intercourse. Additionally, some boys and men report they use condoms as a form of contraception at the behest of their partners.

A middle-aged female nurse not only reveals the willingness of health workers to engage with the issues of HIV prevention at the community level, but she also speaks of the agency of young women in negotiating sexual encounters.

> [Condom use] is up to the daughters and mothers to discuss. When the mother encourages her daughter to go out, she should tell her to take condom. Double-up! Take several condoms when they go out! We need to think more about how to encourage the women to use the condoms with their partners. This idea has been thought about before. After one HIV awareness session that Sister [nurse] gave in a village, an old widow got up and said that there should be notices written in big letters and put up at the market and the trade stores that say: "All single women must be supplied with condoms!" [Interview notes, 11 December 2000]

Such a proposition throws into question the gendered power dynamics of negotiating safe sex, particularly the assumption that while men are responsible for wearing condoms, women are responsible for insisting on protected sex. Significantly, however, the anecdote indicates community receptiveness to the idea of normative condom use, accentuating the importance of community-based approaches for enabling HIV prevention. Apart from the VBA program, such approaches have been undertaken to a limited degree through the IMR research project, which involved the mobilization of community leaders in HIV awareness. Ethel's reflections on the leaders' workshop, and her subsequent experience in promoting condom use among the people in her village, hint at the competing ideologies in HIV prevention and the difficulties of engendering change in sexual practice.

> We talked about all these things at the workshop and we came to learn that the only thing that can prevent the sickness passing from one to another on the whole island is to stick to one sexual partner.
>
> *And is that possible, to stick to one sexual partner?*
> Well, no, it's very hard. Then, because the condom is a new thing on the island, some come to have experience using the condom, and they are happy about it. Especially the village people, the VBA mothers and the health workers let them

know that condoms are the safest way for having sexual intercourse. If you are not faithful to your wife or to your husband or to your partner, condoms are the safest way to prevent HIV from spreading. We have to take it further to help the young ones, our daughters and sons, to think of the grandchildren, the future. It's best that we use condoms to prevent this sickness. Some men complain that it is not good using the condom. They don't like using it. But I told them, if you don't like using it, then be faithful to each other and that's it. But it's very hard. You see, on Saturdays they go, they come with a different partner and the next week you will see them with a different girl. So when they come asking for condoms, I talk to them. Use it wisely and think about the risk of the disease and stay on the safe side when you go out. And I advise them not to throw it around. The children are innocent and they pick them up and try to use them for their balloons. So, you just keep it out of trouble, use it and place it in a proper place, whether burn it with a paper or dig the hole and drop it in and bury it. [Taped interview, 20 June 2003]

As Ethel highlights, the problem of condom disposal is significant in the islands, where latrines are few, where sites of lovemaking are removed from sites designated for defecation and rubbish disposal, and where the potency of bodily substances and personal items and their use in sorcery determine how people handle them. Condoms bring together an individualized, consumable, and disposable materiality with intimate physical acts involving bodily substances, which project symbolic meaning through collective sociality. Perhaps this contradiction in meaning accounts for the careless way people discard condoms after use, contrary to the usual discretion and care taken in handling bodily substances and intimate objects. Several VBAs told me that they stopped distributing condoms in their villages because they were not being disposed of properly. As Ethel pointed out, children think of condoms as balloons and when they find them on the ground they blow them up and play with them. This factor alone was often the biggest objection to condoms voiced by mothers and older women. Diana addressed the issue of disposal with a large gathering of adults and children during the visit to Kuruvitu village, emphasizing the importance of treating used condoms respectfully, not like rubbish. "For condoms, we must think about how this thing has helped you. How can you treat it carelessly, throwing it away anyhow? We must wrap them carefully and burn them. This thing, this bit of rubber is holding part of your body, something that came out of you. It is not the same as waste." (Taped group discussion, 13 November 2003. Translated into English.)

The concern about "proper" condom use and disposal raises the broader issues of the management and control of supplies that frequently thwart effective distribution. During the entire period of my fieldwork in 2003, ten cartons of generic male condoms (each containing 12 boxes of 12 packets, with 12 condoms per packet, making a total of 17,280 condoms), plus one carton of 100 female condoms, sat in the district manager's office at Losuia after being sent by plane from the NACS office in Port Moresby. Most of the cartons remained unopened with only a few individual packets given out informally, but discreetly, to government workers and their associates for personal use. Meanwhile, the VBA condom distribution network, which also functions informally on the basis of social relations but with an inclusive reach into the community, often ran out of the condoms supplied through the health center. I learned that the condoms remained undistributed because the district AIDS committee had to first become functional and draw up a schedule of HIV awareness activities, which would then provide the rationale for distributing the condoms. A view persists among people involved in HIV program implementation that a controlled system of condom distribution will perforce ensure proper usage, whereas random and informal channels of distribution result in careless (meaning promiscuous) use or improper use such as using condoms for fish bait. There are already hundreds if not thousands of sites throughout PNG where condoms are *supposed* to be available free of charge and easily accessible, namely health centers and aid posts, but in many places condoms sit in unopened boxes in government offices because officials either refuse to distribute them or have not established the structures for doing so.

I suggest that the problem of condom inertia, often meaning they are well beyond the use-by date, is partly due to the effects of the "AIDS industry," or the institutional and discursive frameworks that dominate the global response to HIV and the "sites of power" from which resources are mobilized (Altman 1998:235). In PNG, condom supplies tend to be viewed as the property of different programs according to the source of provision, whether NACS or the health system; consequently, they are not viewed in terms of their useful, expedient, and inclusive application. The Trobriand VBA program has been linked to the health system and various donor organizations since its inception, whereas the bureaucratic structures of NACS, including provincial and district committees, have been newly introduced as distinct entities in the government's multisectoral response to the epidemic. Although contrary to the best intentions of the national strategy, one of the consequences of introducing new organizational structures to manage the response to HIV is that established social networks and resources at the local level often get overlooked or excluded.

At a fundamental level, the harboring of cartons of condoms has to do with the politics of control over a fetishized resource. But it also reflects the ensuing problem of breaking the cartons down into individual units for distribution to individual bodies for their own use and subsequent disposal. In this light, perhaps it is helpful to reflect on condom distribution in the context of the traditional exchange system and how material goods and objects circulate on the basis of social relations. The individualized materiality of condoms has been introduced into a distinctly different ethical system of accounting for the circulation of resources in the social world. The relative success of the VBA program in providing the condom distribution network for the Trobriands, and, by extension, the effectiveness of peer education programs in other settings, can be attributed to such programs' responsiveness to the social relations of exchange and reciprocity within which they operate.

The prospect of engendering respectful condom use by building on the values of Trobriand sociality and working through established social relationships is apparent in the sentiments Diana further expressed during the Kuruvitu village session where she talked about condom disposal. Directed to the adults in the group,

Diana's words are especially noteworthy for the way she situates condoms within the ideals of intergenerational reciprocity.

> We should care for the young ones, help them to use condoms. We should help them to use condoms just as the people who have helped us by giving us condoms to use, and the people who invented condoms for prevention have helped us, now it is in our hands to be responsible to use condoms. So if we don't really care about ourselves, whether we have the virus or not, then that's OK with us, but let's think of our new generation because they are the ones who will regenerate in the future. [Taped group discussion, 13 November 2003. Translated into English.]

When Diana says "if we don't really care about ourselves, whether we have the virus or not," she is not expressing the "don't care" attitude toward HIV prevention but instead referring to the fact that voluntary HIV testing is not available in the Trobriands and most people do not have alternative options for finding out their serostatus. Despite the pronounced fear of the unknown and the deadly virus, a surprising number of adults express resignation over the possibility that they may have a slowly progressing viral infection. This seemingly "don't care" attitude is not so much an indication of fatalism but rather reflects the view that with no available testing and treatment services, the usefulness of knowing whether or not one is infected seems inconsequential in the present. Sensitive to this perception, Diana focused her appeal on helping young people to be responsible for using condoms, emphasizing their future role as parents.

The Question Mark of Knowing

What about helping young people to seek voluntary counseling and testing (VCT) for HIV? If testing services become available in the Trobriands as part of the National AIDS Council Secretariat's current efforts to "roll out" VCT services throughout the country,[23] and promises of antiretroviral therapy for those who test positive are realized, how would these services become part of the local landscape of risk and desire? The play that Jowell's troupe performed for World AIDS Day included a scene where a young couple goes to the health center for testing before they get married. Apart from the problematic assumptions about what constitutes "marriage" in the PNG context and the moral framing of VCT services in terms of a monogamous partnership, does such a scenario adequately reflect Trobriand *kubukwabuya* experience, where the path to marriage involves multiple partnering? I asked Jowell how he thought Trobrianders would respond to the opportunity to find out their HIV serostatus if testing were available in the islands.

> For this I would not say yes. People would not go for testing. People are embarrassed to go to health clinics, not only in the Trobriands but elsewhere. You can't really go up to the doctors and say, "Doctor, please can you check my blood to see if I have the virus or not?" For me, I haven't checked my blood yet. Ever since they took me on [as peer educator], I'm not ashamed but it's a bit frightening to think that I could be confirmed to have the virus, you see?

At the moment no one is brave enough to go [and request the test]. That is the main point that our awareness campaign is making. We keep stressing to people that there is no shame; there is no frightening thing about having HIV/AIDS. If I got HIV/AIDS, my cousin-brother can't say, "You don't come and stay with me in my house." There is no frightening thing. It is still OK to stay with him, eat with him, because I can't spread the virus that way. That's the point we are stressing, that people will take away the idea that if anybody gets AIDS it is not a shameful thing, it wasn't their fault that they got the virus. We want to educate people that, to be sure, a son or any relative or any person, if they got the virus, it is just as normal as getting TB, we should look after them properly. [Taped group discussion, 10 October 2003]

Jowell's response is not only personalized, in the predominant discursive style in the Trobriands, but it indicates a concern to alleviate the stigma and shame that surround the virus and normalize the response of caring for those who are sick. Comparing one's HIV status to the "normality" of becoming infected with tuberculosis ironically touches on the synergistic realities of opportunistic infections in PNG's biosocial environment. There is a strong likelihood that the underlying factor in the increasing number of TB patients in the Trobriands is HIV infection, given that TB is a leading cause of death among people with HIV (World Health Organization 2003).

Jowell's prediction about people's reluctance to make use of HIV counseling and testing services if available was echoed by others, many of whom stated that without the prospect of treatment the option of knowing one's HIV status seemed rather pointless. Rose, a community leader and mother of four, explained: "People will just stay at the question mark, *wawoya* [uncertainty], wondering do I have the virus? They won't want the answer from a blood test, not if there isn't any medicine."[24] The area manager for the local government drew a link between people's unwillingness and the fear that has been generated by HIV awareness messages: "People won't be willing to be tested because the awareness campaign was done in such a way to scare people. It is a deadly disease. We can be 100 percent sure that whoever is infected will be dying from AIDS, so people will not want to know this death sentence. Secondly, confidentiality is very difficult in a close place like Trobriands. People will be worried for their personal dignity. They will not accept the option of VCT" (H. Abraham, interview notes, 27 October 2003).

The issue of confidentiality was raised not only in terms of potential stigma but in relation to the obligation for relatives to provide care and support for a sick family member. People talked about the pointlessness, as well as the difficulty, of concealing sickness in close-knit communities. These views point to the moral framing of HIV risk, which conveys a contradiction and disjunction between prevention and care. Prevention emphasizes avoidance and exclusion—protect yourself and your family from AIDS, look after yourself, look after your body, stick to one partner—and the imperative of individualized confidentiality as the code of practice between service provider and "client." Care messages appeal to compassion and inclusion—look after the sick person, do not discriminate against them, do not neglect them—and the imperative of community support. Ruth, a young mother of three small children, posed the question, "How are we supposed to protect ourselves and our children from this disease and at the same time care for the people who have the disease?"[25] Her query indicates the failure of HIV communication to clarify transmission dynamics, often misconstrued as contagion, and to bridge the division between prevention and care in the moral orientation of responses to the epidemic.

The contradictions that trouble people's understandings of the invisible virus and their willingness to know their serostatus might be resolved if and when HIV testing and treatment services become available in the Trobriands. The growing numbers of people accessing VCT services as they become available throughout PNG, at stand-alone sites in communities and at established health facilities, is an encouraging indication of a possible shift in negative perceptions of HIV as a "death sentence" and a disease of sexual deviance. The promotion of VCT services in PNG has used the human rights discourse to encourage access, with the theme for World AIDS Day 2010 being *"Testim na tritim—em rait bilong yu!"* (Tok Pisin for "Get tested and get treated—it's your right!"). The emerging presence of VCT sites has created new relational spaces between individual "clients" and service providers. People are encouraged to access testing services to know their HIV status with the reassurance that results will be kept confidential. Yet the notion of confidentiality, based on individualist modes of service access and provision, has been the source of conceptual discomfort from the beginning of the national response in Papua New Guinea. Opportunities are few for community dialogue on how this translates to local contexts, where secrecy, concealment, and visibility are dialectical forms for strategically managing potent knowledge, agency, and the social relations of exchange. Dissonance occurs between confidentiality as an individual right and the promotion of community participation in HIV prevention, care, and support. Furthermore, the limited capacity within the health system to provide adequate follow-up services and drug treatment to all who need it poses serious ethical contradictions to the rights-based framework. The proposition that testing is a right raises other challenging questions about the effective integration of HIV services within the existing primary health-care system at the community level and about the potential reciprocal benefits of HIV treatment for enhancing prevention efforts.

In the absence of voluntary options in the Trobriands, the main access to HIV testing comes by default as part of the national sentinel surveillance program, which tests pregnant women who attend antenatal clinics at provincial hospitals. Routine surveillance testing generally involves little or no pretest counseling apart from rudimentary information delivered to the assembled group in attendance at the clinic. The policy requires posttest counseling for women (and their partners) whose results are positive, with the possible provision of drug therapy for the prevention of parent-to-child transmission.[26] No follow-up counseling is provided for women whose results are negative, and the procedures for recording and reporting test results seldom comply with the principles of confidentiality.

Because Diana chose to deliver her fourth child at the provincial hospital in Alotau, she involuntarily contributed to the body of statistics that constitutes the national HIV database. Diana shared her experience with the community gathering at Kuruvitu, describing her emotional response.

If you had a blood test and you found that you are positive, you know you will die of AIDS. And you would just think, *nanomekusa*, no solution, your mind moves toward nothing. Then you would think about the kids; who is going to take care of them, clothe them and feed them? I had that sort of feeling when I went to Alotau to have my last-born child. At Alotau, when you go for antenatal clinic, the first thing you have is a blood test for HIV. Not like a malaria test; they use a syringe to get our blood and then transfer it into small bottles. They take the blood, send it to Port Moresby, and when you go back for the next clinic visit, you will be told your result—positive or negative. So I had this in mind when I had the test, how will I react when I hear the result? As I was waiting, lots of things came into my mind. I thought back and had no ending points, no resolutions. Then I went back for the next clinic. Each woman's name was called and she would go up to the desk and mention her name and the nurse would check her result in the book and say positive or negative. When I was called for my turn, while the nurse was still following her finger on the line, I could see my name and I quickly checked with the letter; was it P or N? So when I saw the N—*Auwei!* All that I had in my mind just cooled down. My feeling cooled down. [Taped group discussion, 13 November 2003. Translated into English.]

Diana's story illustrates how the virus is made visible not only by serum testing but also through reflection, underlying the importance of HIV communication that connects with the realities of people's lives. For Diana, the experience of being tested made visible for her new ways to communicate the messages of prevention.

Finding the Right Fit

When I asked Jackie, a young single woman, to tell me what gave her confidence to say no to unwanted sexual advances, I anticipated her answer would touch on gender relations and consensual sex. Jackie simply explained that she follows her monthly fertility cycle and only goes out during her safe period when she is not ovulating, referring to "safe" in relation to pregnancy avoidance rather than disease prevention. "When it comes to the time in the month when it's not safe, then I don't agree to have sex. When it is safe, I agree. If I go out at a time when it is not safe, then I might ask for condom" (Taped group discussion, 12 January 2001).

Jackie's confidence comes from being aware of her fertility cycle, which she said she learned from her mother, as well as her own agency in determining the timing of her sexual activity. How she interpreted my question suggests that coercion is not something she associates with sexual encounters. For her, "unwanted" sex relates to unwanted pregnancy. That Jackie is able to ask her partners to use condoms indicates that young people in the Trobriands are beginning to incorporate condom use as part of the protocol of youth sexuality, further evidence that *kubukwabuya* sexual culture holds important opportunities for HIV prevention.

Jackie's statement also throws into question the usefulness of the "safe sex" vocabulary in HIV communication, mired as it is by evocations of risk, danger, and distrust that evade the values of pleasurable sexuality as well as the importance of regeneration—and fertility management—as part of the embodied expression of sexual agency and desire. Shifting the emphasis in how sex is talked about would help to overcome the "impossibility of condoms" (Hammar 2007:76), including use by married couples and use with other forms of contraception. "Putting sexuality back" into the language of HIV prevention (Boyce et al. 2007), with positive representations of consensual sexual relations and healthy sexual practice, backed by the provision of integrated sexual and reproductive health services for both males and females regardless of marital status, would help to engender normative condom use and increase people's ability to put HIV awareness into action.

Furthermore, HIV communication approaches that work within existing social relations, including intergenerational ties, hold greater promise for effecting change. Within the Trobriand *dala*, mothers, aunts, grandmothers, and maternal uncles have an important role in providing guidance and encouragement to both male and female sexually active youth. Likewise, the relationship between fathers and sons also offers intergenerational support. Encouraging condom use might even be viewed as a form of *buwala*, emphasizing the values of respect and appreciation for sexual partners and the potential for future regeneration. As Diana's words make clear, sexuality also includes the "dimension of cultural survival—investing locally in the future of peoples and clans" (Broughton 2000:65). The cultural values inherent in *dala* identity, matrilineal regeneration, and collective sociality provide a powerful basis for promoting healthy sex to secure cultural viability and vitality.

While the dynamics of Trobriand sociality contribute to the local landscape of risk, sociality also offers resilience and cohesion for mitigating the impact of HIV on Trobriand ways of knowing and being. The language of risk that blames cultural practice for fueling the epidemic is discordant with reflective evaluation of experience and local approaches to prevention. In the Trobriands, as elsewhere, the process of knowing should not forge a divide between cultural practices and HIV prevention—between freedom and fear—but should instead facilitate freedom from fear.

Sustaining Trobriand sociality in the era of AIDS requires the integration of new forms of knowledge and practice with enduring cultural forms. Clement, the STI laboratory technician, pithily expressed this challenge, saying, "We need more condom use so our culture can stand firm." I quickly suppressed my laughter when I realized that no pun was intended by his declaration. The seriousness of his statement has to be met with the same seriousness of intent to address the broader structural factors and dynamic transformations that shape HIV risk, as well as to provide resources that will enable Trobrianders to mitigate the potential devastation of the epidemic on their ways of knowing and living. The challenge lies in reimagining how to talk about risk and prevention in ways that reflect embodied understandings of sexuality and how it is shaped by and situated within social context. The challenge also lies in imagining how HIV testing and treatment services might be integrated with prevention to support coherent local responses as the presence of HIV and AIDS becomes more pronounced in the Trobriands and elsewhere in Papua New Guinea.

Epilogue

Can you imagine the "Islands of Love" with no people on them? That's what it will be like, ten, twenty years' time from now. We must forecast ourselves and think about what is going to happen. The young ones must know they are the future carers for children and grandchildren. If they don't keep this in mind, the islands will be empty.

—Ethel Jacob, community leader, 23 September 2003

The timber walls and doors of Trobriand houses are ledgers of daily life, displaying idle doodling, random musings, creative drawings, and images cut out from newspapers and magazines. Upon my return to the Trobriands for a two-week family visit in January 2007, I was taken by surprise when I noticed a scrawl of chalk on the wall next to the entrance of my mother-in-law's house. The hastily written message in English was simply "AIDS is preventable." I asked household members if they knew who put the message there and everyone just laughed and said "Aiseki!" (Who knows?). I satisfied my curiosity by regarding this parthenogenetic apparition as a sign of good faith to mark my return visit. Like seeing the HIV awareness poster on the *bukumatula*, for me this random message was emblematic of how the discursive presence of HIV has settled into the Trobriand landscape. A subliminal but constant daily reminder—friends reminding friends—at the entrance of a house that welcomes many people for a chat and a chew during the course of the day.

Ethel's statement in the epigraph asserts the importance of being mindful of HIV prevention in the present by imagining a future foretold. Her rhetorical question sharply juxtaposes the idyllic "Islands of Love" with the devastation of HIV, intimating the distinctiveness of the Trobriands in contending not only with imposed representations and models of meaning but with the cultural challenges of prevention. The global HIV pandemic relentlessly imposes paradoxes on local ways of knowing and being (Setel 1999). In the Trobriands, this is acutely apparent in the potential for the decimating virus to manifest through and suffuse the cultural pleasures of fecundity and social regeneration. As an expression of Trobriand sociality, sexuality is a productive resource in building interclan relationships. The life stage of *kubukwabuya*, or unmarried youth, is particularly significant for demonstrating the capacity for social reproduction and, as Ethel forcefully reminds, securing the future.

In what ways can we portray the stories of how people imagine and respond to the unfolding presence of a localized HIV epidemic? Perhaps a vortex into despair is fitting for some realities, as Alex de Waal described during a workshop I attended in 2007.[1] For the Trobriands, I think the spiral of the *wosimwaya* dance, which charts the process of regeneration and the promise of the future by turning back and looking forward to arrive at new levels of understanding, is the appropriate metaphor.

The recursive view of time and retrospective character of growth are central features of a broader Melanesian sociality, which activate ancestral strength and identity to transform the past into the future (Strathern 1988:280). Social action directed toward future outcomes draws on accumulated knowledge through strategic reflection and evaluation. For Malakulans of Vanuatu, the signification and celebration of "custom" are oriented toward "an image of the future . . . as a projection of individual and collective power" (Curtis 2002:241). Similarly, in the Trobriands, exchange as the operative mode of social interaction is based on reflective projections wherein "the future exists as a perspective of the present" (Weiner 1976:82).

Clement's call for condom use to uphold cultural fidelity suggests an image of a future secured by maintaining traditional foundations through the adoption of new practice. Ethel's urgings to "forecast ourselves" grounds the viability of the future firmly in the present. The movement of the *wosimwaya* dance celebrates this capacity by bringing the youngest dancer, trailing at the end of the line, to the fore. The spiral form of the dance evokes the importance of intergenerational relations and how they represent one aspect of the "pivotal moral concept . . . of interdependence" in responding to HIV (Reid 1995:7–8). Ethel expresses a moral concern for the interdependence between generations in this response by emphasizing that future responsibility for nurture and care rests in the present.

The sentiment of interdependence was revealed in many of the discussions during my research, especially by older women who expressed not only concern for the future but a compassionate regret for the present generation of unmarried youth whose *kubukwabuya* freedom is curtailed by the presence of HIV. By reflecting on their own youth, these older women create an empathic connection to the dilemma faced by young people, many of whom do not acknowledge the gravity of the situation when absorbed in the familiar pleasures of immediate experience. "It's difficult to tell our daughters not to go around because of AIDS. They say to us, "You had your time for freedom, now it is our time." It's true, we feel sorry for the young ones that the sickness has come in their time." (Taped group discussion, 23 July 2003. Translated into English.)

Interdependence was also a theme often voiced when people considered how families and clans would meet the demands of debilitating illness. The capacity to draw on the cultural values of support and compassion in responding to the needs of the sick, including support reciprocated through *lubwau* exchanges, is called into question by the potential impact of HIV. "We don't want AIDS to break the love in families. Viewing our customs, we cannot reject the sick one; it is in our custom to help them. If a family member becomes sick, we must fetch firewood, cook the food, and clean the sick person through our love. If one of us gets this sickness, will we forget to act like this?" (United Church pastor, 13 November 2003).

The epidemic trajectory in the Trobriands has not reached a stage where illness and death pervade. However, the cohesion of family and *dala* ties and interclan exchange relations promises a resilient framework for providing care and support to those directly affected by HIV and hopefully for diminishing the negative forces of stigma and blame.

The system of hereditary chieftainship provides the political basis of social cohesion in the Trobriands (see Mosko 1995). The role of chiefs and other community leaders in the local response to HIV holds considerable promise for endorsing and facilitating opportunities for community conversations and, in particular, encouraging the active participation of men in HIV awareness and prevention. Trobriand social cohesion is largely sustained by the reproduction of social relations through wealth creation and circulation. The production and redistribution of exchange items, particularly yams and *doba*, reflect a large degree of gender parity wherein the contribution of men's and women's labor is valued equally, or is equally intrinsic to social viability. The reciprocal exchange system strongly valorizes personal agency and the consensual engagement of participants who act with others in mind. The primary value accorded to maintaining interclan relations and regenerating matrilineal identity through *sagali* transactions is a significant measure of the historical stability and resilience of Trobriand society as it interacts with the effects of modernity (Weiner 1980b; Jolly 1992).[2] Yet the vital significance of *sagali* in providing coherence for Trobriand social relations, by dealing with death and sustaining regeneration through future reciprocations, also gives one pause when considering the potential impact of HIV on the capacity to cope with the demands of social obligation in response to unprecedented disease and death.

Trobrianders apply their cultural models of disease to biomedical representations of HIV, drawing associations between *sovasova* and the "signs and symptoms" of AIDS and expressing confidence that traditional treatments for *sovasova* can be used to treat and cure HIV-related illnesses. While reaffirming cultural knowledge and the efficacy of traditional medicine, this application also allows for complacency among people who believe that AIDS is nothing to worry about if it can be treated with traditional knowledge. Such convergences, or the "mixture of ideas" in the words of the Trobriand health extension officer, involve an interactive process of knowledge production, which holds the potential "to promote mutual respect, communication across boundaries, and exchange where it may be beneficial" (Hahn 1995:2). Indeed, the intrinsic values of reciprocal exchange and difference in Trobriand ideology are highly compatible with a productive medical pluralism. The process of exchange between different interpretive frameworks facilitates shared comprehension and provides the basis for ensuring the coherence of HIV prevention and treatment programs within communities of belonging.

Peter Piot, former executive director of UNAIDS, talks about the "familiarization" of the epidemic (2008), a notion that reflects the continuing transformation of our understanding of HIV and different stages of experience and response within different contexts. Regardless of the debates about how best to categorize epidemic contours in Papua New Guinea—whether isolated, concentrated, clustered, generalized, or feminized—HIV has become familiarized.[3] Buttressed by injections of donor funding and framed by imported models of meaning, PNG's national program of response to the epidemic has undergone several phases and reiterations since the early 1990s in the politically charged process of making HIV visible as an issue for the nation's development. Many parts of the country now have been reached by an array of projects and resources, with growing numbers of people becoming involved in the implementation of various HIV-related activities. Circulating discourses about sexual behavior, risk, and disease have settled into local landscapes and interacted with local ways of knowing. Slowly, but increasingly, the provision of medical treatment, care, and support for people living with HIV is becoming a reality (Kelly et al. 2009). Papua New Guinea's experience of the dynamic epidemic, within and across political borders and borders of being, demonstrates how responding to HIV has become a "form of participation in the modern world" (Swidler 2006:283).

While the presence of HIV is firmly established in the national consciousness, the destructive effects of fear, stigma, and blame continue to plague the response in many places throughout the country. Standardized categories of risk and biased assumptions about the "drivers" of HIV continue to inform program interventions and behavioral surveillance exercises. Aspects of social structure and cultural context remain hidden, while the statistical analysis of individual practice dominates the push for evidence-based program strategies, particularly now that medical interventions have gained importance with the introduction of affordable drug therapies.

For more than two decades, the global response to HIV has been framed not simply as a public health problem but in terms of development. Governments have been encouraged to adopt multisectoral responses to mitigate the social and economic impact of national epidemics (Collins and Rau 2000; Danziger 1994). With the advent of antiretroviral drugs and increased access to these therapies through the Global Fund, national programs are addressing HIV within a biomedical paradigm once again. This shift presents significant challenges for countries like Papua New Guinea, with poorly resourced primary health-care services and limited capacity to provide specialist services. The shift reveals the "paradoxical spiral" of HIV—that of striking a balance between resources for sustained prevention efforts and the commitment to ensure universal access to drug therapies (Bowtell 2007:8). Yet the potential for HIV programs to transform the health-care delivery system and to enhance the relationship between communities and health services holds promise. As Papua New Guinea's national program of response evolves to accommodate changing epidemiology, an expanded program of HIV treatment and care services is expected to enhance the effectiveness of prevention strategies (NAC 2010). Maintaining the momentum for HIV prevention, coupled with the provision of treatment and care for people with HIV, potentially will activate a rights-based movement for improving the range and quality of all health services.

However, until the deep-rooted structural and social inequalities of resource distribution, wealth creation and power, and gender relations are effectively addressed to diminish the transmission of HIV throughout the world, the importance of communication will remain vital to the ongoing response. Effective prevention starts with critical appreciation of the way people make sense of the epidemic. Prominent AIDS theorist and activist Cindy Patton stresses the obligation to "continually reevaluate the concepts through which we understand HIV, looking closely at how the multiple levels of experience and the multiple forms of knowledge interrelate and change over time" (Patton 2002:xxiv). Like sexuality and disease, HIV prevention is above all a social process. Creating spaces for dialogue and reflection allows communication to move beyond the language of intervention and engage meaningfully with local notions of capacity, resilience, and empowerment. Approaches that emerge from the values of social connectedness and collective action have greater potential for effecting change.

Sexual identities and desires are diverse and mutable. The representation of Trobriand sexuality in this book is limited to the heteronormative narrative that dominated group discussions and self-representations. What became quickly apparent during the course of research was the willingness among Trobrianders to participate in reflective and open dialogue and to consider their own susceptibility to HIV in relation to cultural norms and practices. In contrast to other places in Papua New Guinea, where moralistic and religious responses to the epidemic thwart communication about sexuality and HIV prevention (see Butt and Eves, eds. 2008; Dundon 2007; Hammar 2007; Keck 2007), information about HIV is met in the Trobriands by a generally candid receptiveness and a collective interest to address the implications of a looming epidemic. Opportunities for community conversations are accommodated within the established social structures of the village and the church. Furthermore, sexual consensus and mutual pleasure are recurrent themes in people's mediations. Such values provide an important entry point for addressing the range of sexual experience and sexual risk in relation to HIV, as well as addressing gender asymmetries in acting on sexual desire and reciprocating trust. This is especially important where male mobility and infidelity are conjoined, such as during pregnancy and lactation when abstinence defines sexual relations within marriage.

Attention given to HIV as a pressing issue in the Trobriands waxes and wanes in direct response to the irregular flow of resources and program support orchestrated from beyond the islands. In 2010, the paramount chief put a request to the National AIDS Council Secretariat for renewed support for HIV leadership training and for efforts by the national authority to "ascertain the spread of the virus and find ways to help prevent its spread" (Gerawa 2010). The subsequent assessment tour by NACS officials and the NACS-sponsored workshops received national media attention, with reference to the Trobriands' "open lifestyle when it comes to sex and love" and the indictment of "cultural norms" for spreading the virus (Gerawa 2010). The assessment stirred further speculation and rumor about HIV prevalence in the islands, and the official line from NACS was that more testing was required "to state with any accuracy the extent of the spread of HIV" (Gerawa 2010).

The heavy reliance on biomedical technologies of surveillance and testing for building the evidence base for HIV programs raises serious ethical questions about the measurement practices that dominate the global response (Setel 2009). The authority vested in quantitative evidence sets a dangerous precedent for further dislodging sexual practice from cultural meanings and experience and from the social structures and spaces that shape sexual geographies. Responses to HIV require a

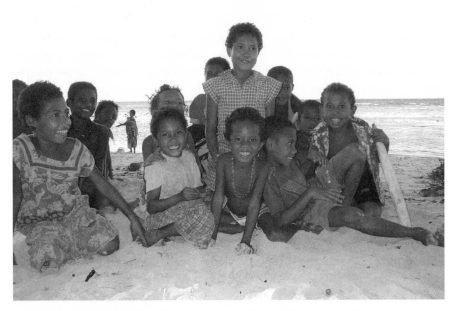

FIGURE 8.1. • Young children on the beach at Kuyawa village, July 2003

move beyond measuring and mapping individual behavior to more closely account for the structural issues of resource distribution and access to opportunities and services, as well as how these factors dynamically influence social risk and the capacity for prevention.

Carol Jenkins's warning during the initial years of Papua New Guinea's response to the impending epidemic was prophetic: "In the rush to develop programmes to diminish the spread of HIV, we must be aware that we could do lasting damage to the image of sexuality we create for ourselves" (1993:55). At this point in the nation's history of responding to HIV, marked by an industry of interventions and technical advice, it is important to reconsider how the discursive power of standardized models of HIV prevention affects the capacity to respond in locally meaningful ways. My involvement in the national response in PNG has made me acutely aware of how the language of prevention can discredit and damage people and communities when it fails to connect with the complexities of lived experience. While my motivation for research comes partially from the fear of a future foretold, I am also deeply apprehensive that an unmediated metanarrative of AIDS will cause people to retract and disengage from messages about HIV prevention in a resistant effort to protect their sense of cultural identity and integrity. By honoring fidelity to the place I feel most at home in PNG, it is my hope that the representation of the Trobriands in this book will help counter the persistent generalizations about people and cultures in PNG that pervade the interventionist response to HIV and will open up space for talking about sexuality in positive, life-affirming ways.

Ethnographic research often is dismissed for not being expedient in producing findings to contribute to the evidence base for informing policies and strategies. In-depth analysis of one particular context also raises questions about the ability to generalize findings, a valued feature of quantitative inquiry in the biomedical paradigm of knowledge production. However, in the rush to respond to the epidemic with statistical evidence, the particulars of place and the importance of process tend to get overlooked. Ethnographic research offers a sound ethical and participatory framework for engaging people in the ongoing process of knowledge production and HIV prevention. The findings from my research suggest that reflective dialogue makes visible the presence of HIV in the collective body of cultural meanings and enables people to act on new knowledge. The Trobriands underscore the importance of cultural specificity in approaches to HIV prevention and, more strategically, challenge the negative assessments of sexuality that dominate the discourse of HIV and AIDS in Papua New Guinea and beyond.

The future is buoyed by Diana's candid appeal to a group of adult men and women during a village awareness session. Her advice to "just relax" is about dissipating the fear of AIDS, not about being disinterested or complacent. Similar to Ethel's entreaty, Diana's insights are especially powerful in the way she positions agency resolutely in the ongoing process of knowing and doing.

> Let's not take regret into our minds. Let's not use this time as a time of regret. These days we should just relax and do our part so that we won't regret in the future. So let's not worry about the question mark. Let's relax and take in the messages and not worry in fear about where AIDS is coming from. So all these things we have heard and learned, we must take them, use them, and claim them as our own. [Taped group discussion, 13 November 2003. Translated into English.]

Glossary

Kiriwina	English
agutoki	thank you
aiseki	who knows
amakawala	what about, how
avaka	what
avakapela	what for, why
baisatuta	now, this instant
baloma	spirit of the dead
besa	that, this, here, there
besobeso	this way and that way, random carelessness, loose
bidalasi	they will regenerate
bidubadu	plenty
bilamapula	physically reciprocal movement between partners during sexual intercourse that results in orgasm
bisila	streamers cut from pandanus leaves
biu	to pull
bobwailila	love, gift, generosity, contribution
bogwa	already, enough, affirmative
bomala	taboo
bubu	relational term used reciprocally between grandparents and grandchildren
bubuna	custom, habit, behavior; also glossed as "culture"
bukumatula	bachelor house
buwa	betel nut
buwala	gift given by boys and men to their sexual partners
buyai	blood
bwagau, bogau	sorcery
bwala	house
bwena	good, yes
dala	subclan or lineage
deli	with, to follow behind, line up one after another; signifies the last series of distributions in sagali
dikwadekuna	itch, sexual pleasure, orgasm
dimdim	white person
doba	bundles of dried banana leaves used for sagali, brightly colored banana and pandanus fiber skirts, skirt

doridori	belt
gala	no
gimwala	buy, sell
ginigini	write, carve
gogebila	to carry on the head
guyau	chief, chiefly clan rank
igau	wait
inamasi	our mother (plural exclusive)
kabisilova	magic used to break off an existing relationship or to cause someone to become estranged from their partner
kabiyamala	contribution, to go with something in hand
kabuyai	menstrual blood
kabweli	apology, appeasement
kadam	his or her maternal uncle
kaidawagu	incised boards used for scraping banana leaves for *doba*
kaikela	leg, feet
kailagila	cooking hearth made with three stones, foundation
kaimelu	main *sagali* distribution to acknowledge the work of all people who provide support
kaimwasila	attraction magic
kaisisu	customary habits, daily routines
kaisosau	large drum
kaiwosi	dance
kakau	deceased's spouse
kalova	to wean
kapikapi	head band
kapisi	sorry
kapu	bereaved parents; signifies deceased's father's line in sagali distributions
kapugula	unmarried female, prime of life, to be sexually active (verb)
karekwa	fabric
karibom	all-night dance promenade during harvest festivities
kariga	death
kasusu	last-born child
katakewa	pole, to carry on the shoulder or on a pole
katoula	illness
katubaiasa	to prepare, to dress
katuigaki	flippant disregard of warning
katuneniya	small drum
katupolusa	hamlet
katupwana	hide
katupwela	to fold
katuvila	to turn over, series of marriage transactions between two families
kaukwau	morning
kaula	food

kauwela	first sagali distribution to repay those who provided food and support throughout the mourning period
kayasa	yam harvest competition
kayta	sexual intercourse
kaytabula	sexual partner from father's clan
kelawodila	trees of the forest, herbal and magical treatments
kepou	singers, drummers, and sponsors in center of circle dance
keyawa	special exchange relations
kivili nanola	to turn the mind, influence, persuade
kokola	fear, afraid
kopoi	to carry baby or dead body during mourning, nurture
kubukwabuya	collective term for unmarried male and female youth
kumila	four ranked matrilineal clans
kuvi	long ceremonial yams
kwaiveka	very big
kwaiwaga	love magic
kwebila	aromatic plant used for dancing and in magic spells
lakwava	(his) wife
liga	tree with small leaves
litulela	children of father; signifies working for father's side in *sagali*
lopogu	my stomach
lubaila	boyfriend and girlfriend, sexual partner
lubwau	soup, distribution of exchange valuables to those who cared for a sick person
lumkola	feeling
makala	like, similar to
mapula	price, equivalent transaction
maunauwela	germs, parasites, worms
meguva	chanted magic
midimidi	streamers
migila	face
milamala	yam harvest season
minumauna	germs, parasites, worms
mitasi	eyes
mokwita	true
momona	semen and vaginal fluids
mosila	shame
mwasawa	game, play
mwau	heaviness, sadness
mweki	go to or visit, poetic synonym for sexual intercourse
nakakau	widow
nanamsa	reflection, thought
nanola	his or her mind
nanomekusa	mind moves toward nothing, no solution
nene	to search

nikoli	knowledge
numwaiya	mature woman
nunu	breasts, breast milk, to suck, term of endearment for deceased mother
nupisi	budding breasts
nupiyakwa	breasts that stand up firm and tight or breasts filled with milk
nutaiya	fallen breasts, whether dry or lactating
ospeta	hospital
paisewa	work
pela	for, because
peta	food basket
pokesa	ulcerous sore, sexually transmitted infection
randasi	around us (from English)
sagali	mortuary exchange feast, general term for distribution of exchange valuables
saimatala	to put into public view
saina	very
sainagaga	very bad
seluva	tying together strips of dried banana leaves to make doba
sepituki	joining or uniting
sepwana	mourning skirts made and worn by clan members of the deceased's spouse and father, special category of doba distribution in sagali
simwakaina	sweet
sovasova	taboo against intraclan sexual relations and marriage between cross-sex siblings, ethnophysiological ailment that results from breach of taboo
susuma	pregnancy
tabu	relational term for ancestral founders of dala, grandparents and grandchildren, father's sister, father's sister's husband, and father's sister's daughter; and from a female ego's standpoint, mother's brother's son and mother's brother's daughter
tabusia	relatives on father's side, third person inclusive
tapiokwa	tapioca, dance chant
tau	boy, male
taytu	yams
tilewai	flattery, compliment
toginigini	student
tokinabogwa	at the beginning of time
toliu'ula	organizing sponsor of an event
toliyouwa	workers at sagali
tomota	people
tomwaiya	old man
toyuvisa	one who untangles, specialist healer
tubukona	moon

tubwa	age group of mixed gender, generation
tomakava	people unrelated
tutabaisa	nowadays
tuvalua	free from shame, confident, brave
ulatile	unmarried male, prime of life, to be sexually active (male)
uliweli	jealousy
ulo	my
u'ula	reason, basis, foundation
vaipaka	divorce
valova	exchanges made to accumulate doba
valu	village
veguwa	valuables
veibibila	arranged marriage
vevai	in-law
veyalela	working sagali for one's own dala
veyola	true kin
vinavana	scented leaves worn for dancing
vivila	girl, female
wawoya	uncertainty
wokuva	empty, to be finished, single-mindedly
wosimwaya	circle dance, traditional dance repertoire
wotia	catch of fish strung together on a rope, special form of exchange
yawala	relational term used reciprocally between parents and their daughters' and sons' spouses; –gu is first-person pronominal suffix; –la is third-person pronominal suffix
yeigu	I, me
yena	fish
yokwa	you (singular)
yakidasi	us, we (plural exclusive)
yopoi	abortion
yowai	fight
yoyowa	witchcraft, witch

Tok Pisin	**English**
asples	place of origin
karamap	to cover up, branded commercial condoms
koap	to go up, sexual intercourse
lainap	group rape or serial intercourse involving a group of men lining up to have sex with a woman
long	to, at, for
marit	marriage
pamuk	prostitute
pasindia meri	passenger woman or prostitute
sanap wantaim	stand up together, unite
tambu	taboo, in-law

Notes

PROLOGUE

1. See Baldwin 1945 for an exegesis on the repertoire of songs used in the *wosimwaya* genre of dance.
2. Figures obtained from the Milne Bay Administration Planning and Coordination Division based on 2000 PNG National Census.
3. *Sagali* is described in more detail in Chapter 4.
4. Personal communication with local agent. The kina is PNG's national currency and was worth about forty cents to the US dollar in 2003.
5. "Islands of Love" is used to describe other islands in Oceania as well, particularly Tahiti and Samoa. The label is historically imbued with European visions of a sexualized Pacific paradise, dating back to the first European voyages and cross-cultural encounters in the eighteenth century (see Jolly, Tcherkézoff, and Tryon, eds. 2009; Tcherkézoff 2004).
6. Journal notes, 16 December 2000.
7. See the ethnographic film *Trobriand Cricket: An Ingenious Response to Colonialism*, produced by Gary Kildea and Jerry Leach, 1974.
8. *Post Courier*, 7 August 2006.
9. Battaglia (1995) provides an account of how the national media in PNG has been used strategically by Trobrianders to communicate the rhetoric of cultural pride, identity, and differentiation while also serving internal political interests.
10. Trobriand word used interchangeably as "custom," "behavior," and "habit"; also glossed as "culture."
11. As hosts to a long succession of anthropologists since the days of Malinowski, Trobrianders are well versed in the purpose and methods of ethnographic fieldwork.
12. The power of geographical delineations to "naturalize" cultural difference has had great influence in anthropology, as acknowledged by Gupta and Ferguson (1997:8). They discuss how "the culture area remains a central disciplinary concept that implicitly structures the way in which we make connections between particular groups of people we study and the groups that other ethnographers study" (9). The name "the Massim," which identifies geographically the numerous and diverse populated islands in the Solomon Sea east of the main island of New Guinea, is an example of anthropological mapping that has no linguistic or cultural salience in the inhabitants' collective identifications.
13. See, for instance, Strathern 1988:1–21 for a discussion of the comparative method in anthropology, which points to the distinction between the theoretical objectives of ethnographies and the people whose cultures are studied and described.

CHAPTER 1

1. This distinctive capacity of HIV is acknowledged particularly in literature on the experience of living with HIV and AIDS. See for example Lather and Smithies 1997.

2. The two main models are the Health Belief Model (Becker, ed. 1974) and the Theory of Reasoned Action (Fishbein and Ajzen 1975).

3. "Prevention of Parent-to-Child Transmission" is the preferred term in PNG to include male partner involvement.

4. The cornerstone of many HIV prevention programs throughout the world, the ABC slogan has been given various reiterations by different organizations but basically stands for "Abstain, Be faithful, use a Condom." The slogan was reportedly first adopted by the Botswanan government in the late 1990s for a national media campaign, utilizing the following message on billboards throughout the country: "Avoiding AIDS as easy as . . . Abstain Be faithful Condomise" (Kanabus and Noble 2005). UNAIDS has revised and elaborated the slogan to highlight "combination prevention" and provides an expanded definition under the following headings: "A means abstinence or delaying sexual initia- tion, B means being safer by staying faithful or reducing the number of sexual partners, and C means correct and consistent condom use" (UNAIDS 2004:73).

5. Access to antiretroviral (ART) drug therapy in PNG is a contentious matter entangled in global policies and issues concerning health disparities and resource inequities, as well as the limited capacity of the PNG health system to deliver services and monitor treatment adherence. ART is still not yet widely available or accessible in PNG, except through a few selected health facilities and, increasingly, through private medical practitioners. The implementation of a pilot project to introduce ART commenced in Port Moresby in 2004 and was phased gradually into other tertiary hospitals in urban centers. Financial and technical support for expanding HIV testing and treatment services is provided through the Global Fund to Fight AIDS, TB and Malaria, and the Clinton Foundation HIV/AIDS Initiative.

6. The concern for cultural relevance was demonstrated in the staging of the 2006 Melane- sian Arts Festival, held in Fiji, with the theme "Living Cultures, Living Traditions." The Fijian Ministry for Health, in collaboration with the Secretariat of the Pacific Commu- nity and other partners, organized various HIV awareness activities during the festival, with the overall message that HIV is a threat to the survival of Melanesian cultures and traditions.

7. See Borrey 2000:110 for a description of how the assertion is reinforced by the rhetoric that PNG customs are consistent with introduced Christian values and, hence, open discussions about sexuality are suppressed on both grounds simultaneously.

8. See, for instance, Abu-Lughod 1991, Brumann 1999, and Moore 1999. But see Schoepf 1995:35 for an analysis of how biomedical approaches to HIV in Africa also have ignored scholarship that critiques the role of anthropology in perpetuating colonial perspectives of African cultural traditions.

9. See Hirsch et al. 2009:28–30 for a discussion of how theoretical turns in the discipline of anthropology have framed ways of thinking about cultural diversity between and within different contexts.

10. Reported data on HIV infection is obtained from sentinel surveillance sites (antenatal, STI, and TB clinics), voluntary counseling and testing sites, screening of blood dona- tions, and clinical diagnoses. Currently, there is no formal notification system for HIV- related deaths in Papua New Guinea (National AIDS Council and National Department of Health 2009).

11. Drug prophylaxis programs for the prevention of mother-to-child transmission com- menced in 2003 but still only reach a small proportion of the HIV-infected pregnant women in the country, with national coverage reported at only 12.2 percent in 2009 (NACS 2006:15, 23; NACS and Partners 2010:26).

12. The gender asymmetry in reported HIV cases in people ages fifteen to twenty-nine years likely reflects greater numbers of women being tested.

13. Female pollution refers to cultural ideologies that view women's sexual and reproductive physiology, including menstruation, pregnancy, and childbirth, as contaminating and dangerous to men, or imbued with sacred and supernatural powers. But see Jolly 2002b:21 for the way female pollution is also conceptualized as "sacred danger" in relation to ancestral power.

14. In a country with more than 850 different languages, Tok Pisin, an English-lexicon creolized language, is one of three official languages spoken in Papua New Guinea, the others being English and Hiri Motu.

15. The NAC was established as a statutory body in 1997 by an act of parliament. Papua New Guinea's first multisectoral strategy was developed over a ten-month period in 1997; it involved broad consultation and the participation of over eighty individuals and organizations comprising six working groups on priority areas for strategic planning (Government of PNG and UNDP 1998). The second multi-sectoral strategy was developed in 2004 and launched in 2006 (Government of PNG and NAC 2006). The third national multisectoral strategy, the National HIV Strategy, 2011–2015, was developed in 2009 (National AIDS Council 2010b).

16. The World Bank (2004:26) reports that the total amount of committed resources provided by various international agencies to support the national response was in excess of US$8 million for 2003–2004 alone. This amount reflects a portion of the AUD$30 million commitment by the Australian Agency for International Development (AusAID) over a five-year period from 2000 to 2005 for the National HIV/AIDS Support Project. Beginning in 2004, the Global Fund to Fight AIDS, Tuberculosis and Malaria has provided funds of more than US$17 million to support the introduction and availability of antiretroviral therapies in PNG (Rudge et al. 2010).

17. Begun in October 2000, the five-year project was funded by AusAID, the leading donor partner in the national response. Managed by an Australian management company, the project supported activities in education and awareness raising, counselling and care, policy development, surveillance systems, clinical services, and strengthening capacity within NACS (AusAID 2006). The second AusAID program of support, called Sanap Wantaim (Tok Pisin for "stand up together"), commenced in 2007.

18. Taped group discussion, 15 October 2003.

19. For examples of media reports and editorials that refer to the "AIDS war" see *Post Courier* 2005a, 2005b and the *National* 2005. See Cullen 2005, 2006 for a historical review of media coverage of the HIV epidemic in Papua New Guinea.

20. See Hammar 2007, 2008, 2010 for discussions of moralistic and alarmist responses to the perceived threat of HIV and AIDS in various communities throughout Papua New Guinea. See also Dundon 2007 and Haley 2010.

21. The concept of "community conversations" is promoted by the United Nations Development Programme (UNDP) as a participatory technique for communities to break the silence surrounding HIV and generate discussion and insights on the social and cultural factors that contribute to its spread.

CHAPTER 2

1. Beginning in 2003, the PNG national response to HIV focused on expanding the provision of testing, treatment, and care services, including a major scaling up of voluntary counseling and testing (VCT) services. By the end of 2009, more than two hundred

VCT facilities throughout the country had been established and accredited for HIV testing, although none were located in the Trobriands. This remains the case at the time of writing. National HIV sero-surveillance sites at antenatal and STI clinics have not included the Trobriands.

2. The first project was a nationwide benchmark study of sexual and reproductive knowledge conducted in 1993, which included the Trobriands in the regional sample (NSRRT and Jenkins 1994). The more recent project was called "Community Based HIV/AIDS and STI Prevention Programs in Trobriand Islands and Karkar Island: Using Traditional and Community Leaders' Initiatives." Research commenced in 2002 with a series of training and recruitment workshops, and involved a baseline knowledge, attitude, and practice (KAP) questionnaire survey, focus group discussions, and individual life-history interviews. For various extraneous reasons, the project ceased before data analysis was completed and written up.

3. I introduce all three women in Chapter 3 and discuss research methodology. Although we share the same surname, Diana and I are not related.

4. The Kiriwina root verb *nikoli* means to understand, to know. The verb conjugation using the prefix *ta-* and suffix *-si* designates plural 3+ inclusive pronoun; the prefix *bi-* denotes incomplete or ongoing action; the prefix *ni-* places emphasis on the immediate time frame.

5. I address the issues of condom supply, distribution, and use in Chapter 7.

6. The "awareness" that the woman refers to was a one-time information session conducted in her village in 2002 by a team of local health workers and community volunteers as part of the community-based research project conducted by the PNG Institute of Medical Research (see note 2, this chapter). It was the only time an HIV awareness session was held at this particular village.

7. The practice of reflexivity, or turning back on oneself to engender critical awareness of the self in relation to others, conveys the social context of the "shared communicative world" of ethnographic research (Mallet 2003:15), where the researcher's standpoint and social position influences the findings. Feminist anthropology has brought to the fore the importance of reflexive engagement in ethnographic encounters and the coproduction of knowledge (Abu-Lughod 1991; Harding 1987; Moore 1999). Reflexivity "enables researchers to critically consider their own cultural biases and negotiate various ways of seeing," and is "particularly sensitive to the socially constructed nature of knowledge production" (Jacobs-Huey 2002:791).

8. See Malinowski 1916, 1929 for descriptions of *milamala*. I return to a discussion of *milamala* in Chapter 7.

9. The suggestion that sexual activity was "taboo" for pubescent girls and boys during an earlier period of time contrasts with Malinowski's account (1929) and colonial administration and missionary reports from the late nineteenth and early twentieth centuries (Reed 1997; Young 1989). Perhaps Bomi's view reflects the influence of several generations of Christian doctrine. Clearly, the supposed taboo is contestable, as suggested by her grandmother's testament. The problematic accounting for behavior change over time and the contestations of taboo were frequent points of discussion during my research. Here I suggest a more nuanced interpretation of her statement concerning continuity and change. I return to this issue in Chapter 5.

10. See Vance 1991:878 for a discussion of how the conventional anthropological approach to sexuality uses a "cultural influence model," which views sex as a universal and natural category of being that is simply influenced, not constructed, by culture.

11. See Lock 1993 for a critical review of how anthropology has theorized the interface between cultural ideology and embodied practice. Margaret Lock observes, "The ques-

tion of the body requires more than reconciling theory with practice. It brings with it the difficulty of people both having and being bodies" (136).

CHAPTER 3

1. These movements between home and field, where ethnographic emplacement is juxtaposed with intimate ties, evoke the notion of "homework" used by anthropologists who engage in research in their own communities of belonging (Jacobs-Huey 2002; Teaiwa 2002; Visweswaran 1994). See Enslin's reflections (1994) on her position of relatedness as a daughter-in-law in the Nepalese community where she does research.

2. *Asples* means place of origin in Tok Pisin. The term was first used in relation to research by the PNG National Sex and Reproduction Research Team (NSRRT), which engaged local researchers to conduct life-history interviews and focus-group discussions in their own languages and communities (NSRRT and Carol Jenkins 1994:8).

3. *Yawala* is the relational term used reciprocally between parents and their daughters' and sons' spouses; *-gu* is first-person pronominal suffix; *-la* is third-person pronominal suffix.

4. Lepani Watson had a long and distinguished public life. He represented the Trobriands as an elected member of the first House of Assembly at pre-independence and was the first premier of Milne Bay Province from 1983 to 1986. He passed away on 17 February 1993, in Vakuta, aged sixty-seven. The Kiriwina word *tomwaiya* is a term of respect.

5. The kinship term *tabu* is complex and holds multiple meanings, as expounded by Weiner (1979:339–40). Broadly, *tabu* refers to the ancestral founders of *dala*; grandparents and grandchildren, reciprocally; father's sister, father's sister's husband, and father's sister's daughter; and from a female ego's standpoint, mother's brother's son and mother's brother's daughter. Linguistically, *tabu* does not convey the notion of taboo, or *bomala* in Kiriwina language.

6. Veitania was an enthusiastic student for several weeks before she opted to be "just a village girl" because she wanted to spend the days with her close friend, Bosewaga, a girl of the same age who was not enrolled in school; Bosewaga later joined my mother-in-law's household for an extended period.

7. See Malinowski 1929, Plate 16. Also refer to pages 49–50 for Malinowski's description of young children's pastimes, including picnic outings.

8. See Senft 1998a:84 for an analysis of this idiom and other Trobriand idioms concerning bodily emotions.

9. Dobu Island is part of the group of islands known collectively as the D'Entrecasteaux, southwest of the Trobriands. Lepani Watson's mother was from Dobu.

10. Although there are only a handful of television sets in the Trobriands, the TV metaphor is not anomalous. Allusions to recorded and televised images and action often pepper stories and jokes. An observation made by a young woman influenced my analogy: "In the village we sit and look at the bushes and sea, people walking, whatever blocks our sight. In Moresby, the television blocks our sight!"

11. See Weiner 1980a for a review of how the term *mapula* is interpreted in the anthropological literature on exchange theory. In the broadest sense, *mapula* refers to an equivalent transaction, or the exchange value of an item. The most salient meaning of the term concerns transactions of wealth items in an ongoing exchange relationship. *Mapula* is also used to designate commercial transactions (e.g., the payment or cost of trade store goods), while the actual process of bartering or buying and selling goods is *gimwala*.

12. See Demian 2000 for what she terms the "aesthetics" of work and how relationships are visibly enacted and evaluated through the effects of labor among Suau speakers on the

southern mainland of Milne Bay Province. See also Kuehling 2005 for an analysis of the moral and aesthetic valence of work in Dobu exchange relations.

13. Research objectivity is inherently partial (Strathern 1991). Donna Haraway espouses a feminist "doctrine and practice of objectivity," which reconceptualizes knowledge as situated, embodied, and partial, "tuned to resonance, not to dichotomy" (1988:584–85, 588). She argues for "politics and epistemologies of location, positioning, and situating, where partiality and not universality is the condition of being heard to make rational knowledge claims" (589).

14. Helan Page defines dialogic process as "any communicative behavior in which the position of self is assessed in relation to the other's expressed position in ways that alter or modify further communication" (1988:164).

15. Lanita Jacobs-Huey observes that in the "choreography of ethnographic inquiry," research participants "affect the people and places to which ethnographers have access during fieldwork, thus influencing their research in substantial ways" (2002:793).

16. See note 2 in Chapter 2.

17. See Luker 2004 for a review of the institutional role of churches in the national response to HIV in PNG.

18. See Keck 2007:46 for an account of a similar response to HIV awareness sessions among Yupno people of the Finisterre Range on the PNG mainland.

19. Mallett (2003:127–28; 2003:66, 99) was aware of how her ethnographic presence on Nuakata was to some extent authorized by perceptions that she was an ally of the medical establishment.

20. Michael Ashkenazi and Fran Markowitz state, "Sexuality must always be a part of the contextualising process by which ethnographers place themselves in a defined and visible position," in relation to research participants and to the readers of the texts produced (1999:14).

21. See, for example, Harding 1987; Gluck and Patai, eds. 1991; and Behar and Gordon, eds. 1995.

22. Early in the global pandemic, Vance observed, "Amid an epidemic, researchers press for rapid results and reject the time, patience, and tolerance for uncertainty that ethnographic and deconstructive techniques seem to require" (1991:881).

CHAPTER 4

1. The title of the film was offensive to a large number of people, while others dismissed it with mild irony. One man who resides in Kaibola village, where much of the filming took place, told me he voiced his concern about the title to the director, who appeared "stunned" and then promptly changed the subject. The man expressed his frustration to me, saying, "Why do they keep insisting on this word 'savage' to tell their story?" (Journal notes, 30 July 2003). An undisputed bonus of the production was a CD recording called *Wosi*, a sampling of Trobriand musical genres, recorded during an open invitation workshop for the film score by the film's music director, David Bridie, for which participants received royalty payments.

2. English translations as given in film subtitles. *Dikwadekuna* literally means "itch" but also refers to orgasm.

3. References to Trobriand conception beliefs and the "virgin birth" conundrum include the following: Seligman 1910; Malinowski 1916, 1932; Rentoul 1931, 1932; Austen 1934; Leach 1967; Powell et al. 1968; Sider 1967; Spiro 1968; Montague 1971; Jorgensen 1983; Delaney 1986; Bashkow 1996; Van Dokkum 1997; Mosko 1998. See Jorgensen 1983:2–4 for a succinct summary of the tone of the tangled debate up to the time of his article and the relevant theoretical issues at stake. See Franklin 1997 for a comprehensive exegesis on the

history of conception theory in anthropology. It is noteworthy that the first recorded observation of Trobriand conception beliefs is provided by Seligman (1910:704), who quotes Bellamy, resident magistrate and medical doctor, as categorically stating, "Intercourse is recognized as the cause of children, although single girls who become pregnant have a curious habit of blaming some or other portion of their diet."

4. Journal notes, 3 September 2003.

5. Interview notes, 15 September 2003.

6. Interview notes, 6 December 2000. Compare Jenkins's analysis of other places in PNG (2007:16–18), and Holly Buchanan-Aruwafu's analysis of other places in the Pacific (2007:114, 117).

7. The consensual and transactional dynamics of Trobriand sexuality find similar expression in other Massim societies. See for instance Battaglia 1990; Kuehling 2005; Lepowsky 1993; and Macintyre 1987. See Braun, Gavey, and McPhillips 2003 on the Western discourse of reciprocity in heterosexual activity.

8. In Kiriwina language, *tau* is male and *vivila* is female. See Malinowski 1929:51 for a listing of gender and age designations. Weiner observes, "Young people are called 'small boys' and 'small girls' until they are in their thirties. Only when villagers are married, have children, and are fully committed to economic and political endeavours will they be considered adults" (1988:67). In using the designations "young boy" and "young girl" to refer to unmarried youth, I am observing Trobrianders' preferred translation and do not imply any disrespect or diminution of agency that such usage may otherwise connote.

9. In Chapter 5, I describe the ethos of *buwala* in more detail and discuss it in relation to the notion of "transactional sex" in HIV discourse.

10. I describe *kwaiwaga* in more detail in Chapter 5.

11. Shame is a common social dynamic throughout Melanesia and is related to the maintenance of social order primarily through avoidance taboos that regulate various kinship and gender relations. See Gibbs and Mondu 2010:31 for a reflection on the notion of shame in PNG in relation to sexuality.

12. In contrast to the substantial ethnographic attention *sovasova* received from Malinowski, Weiner makes no mention of *sovasova* by name or description in her ethnographic accounts (1976, 1979, 1980a, 1988, 1992). This seems anomalous, especially as she focused her extensive interpretive analysis of Trobriand kinship ideology on the brother-sister relationship. Chapter 5 addresses the chronic illness of *sovasova* that results from the breach of the taboo.

13. But see Dowsett 2003 for a critique of how the shift from essentialist views is realigned in HIV discourse, where the incorporation of the gender concept has eclipsed a focus on sexuality. Drawing on the sex/gender dualism, where sex is "nature" and gender is what "culture" does to sexed bodies, the concept reinforces universalistic notions about reproductive sex and the male/female binary while serving as a euphemism for "women."

14. Interview notes, 21 October 2003.

15. Interview notes, 23 October 2003. See Lukere and Jolly 2002 for similar notions throughout the Pacific.

16. Weiner (1976:187) reports a strong preference for marriage partners from within the village population or within neighboring villages that have traditional affiliations. My own observations confirm the tendency for people to marry within the immediate vicinity of their natal village.

17. Melissa Demian discusses how adoption is a "reproductive strategy" among the Suau of Milne Bay Province (2006:136). She states, "As gifts between adults, [children] carry out the objectification of relationships reproduced over time, the creative work required of each generation" (153).

18. The above tableau is based on a *sagali* held on 13 December 2000.

19. "Cousin-brother" is a popular term in Papua New Guinea, which emphasizes the familial kinship ties between male cousins.

20. If the deceased never married because of youth or other circumstances, or if the deceased's father was not from the Trobriands, surrogate *kakau* and *kapu* are nominated to represent the social ties with other *dala*.

21. *Sepwana* is the visual and symbolic essence of *sagali*, providing the organizing framework and regenerative force behind exchange relations. *Sepwana* also refers to the payment of new bundles of *doba* to acknowledge and compensate the mourning of the *kakau* and *kapu*. These *sepwana* piles are the stately hallmark of *sagali* distributions, comprised of carefully stacked fresh *doba* bundles balanced on flat woven baskets and measuring at least one meter in height. Topping the piles of *doba* are new skirts, material, and money. There can be any number of *sepwana* piles at *sagali*, but minimally there have to be two—one for the *kakau* and one for the *kapu*. Additional *sepwana* are made in the name of someone, perhaps a close friend of the deceased, or a favorite nephew or niece, or brothers who work hard for their sisters to acquire *doba* for *sagali*. The women who assemble the *sepwana* piles and carry them to *sagali* on their heads wear new skirts, which are also referred to as *sepwana*. Most *sepwana* skirts these days are sewn out of cotton material, not woven from banana fibers. The skirts are made by the female relatives of the *kakau* and *kapu*, who in turn are the recipients of the *doba* bundles.

22. Kuehling (2005:31, 33) describes the value of work in her ethnography on the ethics of Dobu exchange. Although distinct languages, Dobu and Kiriwina share common words, among them *paisewa* (work) and *tomota* (person). The word *sagali* in Dobu also refers to mortuary exchange distributions, but is markedly different in purpose, structure, and form.

23. In 2000, in preparation for the *sagali* for my mother-in-law's deceased maternal uncle, the last *dala* member of his generation to pass away, Sarah was intensely involved in sewing skirts and dresses. Her personal *doba* inventory included a huge basket measuring two meters in circumference and a meter in height, which contained hundreds of banana leaf bundles. In addition, she had eight banana fiber skirts, forty cotton skirts, twenty-two cotton dresses, four cotton skirts made especially for the *sagali* organizers to wear, twenty pillow cases, and six bolts of material that were cut into two-meter lengths. The daily comings and goings of women with small contributions of *doba* and bits of material to contribute to my mother-in-law's efforts was extraordinary and set the pace for a domestic rhythm that intensified as the day of *sagali* drew closer. She, of course, took careful note of who was supporting her, making a list of names and contributions. *Doba* as a material resource assumes multiple and mutable values depending on how it is put into circulation and how it embodies the labor and intentions of those who activate its value. Women amass bundles of *doba* only when a *dala* death requires them to work for *doba*. At this critical time, when death compels them, women make *doba*, engage in *valova* for *doba*, and receive *doba* from supporters in preparation for a specific *sagali*. No woman would busily produce and store excess *doba* in her house if she is not currently working toward a specific target. To hoard is undesirable and makes one vulnerable to the jealousy of others. For others to view someone as having excess resources when they are not currently working for *doba* in relation to a particular death is the source of great shame. There is a strong continuum of purpose and meaning in the production of *doba* for exchange and in the activity of exchange itself.

24. Journal notes, 9 October 2003. *Deli* is the last series of distributions in *sagali* to inspire ongoing reciprocal support at future *sagali*. The word *deli* is the preposition "with" and also means to "follow behind," or "line up one after another." *Deli* distributions are

paraded in long lines to the recipients. This is the high point in *sagali* when the mourners are "cleaned" by removing their black mourning attire and tying freshly made fiber skirts or cloth material around their hips, and then presented with an array of goods. In addition to skirts, clay pots, woven pandanus mats, and coconut baskets, *deli* items include store merchandise such as cooking pots, plates and cups, cutlery, umbrellas, towels, shirts, and even bras and underpants. With goods and money displayed on poles and cut tree branches, *deli* exudes the consumptive excess of a feast.

25. In Mosko's view, mortuary rituals like *sagali* are ultimately about severing relational ties and obligations, the achieved effect of which he calls "deconception" (1983, 1995). While *sagali* distributions are a form of compensation given to mourners by relatives of the deceased to discharge any further obligations, the overall process involves reconnecting interclan ties. Relational entailments are freed to renew the ongoing process of social reproduction.

26. Chapter 6 addresses witchcraft and sorcery as the underlying causes of illness and death.

27. While the use of the concept is informed by aspects of the Gender and Development (GAD) paradigm, specifically the differential needs and issues facing men and women, and the structural factors that shape inequalities, the term as used in PNG is generally understood in relation to the older Women in Development (WID) theoretical framework, which draws heavily on analysis of the division of labor while focusing on the status of women and the importance of women's rights for achieving equity in development opportunities and benefits (see Parpart, Connelly, and Barriteau, eds. 2000).

28. I acknowledge that, like the WID/GAD debate, "development" is a contested concept with a long genealogy of definitions and approaches. Chambers (1983) was one of the early advocates of a development model that builds on principles of community participation. See Escobar 1991 for a critique of the role of anthropology in development practice.

29. See Zimmer-Tamakoshi 1993 for an argument about how the rhetoric of nationalism in PNG attempts to confine women's gendered identity, and specifically their sexuality, to an idealized notion of the "grassroots" woman who embodies traditional values, as opposed to the educated and liberated modern woman who betrays customary ways for a Western lifestyle. See also Jolly 1996 for a discussion of how women's rights are framed and contested in Vanuatu within ideological tensions between modernity and tradition, individualism and collectivism, and Christian and customary values.

30. I acknowledge the contending discourses on the issue of gender equality. See Jolly 2003 for a discussion of how these discourses relate to questions of sociality, Christianity, and women's activism in Melanesia. See also Strathern 1988:88–92 for an elaboration on the unsuitability of the public/domestic dichotomy for understanding Melanesian sociality.

31. Hirsch et al. (2009:5–8) identify three major shifts in how gender has been conceptualized in public health interventions over the three decades of responding to the HIV pandemic, beginning with acknowledgment of heterosexual transmission, followed by a focus on social inequities between men and women, and, most recently, attention to the ideals of masculinity as a critical aspect of women's HIV risk. However, they argue that the approaches have not adequately addressed the "critical questions of social structure and individual agency" (8). See also Raimondo and Patton 2001.

32. See note 13 in this chapter.

33. Treichler (1999) argues that the ideology of heterosexual superiority, and by inference the primacy of reproductive sex, heavily influenced early scientific models of the virus. She states that homophobia and sexism were "folded imperturbably" into the discourse, which characterized the new disease phenomena as the "gay plague" (xx). Commenting on the silence that surrounded women's susceptibility to HIV during this time, Elizabeth Reid points out that despite early evidence of HIV infection in women, "the characterisa-

tion of the epidemic by gender (male) and sexual orientation (homosexual) remained dominant," and the findings of two critical studies in 1986 "did not elicit a particular concern about women and HIV at the international level" (1996:233).

34. This distinction has been noted widely in the HIV literature. See, for example, Kielmann 1997 and Savage 1996. Representations of prostitution also are cast in terms of victimization, especially in relation to economic and structural constraints, as suggested by the term "survival sex." See Law 2000 for an analysis of how representations of prostitution are undergoing transformation, largely in response to the HIV epidemic, with new emphasis on the agency of the prostitute subject as a "sex worker" in charge of her destiny. Wardlow (2004, 2006) analyzes forms of sex work and female agency in the PNG context.

35. The global pattern of women's susceptibility to HIV infection from intimate partners was acknowledged by the World Health Organization as the key theme for World AIDS Day 2004.

36. The implicit assumption here is that "housewife" refers to a woman in an established and socially recognized relationship with a male partner, whether or not they actually reside together in the same household. It is important to acknowledge that such categories of data collection and analysis do not adequately reflect the fluid and dynamic nature of marital status and household composition in PNG (and elsewhere) and do not necessarily represent women's self-identifications.

37. As quoted from the PowerPoint presentation of findings of the University of Papua New Guinea Public Health knowledge, attitude, and practice study of secondary students in four provinces, National Consensus Workshop, Port Moresby, 17 November 2004.

38. Taped group discussion, 24 October 2003.

39. Weiner concludes her Trobriand monograph by suggesting that to unmask what she calls the Western "myth that denies the fundamental power of women" requires "placing the value of universal womanness within a sociocultural context recognized as powerful within its own right" (1976:236). Her universalistic claim about the inherent value of women's regenerative power has been challenged for perpetuating Western gender dichotomies (see Strathern 1981; Jolly 1992).

40. There are only a few references in the ethnographic literature to traditional methods of contraception used in the Trobriands. Malinowski expresses regret that he did not concentrate attention on this subject, and although he asserts that he had no evidence of any "chemical or mechanical preventives," he was informed that herbal infusions and magical spells were used as abortifacients (1929:167–68). Austen (1934), Bulmer (1971), Weiner (1976), and Pöschl and Pöschl (1985) briefly mention evidence of herbs and magical spells used to induce temporary infertility or abortion. See McDowell, ed. 1988:60–61, 88–90, 108–9, 156, 182–83 and NSRRT and Jenkins 1994:63–67 for overviews of traditional methods of fertility control used in Papua New Guinea. See also Lepowsky 1990:1053 and Mallett 2003:185–89. For regional comparison in the Pacific, see Jolly 2002a:158.

41. Taped group discussion, 31 October 2003.

42. Taped group discussion, 9 January 2001. Fertility control from the perspective of adolescent sexuality and single mothers is discussed further in Chapter 5.

43. The PNG health system promotes family planning services as "birth spacing" for married couples only, with new accepters registered primarily through MCH clinics. Single women generally are dissuaded from seeking family planning services at health centers. Available data from the Family Planning Register Book at Losuia District Health Center reveals only 1,905 new accepters for the period from 1995 to 2003. The majority of registered users from 2000 to 2003 are recorded as married women with at least one live child

(590 of 766), 63 married women have no record of childbirth, and 21 women are recorded as single with no children. The register does not keep records on condom use, nor are condoms discussed as a contraceptive option during MCH clinics. When reviewing the register, I was struck by the number of women who reported having deceased children. While the available data are not adequate for calculating infant mortality rates or interpreting causal factors, the general picture suggests a situation of high infant and child morbidity and mortality, which is consistent with the official figures available for Milne Bay Province from the 2006 Demographic and Health Survey: an infant mortality rate of 69 per 1,000 live births and a child mortality rate for one to four years of age of 28 per 1,000 children (National Statistical Office Papua New Guinea 2010).

44. I received various explanations about the effects of contraceptive herbs on the menstrual cycle (as opposed to herbs for pregnancy termination or sterilization). Some women maintain that herbs suppress menstrual flow while others say that it merely regulates it. Whether ingested herbal methods have a spermicidal effect is not clear. Pöschl and Pöschl (1985:139) report evidence of a particular form of herbal contraceptive that involves inserting into the vagina small balls of plant fibers, which presumably have a spermicidal effect.

45. Papua New Guinea's population policy is a multisectoral framework of action for population and sustainable development, which reflects the ideological emphasis on reproductive rights and responsibilities as articulated in the Programme of Action of the International Conference on Population and Development, held in Cairo in 1994 (Department of Planning and Monitoring 1999). See Basu 1997 for a critique of the paradigmatic shifts in international population policies of the late twentieth century.

46. I return to this issue in Chapter 6.

47. The effect of this strategy is perhaps apparent in the number of children born to Trobriand mission families in the early to mid-twentieth century. I talked to several Trobriand women, aged sixty and over, who were raised on the Oiabia mission station or in the nearby villages of Kavataria and Mulosaida and who report having had over ten siblings born of the same parentage. I have not been able to obtain a current estimate of the fertility rate for the Trobriands; however, the total fertility rate for Milne Bay Province is 5.6 (ages fifteen to forty-nine), according to the PNG 2000 National Census (National Statistical Office 2003).

48. That the fertility puzzle continues to capture attention and curiosity as new waves of students encounter the literature was demonstrated in September 2006 on ASAONET, the Internet listserv of the Association for Social Anthropology in Oceania (www.asao.org/index.html). An anthropology lecturer posted that whenever he teaches Weiner's Trobriand ethnography, his students invariably ask how it is that sexually active young people avoid pregnancy without using contraception. His request for help in explaining the conundrum elicited a voluble and speculative response from more than ten subscribers.

CHAPTER 5

1. See Hammar 2004:1–3 for a critique of HIV terminology, including "sexual debut," which connotes an agency of consent that belies reality for many young girls whose first sexual experience is coerced.

2. *Tubukona* is the celebrated subject of Trobriand folklore, magical chants, and creative expression. The erotic appeal of the human face is metaphorically compared to the radiant glow of the full moon (see Malinowski 1929:296). The agricultural calendar of yam cultivation and harvest follows the seasonal phases of the lunar cycle. Each month

when the sliver of the waxing moon first appears in the sky at dusk, a high-pitched sound resonates throughout the islands as people momentarily stop what they are doing to greet the new moon by singing out, "Woooo," rapidly striking their mouths to produce an ululating effect.

3. Interview notes, 10 October 2003

4. Interview notes, 1 October 2003.

5. The male-to-female sex ratio for the Trobriands is 109 to 87, based on figures from the 2000 National Census. The discrepancy possibly indicates the seriousness of maternal mortality, which at the national level is estimated at 733 per 100,000 live births (National Department of Health 2009). Bellamy's records of vital statistics for 1914 indicate a male-to-female birth ratio of 106 to 100. They also show a distinct gender asymmetry between unmarried males (1412) and unmarried females (856) (Black 1957:237). Bellamy (1990:300–1) suggests that female infanticide occurred in the Trobriands in precolonial times, and he links the practice to customs of yam exchange where a girl would be disadvantaged if she did not have a brother to garden for her. Contemporary reproductive decisions do not indicate a preference for boys over girls. While there seems to be a general preference for the firstborn child to be male, the desire for an equal number of male and female children is widely expressed, as elsewhere in Papua New Guinea (see McDowell 1988:31).

6. Rape is seldom committed in the Trobriands, in contrast to other areas in PNG where high levels of sexual violence are associated not only with rapid social change and urbanization but with customary precedent (see Human Rights Watch 2005; Jenkins 2007; Luker and Dinnen, eds. 2010).

7. Taped group discussion, 22 July 2003.

8. Malinowski concludes *The Sexual Life of Savages* with a transcription and exposition of the *Kumilabwaga* myth, an oral account of the origin of *kwaiwaga*, which Malinowski regards as the "singular rift in traditional doctrine, a dogmatic inconsistency, which makes love and the magic of love derive from brother and sister incest" (1929:451). He explains that the myth "establishes a valid precedent for the efficacy of love magic; it proves that the spells and rites . . . are so powerful that they can even break down the terrible barriers which separate brother and sister and persuade them to commit incest" (459). Weiner (1992:76) interprets the myth as "a celebration of sibling sexuality—the origin of love magic and the more hidden origin of matrilineal reproduction." She uses the myth to make the theoretical claim that sibling intimacy is the basis of matrilineal power, suggesting that Trobrianders believe women are impregnated by ancestral kinsmen (1992:73–74, nn 22, 172) and that "the elaborately ritualized intense sexuality that pervades so much of Trobriand adolescent life is another attempt, unsuccessful at the extreme, to disguise the power of sibling sexuality" (nn 32, 173). I do not think the ethnographic evidence supports such a theoretical interpretation.

9. While the Trobriand phenomenon of *kwaiwaga* provides the most compelling explanation for the surrender of personal sexual autonomy, its cultural logic differs significantly from contexts where the effects of love magic offer an acceptable explanation for unsanctioned or excessive premarital sex (see Bennett 2000).

10. Interview notes, 31 October 2003.

11. Taped interview, 6 August 2003.

12. Interview notes, 1 October 2003.

13. Taped group discussion, 30 June 2003.

14. Lepowsky (1993:103–5) reports that in Vanatinai, *buwa* refers to the initial gift exchange between the matrilines of a young couple prior to marriage.

15. Taped group discussion, 30 June 2003.

16. Taped group discussion, 19 September 2003.

17. Interview notes, 23 June 2003.

18. Taped group discussion, 10 October 2003.

19. However, see Helliwell 1995 for a discussion of how the conflation of "autonomy" and "equality" can seriously misrepresent indigenous understandings of agency and sociality. See Senft 1998a for a linguistic analysis of Trobriand concepts of the mind and body. Compare Lepowsky 1993 on Vanatinai (Sudest Island, Milne Bay).

20. Subsistence productivity is also channeled in response to the challenges of *kayasa*, competitions sponsored by chiefs, which mobilize large-scale efforts toward collective endeavors while rewarding individual achievement (see Malinowski 1922; Battaglia 1986; Campbell 2002).

21. The word *kopoi* means to carry and care for an infant child, as well as to carry a dead person during mortuary rites. Both are valued as performative acts of *paisewa*.

22. Taped group discussion, 15 October 2003. I was told that the practice of *veibibila*, or arranged marriage between cross-cousins, which is largely restricted to chiefly lineages, is not commonly practiced anymore. See Malinowski 1929:80–90.

23. Weiner contends that the "large, communal bachelor houses described by Malinowski (1929) are no longer in existence" (1976:nn 6, 249). Senft also states that during his period of residence in the Trobriands in the 1980s, the institution of *bukumatula* as described by Malinowski was "already history" (1998b:124). It appears there has been a shift from a more collective bachelor house to one that is more personalized. However, younger male siblings will often reside together in an older brother's *bukumatula* until they are ready to construct their own dwellings.

24. Taped group discussion, 9 January 2001. See Lepani 2001:69–70.

25. Interview notes, 1 October 2003.

26. Interview notes, 1 October 2003.

27. See McDowell, ed. 1988 and Lukere and Jolly, eds. 2002 for comparison with other places in PNG and the Pacific.

28. Taped interview, 17 June 2003.

29. The time frame captured by the noun phrase *tutabaisa* (literally, "time-here") is broadly generational. The phrase also is used as a marker of the present in relation to ancestral time, or *tokinabogwa*.

30. Taped group discussion, 31 October 2003. Compare Salomon 2002:87.

31. The matriline's unconditional acceptance of children born to single women is also noted among the Suau (Demian 2006:156–57, n 10).

32. Taped group discussion, 22 July 2003.

33. In both references to *gudukubukwabuya*, Weiner's observations relate to the symbolic significance of the tortoise shell earrings inserted into a baby's pierced earlobes, which are gifts from the child's father. Today the practice of inserting additional shell rings as the child grows is not as common as it was thirty years ago.

34. While not noted by Trobrianders to whom I spoke, these physiological factors are linked as well to evidence of adolescent "subfecundity," which suggests that pubescent females are rarely fully fertile until a year or two after menarche (Whiting, Burbank, and Ratner 1986). See also Nag and Bedford 1969 and Chowning 1969.

35. Taped group discussion, 22 July 2003.

36. The term "unwanted pregnancy" often conflates with "teenage pregnancy" even though unwanted and/or unplanned pregnancies are independent of age and marital status.

37. Compare Burbank and Chisholm 1988.

CHAPTER 6

1. Malinowski (1929) used the spelling *suvosova*. I prefer the spelling used by research participants, which best reflects the contemporary pronunciation of the word in the Kiriwina language and is consistent with the orthography developed by linguist Ralph Lawton (1993).

2. Taped interview, 23 September 2003.

3. Malinowski also used *sovasova* as an analytical device to demonstrate the importance of participant observation fieldwork in unveiling "the polished surface of custom" to reveal contradictions in actual practice (1929:426). He wrote, "What I wish to make clear, by confronting the gist of native statements with the results of direct observation, is that there is a serious discrepancy between the two" (425). In the section on "Exogamy and the Prohibition of Incest" in *The Sexual Life of Savages*, Malinowski launches into a lengthy treatise on the inadequacy of the "technique of question-and-answer" of "modern scientific field-work" to "penetrate to . . . the breach of custom," which he argues can only be attained through language acquisition and prolonged residence (1929:425–29).

4. Interview notes, 16 October 2003.

5. See Tambiah 1983 for a gendered analysis of yoyowa and bwagau.

6. Interview notes, 20 October 2003.

7. Jenny Hughes suggests that in the "saga of oppression and discrimination" that characterized the colonial medical enterprise, Bellamy was "an exception that made other practitioners and officials appear unsympathetic and dictatorial" (1997:234). She also ironically points out that Malinowski makes only two brief references to venereal disease in *The Sexual Life of Savages* (1929:294, 473) and no mention of the extensive treatment program that Bellamy had undertaken. The relationship between Bellamy and Malinowski is discussed by Black (1957:279–80). See also Young (2004:383–87) for a description of the Trobriands at the time of Malinowski's arrival in 1915, which after ten years of Bellamy's administration was "one of the most efficiently governed and healthiest places" in the colonial territory (384).

8. In 1926, Bellamy made a return visit to the Trobriands and prepared a report on vital statistics. He identified two "pandemic waves of influenza" in 1921 and 1925 as being responsible for depopulation during the period from 1919 to 1926 (1990:299). Earlier reports indicate that the population had decreased to 8,500 in 1914 from approximately 10,000 in 1905 (Black 1957:282).

9. The precursor to the existing health center was built in the 1960s on a different site from Bellamy's original lock hospital, which no longer stands.

10. The 2007 estimate of TB prevalence in PNG was 430 per 100,000 population (WHO 2007).

11. Questions on condom use are addressed in Chapter 7.

CHAPTER 7

1. The "Show You Care" poster was one of the first to use photographs of human models rather than cartoon drawings and to shift emphasis away from privileging male protection during sexual "risk-taking" toward promoting consensual, pleasurable sex between partners. See Hammar 2010 for a critique of AIDS awareness materials used in Papua New Guinea.

2. See Hirsch et al. 2009:18–19 for a productive reconceptualization of risk in terms of "social risk," which "highlights how men and women who put themselves 'at risk' of HIV

infection are engaging in behaviors that generally make good sense in a particular social and cultural context."

3. Interview notes, Haydon Abraham, area manager for local level government, 27 October 2003.

4. The "hot spot" metaphor has entered uncritically into PNG's national HIV discourse. In 2003, the PNG National AIDS Council Secretariat embarked on a nationwide social-mapping exercise as the basis for planning HIV programs in provinces and districts and laying the groundwork for the High Risk Settings Strategy (see Lepani 2004 for a critique of this interventionist model). The mapping was heavily framed by assumptions about "high risk" groups and settings, and it marked out "hot spots" of heightened economic and social activity that were viewed as promoting the conditions where "risky" sexual behavior was likely to take place. While the approach sought to identify ways in which risk is socially structured, it was conceptually confined by individualistic and biomedical notions of risk behavior.

5. Unpublished script from HIV/AIDS Community Awareness Theatre Workshop, Alotau, October 2000.

6. Taped group discussion, 10 October 2003.

7. I acknowledge that the freedom to practice culture also involves expectations and pressures on people to behave in normative ways.

8. Taped group discussion, 18 December 2003.

9. Interview notes, 17 June 2003; Taped group discussion, 19 September 2003.

10. Interview notes, 23 October 2003.

11. The "hiding place" translates from *katupwana* (see Chapter 4) and refers here to the secret intimacy of sexual encounters.

12. Recent ethnographic research in the Trobriands by MacCarthy (2010) describes competing discourses among church and community leaders about the "good" and "bad" sides of culture in the context of commercialized tourism and cultural shows.

13. Journal notes, 31 July 2003.

14. Taped group discussion, 10 October 2003.

15. Taped interview, 3 July 2003.

16. The Kiriwina term used for condom in the IMR questionnaire survey was *kapolila kusi*, meaning "wrap the penis." However, I never heard this translation in discussions or interviews. People invariably used "condom" or referred to it indirectly as *miyana vavagi* (literally, "that which is flat," or undefined thing). When I mentioned *kapolila kusi*, people would laugh uproariously and say there was no need to describe the thing in language, adding that they preferred the English word.

17. While resistance to condom use continues to pervade the moralizing discourse in PNG surrounding HIV, important evidence of condom acceptability and use, including female condoms, is reported by various projects involved in HIV prevention activities at the local level. However, the growing acceptance and demand for condoms is directly hampered by a poorly coordinated and managed national system of condom supply and distribution, which has been a persistent issue from the beginning of PNG's strategic response to the epidemic.

18. Taped group discussion, 31 October 2003.

19. Taped group discussion, 19 September 2003.

20. Taped group discussion, 19 September 2003

21. Taped interview, 18 December 2000.

22. Taped group discussion, 18 December 2003.

23. See note 1 in Chapter 2.

24. Interview notes, 14 October 2003.
25. Journal notes, 23 December 2003.
26. Available data for 2008 indicate that only 8.6 percent of all pregnant women in PNG are provided with HIV information, counseling, and testing, and only 4.6 percent of all HIV-positive pregnant women who delivered in health facilities were provided with ART prophylaxis (Inter-Agency Task Team 2009).

EPILOGUE

1. Regional workshop, "HIV/AIDS and Fragile States in Australia's Proximate Region," La Trobe University, Melbourne, 2–3 April 2007, conducted as part of the AIDS, Security and Conflict Initiative.
2. My most recent return visit to Orabesi was in August 2010 to participate in the *sagali* for my mother-in-law, who passed away peacefully in January 2010 at the age of eighty-one. The *sagali* was a massive event that lasted three days and involved more than a thousand participants, including people who traveled home to the Trobriands from urban centers in Papua New Guinea and overseas.
3. Vicki Luker and Sinclair Dinnen (2010:19) prefer the term "endemic" to describe the presence of HIV in PNG because "this reminds us that HIV is here to stay, at least for the foreseeable future."

Bibliography

Abu-Lughod, Lila
    1991   Writing against Culture. In *Recapturing Anthropology: Working in the Present.*
                Edited by Richard G. Fox, pp. 137–62. Santa Fe: School of American Research
                Press.

Adams, Vincanne, and Stacy Leigh Pigg, eds.
    2005   *Sex in Development: Science, Sexuality, and Morality in Global Perspective.*
                Durham, NC: Duke University Press.

Aeno, Herick
    2005   Marriage, Sex, and STDs: Transmission Risks of Papua New Guinea Women as
                Assessed through HIVab Counselling. Paper presented to the Annual Meeting
                of the Association for Social Anthropology in Oceania, Kauai, Hawai'i, 2–5
                February.

Aggleton, Peter, Shalini Bharat, Alex Coutinho, Felecia Dobunaba, Roger Drew, and Tobi Saidel
    2010   Independent Review Group on HIV/AIDS. Report from an assessment visit, 22
                April–5 May 2010, to the PNG National AIDS Council.

Ahearn, Laura M.
    2000   Agency. *Journal of Linguistic Anthropology* 9(1–2):12–15.

Altman, Dennis
    1998   Globalization and the "AIDS" Industry. *Contemporary Politics* 4(3):233–45.

Arney, William Ray, and Bernard J. Bergen
    1984   Power and Visibility: The Invention of Teenage Pregnancy. *Social Science and*
                Medicine 18(1):11–19.

Aruwafu, Holly, Frances Akuani, and Francis Kupe
    2009   *Bio-Behavioral Sentinel Surveillance Survey among Women Attending Port Moresby*
                General Hospital Antenatal (PPTCT) Clinic 2008. Waigani, PNG: Behavioral
                Surveillance Survey Unit, Social and Environmental Studies Division, Papua
                New Guinea National Research Institute.
    2010   *Bio-Behavioral Sentinel Surveillance Survey among Women Attending Lae Friends*
                STI Clinic 2008. Waigani, PNG: Behavioral Surveillance Survey Unit, Social
                and Environmental Studies Division, Papua New Guinea National Research
                Institute.

Ashforth, Adam
    2002   An Epidemic of Witchcraft? The Implications of AIDS for the Post-Apartheid
                State. *African Studies* 61(1):121–43.

Ashkenazi, Michael, and Fran Markowitz
    1999   Introduction: Sexuality and Prevarication in the Praxis of Anthropology. In
                Sex, Sexuality, and the Anthropologist. Edited by Fran Markowitz and Michael
                Ashkenazi, pp. 1–21. Urbana: University of Illinois Press.

Austen, Leo
    1934   Procreation among the Trobriand Islanders. *Oceania* 5:102–18.

Australian Agency for International Development (AusAID)
    2006   *Evaluation of the PNG National HIV/AIDS Support Project.* Evaluation and
            Review Series No. 38. December 2005. Canberra: AusAID.

Baldwin, B.
    1945   *Usituma!* Song of Heaven. *Oceania* 15:201–38.

Ballard, John, and Clement Malau
    2009   Policy Making on AIDS, to 2000. In *Policy Making and Implementation:
            Studies from Papua New Guinea.* Edited by Ron J. May, pp. 369–78. Canberra:
            ANU E Press.

Barnett, Tony, and Justin Parkhurst
    2005   HIV/AIDS: Sex, Abstinence, and Behavior Change. *Lancet Infectious Diseases*
            5(9):590–93.

Barnett, Tony, and Alan Whiteside
    2002   *AIDS in the Twenty-First Century: Disease and Globalization.* New York:
            Palgrave Macmillan.

Bashkow, Ira
    1996   "To Be His Witness If That Was Ever Necessary": Raphael Brudo on
            Malinowski's Fieldwork and Trobriand Ideas of Conception. Footnotes to the
            History of Anthropology. *History of Anthropology Newsletter* 13(1):3–11.

Basu, Alaka M.
    1997   The New International Population Movement: A Framework for a Constructive
            Critique. *Health Transition Review* 7 (Supplement 4):7–31.

Bateson, Mary Catherine
    1994   *Peripheral Visions: Learning along the Way.* New York: HarperCollins.

Battaglia, Debbora
    1986   *"Bringing Home to Moresby": Urban Gardening and Ethnic Pride among Trobriand
            Islanders in the National Capital.* Special Publication 11. Boroko, PNG: Papua
            New Guinea Institute of Applied Social and Economic Research.
    1990   *On the Bones of the Serpent: Person, Memory, and Mortality in Sabarl Island
            Society.* Chicago: University of Chicago Press.
    1995   On Practical Nostalgia: Self-Prospecting among Urban Trobrianders. In
            Rhetorics of Self-Making. Edited by Debbora Battaglia, pp. 77–96. Berkeley:
            University of California Press.
    1997   Ambiguating Agency: The Case of Malinowski's Ghost. *American Anthropologist*
            99(3):505–10.

Bayliss-Smith, Tim
    2006   Fertility and the Depopulation of Melanesia: Childlessness, Abortion, and
            Introduced Disease in Simbo and Ontong Java, Solomon Islands. In *Population,
            Reproduction, and Fertility in Melanesia.* Edited by Stanley J. Ulijaszek, pp. 13–52.
            New York: Berghahn Books.

Becker, Anne E.
    1995   *Body, Self, and Society: The View from Fiji.* Philadelphia: University of
            Pennsylvania Press.

Becker, Marshall H., ed.
    1974   *The Health Belief Model and Personal Health Behavior.* Thorofare, NJ: Charles B.
            Slack.

Behar, Ruth, and Deborah A. Gordon, eds.
  1995   *Women Writing Culture.* Berkeley: University of California Press.

Bell, Diane, Pat Caplan, and Wazir Jahan Karim, eds.
  1993   *Gendered Fields: Women, Men, and Ethnography.* London: Routledge.

Bellamy, R. L.
  1990   Trobriand Vital Statistics in 1926. In *A History of Medicine in Papua New Guinea: Vignettes of an Earlier Period.* Edited by Sir Burton G. Burton-Bradley, pp. 299–310. Kingsgrove, New South Wales: Australasian Medical Publishing.

Bennett, Linda Rae
  2000   Sex, Power and Magic: Constructing and Contesting Love Magic and Premarital Sex in Lombok. Working Paper Series No. 6. Canberra: Gender Relations Center, Australian National University. rspas.anu.edu.au/grc/publications/pdfs/WP_6_Bennett.pdf, accessed 10 August 2008.

Black, Robert H.
  1957   Dr. Bellamy of Papua. *Medical Journal of Australia* 2:189–97, 232–38, 279–84.

Bolton, Ralph
  1992   Mapping Terra Incognita: Sex Research for AIDS Prevention—An Urgent Agenda for the 1990s. In *The Time of AIDS: Social Analysis, Theory, and Method.* Edited by Gilbert Herdt and Shirley Lindenbaum, pp. 124–58. Newbury Park, CA: Sage.

Borrey, Annou
  2000   Sexual Violence in Perspective: The Case of Papua New Guinea. In *Reflections on Violence in Melanesia.* Edited by Sinclair Dinnen and Allison Ley, pp. 105–18. Leichhardt, New South Wales: Hawkins Press.

Bowtell, Bill
  2007   *HIV/AIDS: The Looming Asia Pacific Pandemic.* Lowy Institute Policy Brief. Sydney: Lowy Institute for International Policy.

Boyce, P., M. Huang Soo Lee, C. Jenkins, S. Mohamed, C. Overs, V. Paiva, E. Reid, M. Tan, and P. Aggleton
  2007   Putting Sexuality (Back) into HIV/AIDS: Issues, Theory and Practice. *Global Public Health* 2(1):1–34.

Braun, Virginia, Nicola Gavey, and Kathryn McPhillips
  2003   The "Fair Deal"? Unpacking Accounts of Reciprocity in Heterosex. *Sexualities* 6(2):237–61.

Brison, Karen J.
  1992   *Just Talk: Gossip, Meetings, and Power in a Papua New Guinea Village.* Berkeley: University of California Press.

Broughton, Bernard
  2000   Safe Sex or Healthy Sex? *Development Bulletin* 52:64–52.

Brumann, Christoph
  1999   Writing for Culture: Why a Successful Concept Should Not Be Discarded. Supplement: Theme Issue, "Culture: A Second Chance?" *Current Anthropology* 40:S1–S27.

Brummelhuis, Han Ten, and Gilbert Herdt
  1995   Introduction: Anthropology in the Context of AIDS. In *Culture and Sexual Risk: Anthropological Perspectives on AIDS.* Edited by Han Ten Brummelhuis and Gilbert Herdt, pp. ix–xxiv. Amsterdam: Gordon and Breach.

Brummelhuis, Han Ten, and Gilbert Herdt, eds.
  1995   *Culture and Sexual Risk: Anthropological Perspectives on AIDS*. Amsterdam: Gordon and Breach.

Buchanan-Aruwafu, Holly
  2007   Youth Vulnerability to HIV in the Pacific. In *Cultures and Contexts Matter: Understanding and Preventing HIV in the Pacific*. Edited by Carol Jenkins and Holly Buchanan-Aruwafu, pp. 71–154. Manila: Asia Development Bank. www.adb.org/documents/Books/Cultures-Contexts-Matter/Cultures-Contexts-Matter.pdf, accessed 8 March 2012.

Buchanan-Aruwafu, Holly, and Rose Maebiru
  2008   Smoke from Fire: Desire and Secrecy in Auki, Solomon Islands. In *Making Sense of AIDS: Culture, Sexuality, and Power in Melanesia*. Edited by Leslie Butt and Richard Eves, pp. 168–86. Honolulu: University of Hawaii Press.

Bucholtz, Mary
  2002   Youth and Cultural Practice. *Annual Review of Anthropology* 31:525–52.

Bujra, Janet
  2000   Risk and Trust: Unsafe Sex, Gender, and AIDS in Tanzania. In *Risk Revisited*. Edited by Patricia Caplan, pp. 59–84. London: Pluto Press.

Bulmer, R. N. H.
  1971   Traditional Forms of Family Limitation in New Guinea. In *Population Growth and Socio-Economic Change*. Edited by M. W. Ward, pp. 137–62. Papers from the Second Demography Seminar, Port Moresby, 1970. *New Guinea Research Bulletin* 42.

Burbank, Victoria K., and James S. Chisholm
  1998   Adolescent Pregnancy and Parenthood in an Australian Aboriginal Community. In *Adolescence in Pacific Island Societies*. Edited by Gilbert Herdt and Stephen C. Leavitt, pp. 55–70. ASAO Monograph No. 16. Pittsburgh: University of Pittsburgh Press.

Butler, Judith
  1995   Excerpt from Introduction to *Bodies That Matter: On the Discursive Limits of "Sex."* In *The Gender/Sexuality Reader: Culture, History, Political Economy*. Edited by Roger N. Lancaster and Micaela di Leonardo, pp. 532–42. New York: Routledge.

Butt, Leslie, and Richard Eves, eds.
  2008   *Making Sense of AIDS: Culture, Sexuality, and Power in Melanesia*. Honolulu: University of Hawai'i Press.

Butt, Leslie, and Jenny Munro
  2007   Rebel Girls? Unplanned Pregnancy and Colonialism in Highlands Papua, Indonesia. *Culture, Health and Sexuality* 9(6):585–98.

Butt, Leslie, Gerdha Numbery, and Jake Morin
  2002   The Smokescreen of Culture. *Pacific Health Dialog* 9(2):283–89.

Byford, Julia
  1999   Dealing with Death Beginning with Birth: Women's Health and Childbirth on Misima Island, Papua New Guinea. PhD diss., Australian National University.

Caldwell, John C.
  2000   AIDS in Melanesia. Paper prepared for AusAID Special Seminar, *It's Everyone's Problem: HIV/AIDS and Development in Asia and the Pacific,* 22 November. Commonwealth of Australia.

Campbell, Catherine
2003   *"Letting Them Die": Why HIV/AIDS Prevention Programmes Fail.* International African Institute. Bloomington: Indiana University Press.

Campbell, Shirley F.
2002   *The Art of Kula.* Oxford: Berg.

Carovano, Kathryn
1991   More than Mothers and Whores: Redefining the AIDS Prevention Needs of Women. *International Journal of Health Services* 21(1):131–42.

Cassell, Joan, ed.
1987   *Children in the Field: Anthropological Experiences.* Philadelphia: Temple University Press.

Chambers, Robert
1983   *Rural Development: Putting the Last First.* London: Longman.

Chowning, Ann
1969   The Fertility of Melanesian Girls, Laboratory Mice, and Prostitutes: A Comment on the "Bruce Effect." *American Anthropologist* 71(6):1122–25.

Clark, Jeffrey, and Jenny Hughes
1995   A History of Sexuality and Gender in Tari. In *Papuan Borderlands: Huli, Duna, and Ipili Perspectives on the Papua New Guinea Highlands.* Edited by Aletta Biersack, pp. 315–40. Ann Arbor: University of Michigan Press.

Clatts, Michael
1995   Disembodied Acts: On the Perverse Use of Sexual Categories in the Study of High-Risk Behavior. In *Culture and Sexual Risk: Anthropological Perspectives on AIDS.* Edited by Han Ten Brummelhuis and Gilbert Herdt, pp. 241–56. Amsterdam: Gordon and Breach.

Clifford, James
1997   *Routes: Travel and Translation in the Late Twentieth Century.* Cambridge, MA: Harvard University Press.

Collins, Joseph, and Bill Rau
2000   *AIDS in the Context of Development.* Paper No. 4, Programme on Social Policy and Development. United Nations Research Institute on Social Development.

Connelly, Andrew James
2007   Counting Coconuts: Patrol Reports from the Trobriand Islands, Part I: 1907– 1934. MA thesis, California State University, Sacramento.

Corder, Mike
2005   AIDS is "Galloping" through PNG. Associated Press, 23 October.

Craddock, Susan
2000   Disease, Social Identity, and Risk: Rethinking the Geography of AIDS. *Transactions of the Institute of British Geographers,* New Series 25:153–68.
2004   Introduction. Beyond Epidemiology: Locating AIDS in Africa. In *HIV and AIDS in Africa: Beyond Epidemiology.* Edited by Ezekiel Kalipeni, Susan Craddock, Joseph R. Oppong, and Jayati Ghosh, pp. 1–10. Malden, MA: Blackwell.

Csordas, Thomas J.
1990   Embodiment as a Paradigm for Anthropology. *Ethos* 18(1):5–47.

Cullen, Trevor
2005   Press Coverage of HIV/AIDS in PNG: Is It Sufficient to Report Only the News? *Australian Studies in Journalism* 15:133–50.

2006   HIV/AIDS in Papua New Guinea: A Reality Check. *Pacific Journalism Review* 12(1):153–65.

Curtis, Tim
2002   Talking about Place: Identities, Histories and Powers among the Na'hai Speakers of Malakula (Vanuatu). PhD diss., Australian National University.

Damon, Frederick H.
1989   Introduction. In *Death Rituals and Life in the Societies of the Kula Ring*. Edited by Frederick H. Damon and Roy Wagner, pp. 3–19. DeKalb: Northern Illinois University Press.

Damon, Frederick H., and Roy Wagner, eds.
1989   *Death Rituals and Life in the Societies of the Kula Ring*. DeKalb: Northern Illinois University Press.

Danziger, Renee
1994   The Social Impact of HIV/AIDS in Developing Counties. *Social Science and Medicine* 39(7):905–17.

Dekuku, R. Chris, and Joseph Anang
2003   Attempts at Gaining Some Understanding of the Possible Factors that Promote HIV/AIDS Spread in Papua New Guinea. *Papua New Guinea Journal of Agriculture, Forestry and Fisheries* 46(1–2):31–39.

Delaney, Carole
1986   The Meaning of Paternity and the Virgin Birth Debate. *Man* 21(3):494–513.

Demian, Melissa
2000   Longing for Completion: Toward an Aesthetics of Work in Suau. *Oceania* 71(2):94–109.
2006   "Emptiness" and Complementarity in Suau Reproductive Strategies. In *Population, Reproduction and Fertility in Melanesia*. Edited by Stanley J. Ulijaszek, pp. 136–58. New York: Berghahn Books.

Denoon, Donald with Kathleen Dugan and Leslie Marshall
1989   *Public Health in Papua New Guinea: Medical Possibility and Social Constraint, 1884–1984*. Cambridge: Cambridge University Press.

Department of Planning and Monitoring
1999   *Papua New Guinea National Population Policy, 2000–2010*. Waigani, PNG: Population and Human Resources Branch, Department of Planning and Monitoring.

Dixon-Mueller, Ruth
1993   "Population Controllers" and the Feminist Critique. In *Population Policy and Women's Rights: Transforming Reproductive Choice*. Edited by Ruth Dixon-Mueller, pp. 31–53. Westport, CT: Praeger.

Douglas, Mary
1990   Risk as a Forensic Resource. *Daedalus* 199(4):1–16.

Dowsett, Gary W.
2003   Some Considerations on Sexuality and Gender in the Context of AIDS. *Reproductive Health Matters* 11(22):21–29.

Dundon, Alison
2007   Warrior Women, the Holy Spirit and HIV/AIDS in Rural Papua New Guinea. Special Issue, "HIV/AIDS in Rural Papua New Guinea," edited by Alison Dundon and Charles Wilde. *Oceania* 77(1):29–42.

Eime, Roderick
  2006   Seduced by Islands of Love. *Sunday Telegraph,* 12 March. www.news.com.au/
          seduced-by-islands-of-love/story-0-1111112115512, accessed 8 March 2012.

Elliot, Tirah, Russel Kitau, and Joachim Pantumari
  2006   Why Sexually Transmitted Infections Are High in Trobriand Islands. Paper
          presented at the Eighteenth Annual Australasian Society for HIV Medicine
          Conference, Melbourne, 11–14 October.

Enslin, Elizabeth
  1994   Beyond Writing: Feminist Practice and the Limitations of Ethnography. *Cultural
          Anthropology* 9(4):537–68.

Escobar, Arturo
  1991   Anthropology and the Development Encounter: The Making and Marketing of
          Development Anthropology. *American Ethnologist* 18(4):658–82.

Eves, Richard
  2003   AIDS and Apocalypticism: Interpretations of the Epidemic from Papua New
          Guinea. *Culture, Health and Sexuality* 5(3):249–64.

Eves, Richard, and Leslie Butt
  2008   Introduction. In *Making Sense of AIDS: Culture, Sexuality and Power in
          Melanesia.* Edited by Leslie Butt and Richard Eves, pp. 1–23. Honolulu:
          University of Hawai'i Press.

Fabian, Johannes
  1983   *Time and the Other: How Anthropology Makes Its Object.* New York: Columbia
          University Press.
  2001   *Anthropology with an Attitude: Critical Essays.* Stanford, CA: Stanford
          University Press.

Farmer, Paul
  1990   Sending Sickness: Sorcery, Politics, and Changing Concepts of AIDS in Rural
          Haiti. Theme Issue, "Culture and Behavior in the AIDS Epidemic," *Medical
          Anthropology Quarterly,* New Series 4(1):6–27.
  1992a   *AIDS and Accusation: Haiti and the Geography of Blame.* Berkeley: University of
          California Press.
  1992b   New Disorder, Old Dilemmas: AIDS and Anthropology in Haiti. In *The Time of
          AIDS: Social Analysis, Theory, and Method.* Edited by Gilbert Herdt and Shirley
          Lindenbaum, pp. 287–318. Newbury Park, CA: Sage.
  1994   AIDS-Talk and the Constitution of Cultural Models. *Social Science and Medicine*
          38(6):801–9.
  1997   AIDS and Anthropologists: Ten Years Later. *Medical Anthropology Quarterly*
          11:516–25.
  1999   *Infections and Inequalities: The Modern Plagues.* Berkeley: University of
          California Press.

Farmer, Paul, Margaret Conners, Kenneth Fox, and Jennifer Furin, eds.
  1996   Rereading Social Science. In *Women, Poverty, and AIDS: Sex, Drugs, and
          Structural Violence.* Edited by Paul Farmer, Margaret Conners, and Janie
          Simmons, pp. 147–205. Cambridge, MA: Partners in Health, Institute for
          Health and Social Justice.

Fishbein, Martin, and Icek Ajzen
  1975   *Belief, Attitude, Intention and Behavior: An Introduction to Theory and Research.*
          Reading, MA: Addison-Wesley.

Foster, George M.
    1976   Disease Etiologies in Non-Western Medical Systems. *American Anthropologist*
            78(4):773–82.

Foster, Robert J.
    2002   *Materializing the Nation: Commodities, Consumption, and Media in Papua New
            Guinea.* Bloomington: Indiana University Press.

Foster, Susan, ed.
    1996   *Corporealities: Dancing Knowledge, Culture and Power.* London: Routledge.

Frankel, Stephen, and Gilbert Lewis, eds.
    1989   *A Continuing Trial of Treatment: Medical Pluralism in Papua New Guinea.*
            Dordrecht, Netherlands: Kluwer Academic.

Franklin, Sarah
    1997   *Embodied Progress: A Cultural Account of Assisted Conception.* London: Routledge.

Friedl, Ernestine
    1994   Sex the Invisible. *American Anthropologist* 96(4):833–44.

Gammage, Bill
    2006   Sorcery in New Guinea, 1938 and 1988. *Journal of Pacific History* 41(1):87–96.

Garap, Sarah
    2000   Struggle of Women and Girls—Simbu Province, Papua New Guinea. In
            Reflections on Violence in Melanesia. Edited by Sinclair Dinnen and Allison Ley,
            pp. 159–71. Leichhardt, New South Wales: Hawkins Press.

Gerawa, Maureen
    2010   Cultural Norms Spreading HIV/AIDS. *Post Courier,* 19 April.

Gibbs, Philip, and Marie Mondu
    2010   *Sik Nogut o Nomol Sik: A Study into the Socio-cultural Factors Contributing
            to Sexual Health in the Southern Highlands and Simbu Provinces, Papua New
            Guinea.* Alexandria, New South Wales: Caritas Australia.

Gluck, Sherma Berger, and Daphne Patai, eds.
    1991   *Women's Words: The Feminist Practice of Oral History.* New York: Routledge.

Gordon, Deborah R.
    1988   Tenacious Assumptions in Western Medicine. In *Biomedicine Examined.* Edited
            by Margaret Lock and Deborah Gordon, pp. 19–56. London: Kluwer Academic.

Government of Papua New Guinea
    2004   *Medium Term Development Strategy, 2005–2010.* Waigani, PNG: Department of
            Planning and Development.
    2010   *National Health Plan 2011–2020,* Volume 2, Part A: Reference Data and National
            Health Profile, June 2010.

Government of Papua New Guinea and National AIDS Council
    2006   *PNG National Strategic Plan on HIV/AIDS, 2006–2010.* Waigani, PNG: National
            AIDS Council Secretariat.

Government of Papua New Guinea and United Nations Development Programme
    1998   *PNG National HIV/AIDS Medium Term Plan, 1998–2002.* Port Moresby,
            PNG: Government of Papua New Guinea and United Nations Development
            Programme.

Greenfield, Sidney
    1968   The Bruce Effect and Malinowski's Hypothesis on Mating and Fertility.
            American Anthropologist 70(4):759–61.

Gregory, Chris
　　1982　　*Gifts and Commodities*. London: Academic Press.

Gupta, Akhil, and James Ferguson
　　1992　　Beyond "Culture": Space, Identity and the Politics of Difference. *Cultural Anthropology* 7(1):6–23.
　　1997　　Discipline and Practice: "The Field" as Site, Method, and Location in Anthropology. In *Anthropological Locations: Boundaries and Grounds of a Field Science*. Edited by Akhil Gupta and James Ferguson, pp. 1–46. Berkeley: University of California Press.

Gupta, Geeta Rao
　　2000　　Gender, Sexuality, and HIV/AIDS: The What, the Why, and the How. Plenary address to the XIIIth International AIDS Conference, Durban, South Africa, 12 July. Washington, DC: International Center for Research on Women.

Hahn, Robert A.
　　1995　　*Sickness and Healing: An Anthropological Perspective*. New Haven, CT: Yale University Press.

Hahn, Robert A., and Marcia C. Inhorn
　　2009　　*Anthropology and Public Health: Bridging Differences in Culture and Society*. New York: Oxford University Press.

Haley, Nicole
　　2008　　When There's No Accessing Basic Health Care: Local Politics and HIV/AIDS at Lake Kopiago, Papua New Guinea. In *Making Sense of AIDS: Culture, Sexuality, and Power in Melanesia*. Edited by Leslie Butt and Richard Eves, pp. 24–40. Honolulu: University of Hawai'i Press.
　　2010　　Witchcraft, Torture and HIV. In *Civic Insecurity: Law, Order and HIV in Papua New Guinea*. Edited by Vicki Luker and Sinclair Dinnen, pp. 219–35. State, Society and Governance in Melanesia Program, Studies in State and Society in the Pacific, No. 6. Canberra: ANU E Press. epress.anu.edu.au/titles/state-society-and-governance-in-melanesia/civic_insecurity_citation/pdf-download, accessed 8 March 2012.

Hammar, Lawrence
　　1998a　　AIDS, STDs, and Sex Work in Papua New Guinea. In *Modern Papua New Guinea*. Edited by Laura Zimmer-Tamakoshi, pp. 257–96. Kirksville, MO: Thomas Jefferson University Press.
　　1998b　　Sex Industries and Sexual Networking in Papua New Guinea: Public Health Risks and Implications. *Pacific Health Dialog* 5(1):47–53.
　　2004　　Editorial. Sexual Health, Sexual Networking and AIDS in Papua New Guinea and West Papua. *Papua New Guinea Medical Journal* 47(1–2):1–12.
　　2007　　Epilogue: Homegrown in PNG—Rural Responses to HIV and AIDS. Special Issue, "HIV/AIDS in Rural Papua New Guinea," edited by Alison Dundon and Charles Wilde. *Oceania* 77(1):72–94.
　　2008　　Fear and Loathing in Papua New Guinea: Sexual Health in a Nation under Siege. In *Making Sense of AIDS: Culture, Sexuality, and Power in Melanesia*. Edited by Leslie Butt and Richard Eves, pp. 60–79. Honolulu: University of Hawai'i Press.
　　2010　　*Sin, Sex and Stigma: A Pacific Response to HIV and AIDS*. Anthropology Matters, Volume 4. London: Sean Kingston Publishing.

Haraway, Donna
　　1988　　Situated Knowledges: The Science Question in Feminism and the Privilege of the Partial Perspective. *Feminist Studies* 14(3):575–99.

Harding, Sandra, ed.
    1987   *Feminism and Methodology: Social Science Issues.* Bloomington: Indiana
            University Press.

Heise, Lori L., and Christopher Elias
    1995   Transforming AIDS Prevention to Meet Women's Needs: A Focus on
            Developing Countries. *Social Science and Medicine* 40(7):931–43.

Helliwell, Christine
    1995   Autonomy as Natural Equality: Inequality in "Egalitarian" Societies. *Journal of*
            the Royal Anthropological Institute 1(2):359–75.

Helman, Cecil G.
    1994   *Culture, Health and Illness: An Introduction for Health Professionals.* 3rd ed.
            Oxford: Butterworth-Heinemann.

Herdt, Gilbert
    1992   Introduction. In *The Time of AIDS: Social Analysis, Theory, and Method.* Edited
            by Gilbert Herdt and Shirley Lindenbaum, pp. 3–26. Newbury Park, CA: Sage.
    1997   Sexual Cultures and Population Movement: Implications for AIDS/STDs.
            In *Sexual Cultures and Migration in the Era of AIDS: Anthropological and*
            Demographic Perspectives. Edited by Gilbert Herdt, pp. 3–22. Oxford: Clarendon.
    1999   Clinical Ethnography and Sexual Culture. *Annual Review of Sex Research*
            10:100–19.
    2001   Stigma and the Ethnographic Study of HIV: Problems and Prospects. *AIDS*
            and Behavior 5(2):141–49.

Herdt, Gilbert H., ed.
    1984   *Ritualized Homosexuality in Melanesia.* Berkeley: University of California Press.
    1992   *Rituals of Manhood: Male Initiation in Papua New Guinea.* Berkeley: University
            of California Press.

Herdt, Gilbert, and Stephen C. Leavitt, eds.
    1998   Introduction: Studying Adolescence in Contemporary Pacific Island
            Communities. In *Adolescence in Pacific Island Societies.* Edited by Gilbert Herdt
            and Stephen C. Leavitt, pp. 3–26. ASAO Monograph No. 16. Pittsburgh:
            University of Pittsburgh Press.

Herdt, Gilbert, and Shirley Lindenbaum, eds.
    1992   *The Time of AIDS: Social Analysis, Theory, and Method.* Newbury Park, CA: Sage.

Herring, Ann, and Alan Swedlund, eds.
    2010   *Plagues and Epidemics: Infected Spaces Past and Present.* Wenner-Gren Foundation
            Monograph Series. Oxford: Berg.

Hirsch, Eric
    2002   Guest Editorial. Malinowski's Intellectual Property. *Anthropology Today*
            18(2):1–2.

Hirsch, Jennifer S., Holly Wardlow, Daniel Jordan Smith, Harriet M. Phinney,
Shanti Parikh, and Constance A. Nathanson
    2009   *The Secret: Love, Marriage, and HIV.* Nashville, TN: Vanderbilt University Press.

Hughes, Jenny
    1997   A History of Sexually Transmitted Diseases in Papua New Guinea. In *Sex,*
            Disease, and Society: A Comparative History of Sexually Transmitted Diseases and
            HIV/AIDS in Asia and the Pacific. Edited by Milton Lewis, Scott Bamber, and
            Michael Waugh, pp. 231–48. Westport, CT: Greenwood.

Human Rights Watch
    2005   *"Making Their Own Rules": Police Beatings, Rape, and Torture of Children in Papua New Guinea*. New York: Human Rights Watch.

Hutchins, Edwin
    1978   Reasoning in Discourse: An Analysis of Trobriand Land Litigation. PhD diss., University of California, San Diego.

Hutchinson, Janis F.
    2003   HIV and the Evolution of Infectious Diseases. In *Learning from HIV and AIDS*. Edited by George Ellison, Melissa Parker, and Catherine Campbell, pp. 32–58. Cambridge: Cambridge University Press.

Ingham, Roger, and Peter Aggleton
    2006   *Promoting Young People's Sexual Health: International Perspectives*. London: Routledge.

Ingstad, Benedicte
    1990   The Cultural Construction of AIDS and Its Consequences for Prevention in Botswana. Special Issue, "Culture and Behavior in the AIDS Epidemic," *Medical Anthropology Quarterly,* New Series 4(1):28–40.

Inter-Agency Task Team
    2009   Papua New Guinea Prevention of Parent to Child Transmission of HIV (PPTCT) and Paediatrics Review, March 9–16, Joint Mission Report and Recommendations, Version 3.

Jacobs-Huey, Lanita
    2002   The Natives are Gazing and Talking Back: Reviewing the Problematics of Positionality, Voice, and Accountability among "Native" Anthropologists. *American Anthropologist* 104(3):791–804.

Jenkins, Carol
    1993   Culture and Sexuality: Papua New Guinea and the Rest of the World. *Venereology* 6:55.
    1996a   Editorial. AIDS in Papua New Guinea. *Papua New Guinea Medical Journal* 39:164–65.
    1996b   The Homosexual Context of Heterosexual Practice in Papua New Guinea. In *Bisexualities and AIDS: International Perspectives*. Edited by Peter Aggleton, pp. 191–206. London: Taylor and Francis.
    1997   *Youth in Danger: AIDS and STDs among Young People in Papua New Guinea*. Port Moresby: Papua New Guinea Institute of Medical Research and United Nations Population Fund.
    2000   *Female Sex Worker HIV Prevention Projects: Lessons Learnt from Papua New Guinea, India and Bangladesh*. UNAIDS Case Study. Geneva: UNAIDS.
    2002   HIV/AIDS and Culture: Implications for Policy. Discussion paper for the World Bank. Washington, DC: World Bank.
    2004   Male Sexuality, Diversity and Culture: Implications for HIV Prevention and Care. Paper for UNAIDS. www.thailadyboyskatoeys.com/PDF-ladyboys-gay-lesbian-bisexual-transgender/1-Male-Sexual-Diversity.pdf, accessed 15 June 2012.
    2007   HIV/AIDS, Culture, and Sexuality in Papua New Guinea. In *Cultures and Contexts Matter: Understanding and Preventing HIV in the Pacific*. Edited by Carol Jenkins and Holly Buchanan-Aruwafu, pp. 5–69. Manila: Asia Development Bank. www.adb.org/documents/Books/Cultures-Contexts-Matter/Cultures-Contexts-Matter.pdf, accessed 8 March 2012.

Jenkins, Carol, and Megan Passey
    1998   Papua New Guinea. In *Sexually Transmitted Diseases in Asia and the Pacific*.

Edited by Tim Brown, Brian Mulhall, Rabin Sarda, and Doris Mugrditchian, pp. 231–52. Armidale, New South Wales: Venereology Publishing.

Jolly, Margaret
    1992   Banana Leaf Bundles and Skirts: A Pacific Penelope's Web? In *History and Tradition in Melanesian Anthropology.* Edited by James G. Carrier, pp. 38–63. Berkeley: University of California Press.
    1996   *Woman ikat raet long human raet o no?:* Women's Rights, Human Rights and Domestic Violence in Vanuatu. *Feminist Review* 52:169–90.
    2001a   Damming the Rivers of Milk? Fertility, Sexuality, and Modernity in Melanesia and Amazonia. In *Gender in Amazonia and Melanesia.* Edited by Thomas A. Gregor and Donald Tuzin, pp. 175–206. Berkeley: University of California Press.
    2001b   Infertile States: Person and Collectivity, Region and Nation in the Rhetoric of Pacific Population. In *Borders of Being: Citizenship, Fertility, and Sexuality in Asia and the Pacific.* Edited by Margaret Jolly and Kalpana Ram, pp. 262–306. Ann Arbor: University of Michigan Press.
    2002a   From Darkness to Light? Epidemiologies and Ethnographies of Motherhood in Vanuatu. In *Birthing in the Pacific: Beyond Tradition and Modernity?* Edited by Vicki Lukere and Margaret Jolly, pp. 148–77. Honolulu: University of Hawai'i Press.
    2002b   Introduction: Birthing beyond the Confinements of Tradition and Modernity? In *Birthing in the Pacific: Beyond Tradition and Modernity?* Edited by Vicki Lukere and Margaret Jolly, pp. 1–30. Honolulu: University of Hawai'i Press.
    2003   Epilogue. Special Issue, "Women's Groups and Everyday Modernity in Melanesia," edited by Bronwen Douglas. *Oceania* 74(1–2):134–47.
    2005   Beyond the Horizon? Nationalisms, Feminisms, and Globalization in the Pacific. *Ethnohistory* 52(1):137–66.

Jolly, Margaret, and Martha Macintyre
    1989   Introduction. In *Family and Gender in the Pacific: Domestic Contradictions and the Colonial Impact.* Edited by Margaret Jolly and Martha Macintyre, pp. 1–18. Cambridge: Cambridge University Press.

Jolly, Margaret, and Lenore Manderson
    1997   Introduction: Sites of Desire/Economies of Pleasure in Asia and the Pacific. In *Sites of Desire, Economies of Pleasure: Sexualities in Asia and the Pacific.* Edited by Lenore Manderson and Margaret Jolly, pp. 1–26. Chicago: University of Chicago Press.

Jolly, Margaret, and Kalpana Ram, eds.
    2001   *Borders of Being: Citizenship, Fertility, and Sexuality in Asia and the Pacific.* Ann Arbor: University of Michigan Press.

Jolly, Margaret, and Nicholas Thomas, eds.
    1992   Special Issue, "Politics of Tradition in the Pacific." *Oceania* 62(4).

Jolly, Margaret, Serge Tcherkézoff, and Darrell Tryon, eds.
    2009   *Oceanic Encounters: Exchange, Desire, Violence.* Canberra, Australia: ANU E Press. epress.anu.edu.au/oceanic_encounters_citation.html, accessed 7 January 2010.

Jorgensen, Dan
    1983   Introduction: The Facts of Life, Papua New Guinea Style. *Mankind* 14(1):1–12.

Josephides, Lisette
    1985   *The Production of Inequality: Gender and Exchange among the Kewa.* London: Tavistock.

Kalipeni, Ezekiel, Susan Craddock, Joseph R. Oppong, and Jayati Ghosh, eds.
    2004   *HIV and AIDS in Africa: Beyond Epidemiology.* Malden, MA: Blackwell.

Kalipeni, Ezekiel, Joseph Oppong, and Assata Zerai
    2007   HIV/AIDS, Gender, Agency and Empowerment Issues in Africa. *Social Science and Medicine* 64(5):1015–18.

Kanabus, Annabel, and Rob Noble
    2005   The ABC of HIV Prevention. AVERT. Electronic document, www.avert.org/abc-hiv.htm, accessed 15 July 2005.

Keck, Verena
    2007   Knowledge, Morality, and "Kastom": "*SikAIDS*" among Young Yupno People, Finisterre Range, Papua New Guinea. Special Issue, "HIV/AIDS in Rural Papua New Guinea," edited by Alison Dundon and Charles Wilde. *Oceania* 77(1):43–57.

Kelly, Angela, Andrew Frankland, Martha Kupul, Barbara Kepa, Brenda Cangah, Somu Nosi, Rebecca Emori, Lucy Walizopa, Agnes Mek, Lawrencia Pirpir, Frances Akuani, Rei Frank, Heather Worth, and Peter Siba
    2009   *The Art of Living: The Social Experience of Treatments for People Living with HIV in Papua New Guinea.* Goroka: PNG Institute of Medical Research.

Kelly, Angela, Heather Worth, Frances Akuani, Barbara Kepa, Martha Kupul, Lucy Walizopa, Rebecca Emori, Brenda Cangah, Agnes Mek, Somu Nosi, Lawrencia Pirpir, Kritoe Keleba, and Peter Siba
    2010   Gendered Talk about Sex, Sexual Relationships and HIV among Young People in Papua New Guinea. *Culture, Health and Sexuality* 12(3):221–32.

Ketobwau, Ignatius Towabu
    1994   Tuma—The Trobriand Heaven: A Study toward the Value of Traditional Trobriand Understanding of Tuma as Heaven. BA thesis, Rarongo Theological College, Rabaul, Papua New Guinea.

Kielmann, Karina
    1997   "Prostitution," "Risk," and "Responsibility": Paradigms of AIDS Prevention and Women's Identities in Thika, Kenya. In *The Anthropology of Infectious Disease: International Health Perspectives.* Edited by Marcia C. Inhorn and Peter J. Brown, pp. 375–411. Amsterdam: Gordon and Breach.

Kippax, Susan, and June Crawford
    1993   Flaws in the Theory of Reasoned Action. In *The Theory of Reasoned Action: Its Application to AIDS-Preventive Behavior.* Edited by Deborah J. Terry, Cynthia Gallois, and Malcolm McCamish, pp. 253–69. Oxford: Pergamon.

Knauft, Bruce M.
    1994   Foucault Meets South New Guinea: Knowledge, Power, Sexuality. *Ethos* 22(4):391–438.
    1997   Gender Identity, Political Economy and Modernity in Melanesia and Amazonia. *Journal of the Royal Anthropological Institute* 3(2):233–59.
    2003   What Ever Happened to Ritualized Homosexuality? Modern Sexual Subjects in Melanesia and Elsewhere. *Annual Review of Sex Research* 14:137–59.

Kuehling, Susanne
    2005   *Dobu: Ethics of Exchange on a Massim Island, Papua New Guinea.* Honolulu: University of Hawai'i Press.

Kulick, Don, and Margaret Willson, eds.
    1995   *Taboo: Sex, Identity, and Erotic Subjectivity in Anthropological Fieldwork.* London: Routlege.

Lather, Patti, and Chris Smithies
    1997   *Troubling the Angels: Women Living with HIV/AIDS.* Boulder, CO: Westview.

Law, Lisa
    2000   *Sex Work in Southeast Asia: The Place of Desire in a Time of AIDS*. London: Routledge.

Lawton, Ralph
    1993   *Topics in the Description of Kiriwina*. Pacific Linguistics Series D-84. Canberra: Department of Linguistics, Research School of Pacific Studies, Australian National University.

Leach, Edmund R.
    1967   Virgin Birth. Proceedings of the Royal Anthropological Institute, 1966, pp. 39–50.

Leach, Jerry W., and Edmund Leach, eds.
    1983   *The Kula: New Perspectives in Massim Exchange*. Cambridge: Cambridge University Press.

Lepani, Katherine
    2001   Negotiating "Open Space": The Importance of Cultural Context in HIV/AIDS Communication Models. A Qualitative Study of Gender, Sexuality, and Reproduction in the Trobriand Islands of Papua New Guinea. MPH thesis, University of Queensland, Brisbane, Australia.
    2004   Concept Paper on HIV/AIDS High Risk Settings Strategy, Focal Point Project Analysis. Goroka: Save the Children in Papua New Guinea.

Lepowsky, Maria
    1990   Sorcery and Penicillin: Treating Illness on a Papua New Guinea Island. *Social Science and Medicine* 30(10):1049–63.
    1993   *Fruit of the Motherland: Gender in an Egalitarian Society*. New York: Columbia University Press.

Lévi-Strauss, Claude
    1969 [1949]   *The Elementary Structures of Kinship*. Boston: Beacon.

Lewis, Gilbert
    1993   Double Standards of Treatment Evaluation. In *Knowledge, Power, and Practice: The Anthropology of Medicine and Everyday Life*. Edited by Shirley Lindenbaum and Margaret Lock, pp. 189–218. Berkeley: University of California Press.

Lewis, I., B. Maruia, D. Mills, and S. Walker
    2007   Final Report on Links between Violence against Women and Transmission of HIV in 4 Provinces of PNG. Canberra, Australia: University of Canberra.

Lindenbaum, Shirley
    1979   *Kuru Sorcery: Disease and Danger in the New Guinea Highlands*. Palo Alto, CA: Mayfield.
    1991   Review of *A Continuing Trial of Treatment: Medical Pluralism in Papua New Guinea,* edited by Stephen Frankel and Gilbert Lewis. *Medical Anthropology Quarterly,* New Series 5(2):175–77.
    2001   Kuru, Prions, and Human Affairs: Thinking about Epidemics. *Annual Review of Anthropology* 30:363–85.

Lock, Margaret
    1988   Introduction. In *Biomedicine Examined*. Edited by Margaret Lock and Deborah Gordon, pp. 3–10. London: Kluwer Academic.
    1993   Cultivating the Body: Anthropology and Epistemologies of Bodily Practice and Knowledge. *Annual Review of Anthropology* 22:133–55.

Loizos, Peter, and Patrick Heady
    1999   Introduction. In *Conceiving Persons: Ethnographies of Procreation, Fertility, and Growth*. Edited by Peter Loizos and Patrick Heady, pp. 1–17. London: Athlone.

Long, Lynellyn D., and E. Maxine Ankrah, eds.
1996   *Women's Experiences with HIV/AIDS: An International Perspective.* New York: Columbia University Press.

Luke, Nancy, and Kathleen M. Kurz
2002   Cross-Generational and Transactional Sexual Relations in Sub-Saharan Africa: Prevalence of Behavior and Implications for Negotiating Safer Sexual Practices. Paper prepared by ICRW in collaboration with PSI as part of the AIDSMark project, funded by Office of HIV/AIDS, Global Bureau, and Office of Sustainable Development, Africa Bureau, U.S. Agency for International Development, Population Services International, International Center for Research on Women.

Luker, Vicki
2002   Gender, Women and Mothers: HIV/AIDS in the Pacific. Working Paper No. 7, Gender Relations Center, Research School of Pacific and Asian Studies, Australian National University. rspas.anu.edu.au/grc/publications/pdfs/ LukereHIV.pdf, accessed 10 August 2007.
2004   Civil Society, Social Capital and the Churches: HIV/AIDS in Papua New Guinea. State, Society and Governance in Melanesia Project Working Paper 1/2004. ips.cap.anu.edu.au.virtual.anu.edu.au/ssgm/papers/working_papers/ LukerCivilSocietyFeb04.pdf, accessed 15 June 2012.

Luker, Vicki, and Sinclair Dinnen, eds.
2010   *Civic Insecurity: Law, Order and HIV in Papua New Guinea.* State, Society and Governance in Melanesia Program, Studies in State and Society in the Pacific, No. 6. Canberra, Australia: ANU E Press. epress.anu.edu.au/titles/state-society-and-governance-in-melanesia/civic_insecurity_citation/pdf-download, accessed 8 March 2012.

Lukere, Vicki, and Margaret Jolly, eds.
2002   *Birthing in the Pacific: Beyond Tradition and Modernity?* Honolulu: University of Hawai'i Press.

Lyttleton, Chris
2000   *Endangered Relations: Negotiating Sex and AIDS in Thailand.* Amsterdam: Harwood Academic.

MacCarthy, Michelle
2010   Judging "Culture": Contesting Views of the "Islands of Love." Paper presented at the American Anthropological Association Annual Conference, New Orleans, Louisiana, November 2010.

Macintyre, Martha
1987   Flying Witches and Leaping Warriors: Supernatural Origins of Power and Matrilineal Authority in Tubetube Society. In *Dealing with Inequality: Analysing Gender Relations in Melanesia and Beyond.* Edited by Marilyn Strathern, pp. 207–29. Cambridge: Cambridge University Press.
1998   The Persistence of Inequality: Women in Papua New Guinea since Independence. In *Modern Papua New Guinea.* Edited by Laura Zimmer-Tamakoshi, pp. 211–28. Kirksville, MO: Thomas Jefferson University Press.

Maclean, Neil
1994   Freedom or Autonomy: A Modern Melanesian Dilemma. *Man,* New Series 29(3):667–88.

Maddocks, Ian
1975   Medicine and Colonialism. *Australian and New Zealand Journal of Sociology* 11(3):27–33.

Malau, Clement, and Sue Crockett
    2000   HIV and Development the Papua New Guinea Way. *Development Bulletin*
            52:58–60.

Malinowski, Bronislaw
    1916   *Baloma:* Spirits of the Dead in the Trobriand Islands. *Journal of the Royal
            Anthropological Institute* 46:354–430.
    1922   *Argonauts of the Western Pacific.* London: Routledge.
    1929   *The Sexual Life of Savages in North-Western Melanesia: An Ethnographic Account
            of Courtship, Marriage and Family Life among the Natives of the Trobriand Islands,
            British New Guinea.* 3rd ed., 1932. London: Routledge and Kegan Paul.
    1932   Pigs, Papuans, and Police Court Perspective. *Man* 32:33–38.
    1934   Introduction. In *Law and Order in Polynesia.* By H. Ian Hogbin, pp. xxxi–lxxii.
            New York: Harcourt Brace.
    1939   The Group and the Individual in Functional Analysis. *American Journal of
            Sociology* 44(6):938–64.
    1953   *Sex and Repression in Savage Society.* 4th ed. London: Routledge and Kegan Paul.
    1974   Parenthood, the Basis of Social Structure. In *The Family: Its Structures and
            Functions.* 2nd ed. Edited by Rose Laub Coser, pp. 51–63. New York: St. Martin's
            Press.

Mallett, Shelley
    2003   *Conceiving Cultures: Reproducing People and Places on Nuakata, Papua New
            Guinea.* Ann Arbor: University of Michigan Press.

Manderson, Lenore, and Margaret Jolly, eds.
    1997   *Sites of Desire, Economies of Pleasure: Sexualities in Asia and the Pacific.* Chicago:
            University of Chicago Press.

Mane, Purnima, and Peter Aggleton
    2001   Gender and HIV/AIDS: What Do Men Have to Do with It? *Current Sociology*
            49(6):23–37.

Mann, Jonathan, and Daniel Tarantola
    1998   Responding to HIV/AIDS: A Historical Perspective. *Health and Human Rights*
            2(4):5–8.

Mannheim, Bruce, and Dennis Tedlock
    1995   Introduction. In *The Dialogic Emergence of Culture.* Edited by Dennis Tedlock
            and Bruce Mannheim, pp. 1–31. Urbana: University of Illinois Press.

Markowitz, Fran, and Michael Ashkenazi, eds.
    1999   *Sex, Sexuality, and the Anthropologist.* Urbana: University of Illinois Press.

McDowell, Nancy, ed.
    1988   *Reproductive Decision Making and the Value of Children in Rural Papua New
            Guinea.* Monograph 27. Waigani: Papua New Guinea Institute of Applied Social
            and Economic Research.

McPherson, Naomi M.
    2008   *SikAIDS:* Deconstructing the Awareness Campaign in Rural West New Britain,
            Papua New Guinea. In *Making Sense of AIDS: Culture, Sexuality, and Power
            in Melanesia.* Edited by Leslie Butt and Richard Eves, pp. 224–45. Honolulu:
            University of Hawaii Press.

Meigs, Anna, and Kathleen Barlow
    2002   Beyond the Taboo: Imagining Incest. *American Anthropologist* 104(1):38–49.

Merry, Sally Engle
    2011   Measuring the World: Indicators, Human Rights, and Global Governance.

Special Issue, "Corporate Lives: New Perspectives on the Social Life of the Corporate Form," edited by Damani J. Partridge, Marina Walker, and Rebecca Hardin. *Current Anthropology* 52(S3):S83–S95.

Milne Bay Tourism Bureau
2003   Milamala Festival, July 29th to August 1st, 2003. Brochure and daily program.

Montague, Susan
1971   Trobriand Kinship and the Virgin Birth Controversy. *Man* 6(3):353–68.

Moore, Henrietta L.
1994   *A Passion for Difference*. Bloomington: Indiana University Press.
1999   Anthropological Theory at the Turn of the Century. In *Anthropological Theory Today*. Edited by Henrietta L. Moore, pp. 1–23. Cambridge: Polity Press.

Moore, Susan, and Doreen Rosenthal
2006   *Sexuality in Adolescence: Current Trends*. New York: Routledge.

Mosko, Mark. S.
1983   Conception, De-conception and Social Structure in Bush Mekeo Culture. *Mankind* 14:24–32.
1995   Rethinking Trobriand Chieftainship. *Journal of the Royal Anthropological Institute,* New Series 1:763–85.
1998   On "Virgin Birth," Comparability, and Anthropological Method. *Current Anthropology* 39(5):685–87.
2000   Inalienable Ethnography: Keeping-while-Giving and the Trobriand Case. *Journal of the Royal Anthropological Institute,* New Series 6:377–96.
2002   Totem and Transaction: The Objectification of "Tradition" among North Mekeo. *Oceania:* 73(2):89–109.
2005   Sex, Procreation and Menstruation: North Mekeo and the Trobriands. In *A Polymath Anthropologist: Essays in Honour of Ann Chowning*. Edited by Claudia Gross, Harriet D. Lyons, and Dorothy A. Counts, pp. 55–61. Research in Anthropology and Linguistics Monograph No. 6. Aukland, New Zealand: Department of Anthropology, University of Auckland.

Nag, Moni, and J. Michael Bedford
1969   Promiscuity and Fertility: Comments on Greenfield's "The Bruce Effect and Malinowski's Hypothesis on Mating and Fertility." *American Anthropologist* 71(6):1119–22.

Narayan, Kirin
1993   How Native Is a "Native" Anthropologist? *American Anthropologist* 95(3):671–86.

Nash, Jill
1981   Sex, Money, and the Status of Women in Aboriginal South Bougainville. *American Ethnologist* 8(1):107–26.

National
2005   WWIII Ready to Invade PNG, 24 February.
2010   Editorial: Condoms Promote Promiscuity, 5 February.

National AIDS Council (NAC)
2006   *National Gender Policy and Plan on HIV and AIDS, 2006–2010*. Waigani, PNG: National AIDS Council.
2010a   *National HIV and AIDS Strategy 2011–2015*. Waigani, PNG: National AIDS Council.
2010b   *National HIV Prevention Strategy, 2011–2015*. Waigani, PNG: National AIDS Council.

National AIDS Council and National Department of Health
    2004   The Report of the 2004 National Consensus Workshop of Papua New Guinea.
              Waigani, PNG: National AIDS Council Secretariat and National Department of
              Health.
    2009   The 2008 STI, HIV and AIDS Annual Surveillance Report. Port Moresby, PNG:
              National Department of Health.

National AIDS Council and UNAIDS
    2006   Report on the First National HIV Prevention Summit. Port Moresby, PNG:
              UNAIDS.

National AIDS Council Secretariat (NACS)
    2002   Government Launches Second National HIV/AIDS Media Campaign to
              Promote Condom Use in PNG. Media Release, 12 September.
    2006   *Monitoring the Declaration of Commitment on HIV/AIDS, January 2004–*
              December 2005. Country Report to the United Nations General Assembly Special
              Session on HIV/AIDS.

National AIDS Council Secretariat and Partners
    2010   *2010 Country Progress Report Papua New Guinea.* United Nations General
              Assembly Special Session on HIV/AIDS.

National Department of Health (NDOH)
    2009   Ministerial Taskforce on Maternal Health Papua New Guinea Report. Waigani,
              PNG: NDOH.
    2010   Papua New Guinea HIV Prevalence: 2009 Estimates. Waigani, PNG: NDOH.

National Sex and Reproduction Research Team (NSRRT) and Carol Jenkins
    1994   *National Study of Sexual and Reproductive Knowledge and Behavior in Papua New*
              Guinea. Monograph No. 10. Goroka: PNG Institute of Medical Research.

National Statistical Office Papua New Guinea
    2003   *PNG National Census.* Waigani: National Statistical Office Papua New Guinea.
    2010   *Demographic and Health Survey 2006.* Waigani: National Statistical Office Papua
              New Guinea.

O'Keefe, Michael
    2011   Contextualising the AIDS Epidemic in the South Pacific: Orthodoxies,
              Estimates and Evidence. *Australian Journal of International Affairs* 65(2):185–202.

Ortner, Sherry B.
    1996   *Making Gender: The Politics and Erotics of Culture.* Boston: Beacon.

Overseas Development Institute
    2008   Gender and the MDGs. Briefing Paper 42. September 2008. www.odi.org.uk/
              resources/download/2386.pdf, accessed 7 July 2009.

Page, Helan E.
    1988   Dialogic Principles of Interactive Learning in the Ethnographic Relationship.
              Journal of Anthropological Research 44(2):163–81.

Parker, Richard
    1995   The Social and Cultural Construction of Sexual Risk, or How to Have (Sex)
              Research in an Epidemic. In *Culture and Sexual Risk: Anthropological Perspectives*
              on AIDS. Edited by Han Ten Brummelhuis and Gilbert Herdt, pp. 257–69.
              Amsterdam: Gordon and Breach.
    2001   Sexuality, Culture, and Power in HIV/AIDS Research. *Annual Review of*
              Anthropology 30:163–79.
    2009   Sexuality, Culture and Society: Shifting Paradigms in Sexuality Research.
              Culture, Health and Sexuality 11(3):251–66.

Parker, Richard, and Delia Easton
  1998   Sexuality, Culture, and Political Economy: Recent Developments in
            Anthropological and Cross-Cultural Sex Research. *Annual Review of Sex Research*
            9:1–19.

Parker, Richard, and Anke A. Ehrhardt
  2001   Through an Ethnographic Lens: Ethnographic Methods, Comparative Analysis,
            and HIV/AIDS Research. *AIDS and Behavior* 5(2):105–14.

Parker, Richard G., and John H. Gagnon, eds.
  1995   *Conceiving Sexuality: Approaches to Sex Research in a Postmodern World*. New York:
            Routledge.

Parikh, Shanti
  2005   From Auntie to Disco: The Bifurcation of Risk and Pleasure in Sex Education
            in Uganda. In *Sex in Development: Science, Sexuality, and Morality in Global
            Perspective*. Edited by Vincanne Adams and Stacy Leigh Pigg, pp. 125–58. Durham,
            NC: Duke University Press.

Parpart, Jane L., M. Patricia Connelly, and V. Eudine Barriteau, eds.
  2000   *Theoretical Perspectives on Gender and Development*. Ottawa: International
            Development Research Center.

Passey, Megan
  1996   Issues in the Management of Sexually Transmitted Diseases in Papua New
            Guinea. *Papua New Guinea Medical Journal* 39:252–60.

Patton, Cindy
  1990   What Science Knows: Formation of AIDS Knowledges. In *AIDS: Individual,
            Cultural and Policy Dimensions*. Edited by Peter Aggleton, Peter Davies, and
            Graham Hart, pp. 1–17. London: Falmer Press.
  1994   *Last Served? Gendering the HIV Pandemic*. London: Taylor and Francis.
  2002   *Globalizing AIDS*. Minneapolis: University of Minnesota Press.

Peirano, Mariza G. S.
  1998   When Anthropology Is at Home: The Different Contexts of a Single Discipline.
            Annual Review of Anthropology 27:105–28.

Pelto, Pertti J., and Gretel H. Pelto
  1997   Studying Knowledge, Culture, and Behavior in Applied Medical Anthropology.
            Medical Anthropology Quarterly 11(2):147–63.

Perez Hattori, Anne
  2004   *Colonial Dis-ease: U.S. Navy Health Policies and the Chamorros of Guam, 1898–1941*.
            Pacific Islands Monograph Series No. 19. Honolulu: University of Hawai'i Press.

Petersen, Alan
  1997   Risk, Governance and the New Public Health. In *Foucault, Health and Medicine*.
            Edited by Alan Petersen and Robin Bunton, pp. 189–206. London: Routledge.

Pigg, Stacy Leigh
  2001a   Expecting the Epidemic: A Social History of the Representation of Sexual Risk in
            Nepal. *Feminist Media Studies* 2(1):97–125.
  2001b   Languages of Sex and AIDS in Nepal: Notes on the Social Production of
            Commensurability. *Cultural Anthropology* 16(4):481–541.

Piot, Peter
  2008   AIDS: Exceptionalism Revisited. Lecture delivered at London School
            of Economics and Political Science, 15 May. data.unaids.org/pub/
            SpeechEXD/2008/20080526_pp_lse_lecture_en.pdf, accessed 15 October 2010.

Pirkle, Catherine M
    2009   Epidemiological Fallacies: Beyond Methodological Individualism. Working
                Paper. *The Fourth Wave: Violence, Gender, Culture and HIV in the Twenty-
                First Century.* Edited by Vinh-Kim Nguyen and Jennifer F. Klot. UNESCO
                and Social Science Research Council. blogs.ssrc.org/fourthwave/, accessed 10
                September 2010.

Poole, Fitz John P., and Gilbert H. Herdt, eds.
    1982   Sexual Antagonism, Gender, and Social Change in Papua New Guinea. *Social
                Analysis,* Special Issue 12.

Pöschl, Rupert, and Ulrike Pöschl
    1985   Childbirth on Kiriwina, Trobriand Islands, Milne Bay Province. *Papua New
                Guinea Medical Journal* 28:137–45.

Post Courier
    2005a   Leaderless War, 1 June.
    2005b   AIDS War into Top Gear, 24 February.
    2006   Government Hit over HIV Funding, 7 August.

Powell, H. A., R. M. W. Dixon, K. O. L. Burridge, E. Leach, and M. E. Spiro
    1968   Virgin Birth. *Man* 3(4):651–56.

Raimondo, Meredith, and Cindy Patton
    2001   Guest Editors' Introduction. *Feminist Media Studies* 2(1):5–18.

Reed, Adam
    1997   Contested Images and Common Strategies: Early Colonial Sexual Politics in
                the Massim. In *Sites of Desire, Economies of Pleasure: Sexualities in Asia and the
                Pacific.* Edited by Lenore Manderson and Margaret Jolly, pp. 48–71. Chicago:
                University of Chicago Press.

Reid, Elizabeth
    1994   *Approaching the Epidemic.* Issues paper No. 14. HIV and Development
                Programme. New York: United Nations Development Programme.
    1995   Introduction. In *HIV and AIDS: The Global Inter-connection.* Edited by
                Elizabeth Reid, pp. 1–12. West Hartford, CT: Kumarian Press.
    1996   Young Women: Silence, Susceptibility and the HIV Epidemic. *Pacific Health
                Dialog* 3(2):233–39.
    2004   Human Rights and HIV in Settings of Poverty: Putting People at the Heart of
                the Epidemic. *HIV Australia* 3(2):33–37.
    2009   *Interrogating a Statistic: HIV Prevalence in PNG.* Discussion Paper, 2009/1. State,
                Society and Governance in Melanesia Project, Research School of Pacific and
                Asian History. Canberra: Australian National University.
    2010   Putting Values into Practice in PNG: The Poro Sapot Project and Aid
                Effectiveness. *Pacific Currents* 1(2) and 2(1). intersections.anu.edu.au/
                pacificurrents/reid.htm, accessed 12 January 2011.

Rentoul, Alex C.
    1931   Physiological Paternity and the Trobrianders. *Man* 31:152–54.
    1932   Papuans, Professors, and Platitudes. *Man* 32:274–76.

Riessman, Catherine Kohler
    1993   *Narrative Analysis.* Newbury Park, CA: Sage.

Rival, Laura, Don Slater, and Daniel Miller
    1998   Sex and Sociality: Comparative Ethnography of Sexual Objectification. *Theory,
                Culture and Society* 15(3–4):295–321.

Robertson, Sarah
    2007   Research Interests. Discipline of Obstetrics and Gynaecology, University of
             Adelaide. health.adelaide.edu.au/og/people/robertsons.html, accessed 8 March
             2012.

Rodman, Margaret C.
    1992   Empowering Place: Multilocality and Multivocality. *American Anthropologist,*
             New Series 94(3):640–56.

Rudge, James W., Suparat Phuanakoonon, K. Henry Nema, Sandra Mounier-Jack, and
Richard Coker
    2010   Critical Interactions between Global Fund–Supported Programmes and Health
             Systems: A Case Study in Papua New Guinea. *Health Policy and Planning*
             25:148–152.

Salomon, Christine
    2002   Obligatory Maternity and Diminished Reproductive Autonomy in A'jië and
             Paicî Kanak Societies: A Female Perspective. In *Birthing in the Pacific: Beyond*
             Tradition and Modernity? Edited by Vicki Lukere and Margaret Jolly, pp. 79–99.
             Honolulu: University of Hawaii Press.

Savage, Angela
    1996   "Vectors" and "Protectors": Women and HIV/AIDS in the Lao People's
             Democratic Republic. In *Maternity and Reproductive Health in Asian Societies.*
             Edited by Pranee Liamputtong Rice and Lenore Manderson, pp. 277–99.
             Amsterdam: Harwood Academic.

Scheper-Hughes, Nancy, and Margaret Lock
    1987   The Mindful Body: A Prolegomenon to Future Work in Medical Anthropology.
             Medical Anthropology Quarterly, New Series 1(1):6–41.

Schneider, David
    1984   *A Critique of the Study of Kinship.* Ann Arbor: University of Michigan Press.

Schoepf, Brooke G.
    1992   Sex, Gender, and Society in Zaire. In *Sexual Behavior and Networking:*
             Anthropological and Socio-Cultural Studies on the Transmission of HIV. Edited by
             Tim Dyson, pp. 353–75. Liège, Belgium: Editions Derouaux Ordina.
    1995   Culture, Sex Research and AIDS Prevention in Africa. In *Culture and Sexual*
             Risk: Anthropological Perspectives on AIDS. Edited by Han Ten Brummelhuis and
             Gilbert Herdt, pp. 29–51. Amsterdam: Gordon and Breach.
    2001   International AIDS Research in Anthropology: Taking a Critical Perspective on
             the Crisis. *Annual Review of Anthropology* 30:335–61.
    2004   AIDS, History, and Struggles over Meaning. In *HIV and AIDS in Africa: Beyond*
             Epidemiology. Edited by Ezekiel Kalipeni, Susan Craddock, Joseph R. Oppong,
             and Jayati Ghosh, pp. 15–28. Malden, MA: Blackwell.

Secretariat of the Pacific Community
    2005   *The Pacific Regional Strategy on HIV/AIDS 2004–2008.* Noumea, New Caledonia:
             Secretariat of the Pacific Community.

Seidel, Gill, and Laurent Vidal
    1997   The Implications of "Medical," "Gender and Development" and "Culturist"
             Discourses for HIV/AIDS Policy in Africa. In *Anthropology of Policy: Critical*
             Perspectives on Governance and Power. Edited by Shore Cris and Susan Wright,
             pp. 59–87. London: Routledge.

Seligman, Charles. G.
    1910   *The Melanesians of British New Guinea.* Cambridge: Cambridge University Press.

Senft, Gunter
    1998a   Body and Mind in the Trobriand Islands. *Ethos* 26(1):73–104.
    1998b   "Noble Savages" and the "Islands of Love": Trobriand Islanders in "Popular
             Publications." In *Pacific Answers to Western Hegemony: Cultural Practices of
             Identity Construction*. Edited by Jürg Wassmann, pp. 119–40. Oxford: Berg.

Sepoe, Orovu. V.
    2000   *Changing Gender Relations in Papua New Guinea: The Role of Women's
             Organizations*. New Delhi, India: UBS Publishers' Distributors.

Setel, Philip W.
    1999   *A Plague of Paradoxes: AIDS, Culture and Demography in Northern Tanzania*.
             Chicago: University of Chicago Press.
    2009   Cultures of Measurement: Introductory Essay. Working paper. *The Fourth
             Wave: Violence, Gender, Culture and HIV in the Twenty-First Century*. Edited by
             Vinh-Kim Nguyen and Jennifer F. Klot. UNESCO and Social Science Research
             Council. blogs.ssrc.org/fourthwave/, accessed 10 September 2010.

Sider, Karen Blu
    1967   Kinship and Culture: Affinity and the Role of the Father in the Trobriands.
             Southwest Journal of Anthropology 23(1):90–109.

Singer, Merrill, and Scott Clair
    2003   Syndemics and Public Health: Reconceptualizing Disease in Bio-Social Context.
             Medical Anthropology Quarterly 17(4):423–41.

Skolbekkan, John-Arne
    1995   The Risk Epidemic in Medical Journals. *Social Science and Medicine*
             40(3):291–305.

Smith, Daniel Jordan
    2004   Premarital Sex, Procreation, and HIV Risk in Nigeria. *Studies in Family Planning*
             35(4):223–35.
    2009   Gender Inequality, Infidelity, and the Social Risks of Modern Marriage in
             Nigeria. In *The Secret: Love, Marriage, and HIV*. By Jennifer S. Hirsch, Holly
             Wardlow, Daniel Jordan Smith, Harriet M. Phinney, Shanti Parikh, and
             Constance A. Nathanson, pp. 84–107. Nashville, TN: Vanderbilt University
             Press.

Sobo, Elisa J.
    1993   Bodies, Kin, and Flow: Family Planning in Rural Jamaica. *Medical Anthropology
             Quarterly* 7(1):50–73.
    1995   *Choosing Unsafe Sex: AIDS Risk Denial among Disadvantaged Women*.
             Philadelphia: University of Pennsylvania Press.

Spencer, Margaret
    1999   *Public Health in Papua New Guinea, 1870–1039*. Brisbane: Australian Centre for
             International and Tropical Health and Nutrition, University of Queensland.

Spiro, Melford E.
    1968   Virgin Birth, Parthenogenesis and Physiological Paternity: An Essay in Cultural
             Interpretation. *Man* 3:242–61.

Squire, Corrine
    1993   Introduction. In *Women and AIDS: Psychological Perspectives*. Edited by Corrine
             Squire, pp. 1–15. London: Sage.

Stillwaggon, Eileen
    2003   Racial Metaphors: Interpreting Sex and AIDS in Africa. *Development and
             Change* 34(5):809–32.

2006   *AIDS and the Ecology of Poverty*. New York: Oxford University Press.

Strathern, Marilyn
    1981   Culture in a Net Bag: The Manufacture of a Subdiscipline in Anthropology. *Man,* New Series 16:665–88.
    1987   Conclusion. In *Dealing with Inequality: Analysing Gender Relations in Melanesia and Beyond*. Edited by Marilyn Strathern, pp. 278–302. Cambridge: Cambridge University Press.
    1988   *The Gender of the Gift: Problems with Women and Problems with Society in Melanesia*. Berkeley: University of California Press.
    1991   *Partial Connections*. Savage, MD: Rowman and Littlefield.
    1999   *Property, Substance and Effect: Anthropological Essays on Persons and Things*. London: Athlone Press.

Street, Alice
    2010   Belief as Relational Action: Christianity and Cultural Change in Papua New Guinea. *Journal of the Royal Anthropological Institute* 16:260–78.

Swidler, Ann
    2006   Syncretism and Subversion in AIDS Governance: How Locals Cope with Global Demands. *International Affairs* 82(2):269–84.

Swidler, Ann, and Susan Cotts Watkins
    2006   Ties of Dependence: AIDS and Transactional Sex in Rural Malawi. On-Line Working Paper Series. California Center for Population Research. University of California, Los Angeles. escholarship.org/uc/item/7jp02onm#page-8, accessed 15 June 2012.

Tambiah, Stanley J.
    1983   On Flying Witches and Flying Canoes: The Coding of Male and Female Values. In *The Kula: New Perspectives in Massim Exchange*. Edited by Jerry W. Leach and Edmund Leach, pp. 171–200. Cambridge: Cambridge University Press.

Tawfika, Linda, and Susan Cotts Watkins
    2007   Sex in Geneva, Sex in Lilongwe, and Sex in Balaka. *Social Science and Medicine* 64:1090–1101.

Taylor, Christopher
    1988   The Concept of Flow in Rwandan Popular Medicine. *Social Science and Medicine* 27:1343–48.

Tcherkézoff, Serge
    2004   *"First Contacts" in Polynesia: The Samoan Case (1722–1848). Western Misunderstandings about Divinity and Sexuality*. Canberra, Australia: Journal of Pacific History. Christchurch, New Zealand: Macmillan Brown Center for Pacific Studies.

Teaiwa, Katerina
    2002   Visualizing te Kainga, Dancing te Kainga: History and Culture between Rabi, Banaba and Beyond. PhD diss., Australian National University.

Tedlock, Barbara
    1991   From Participant Observation to the Observation of Participation: The Emergence of Narrative Ethnography. *Journal of Anthropological Research* 47:69–94.

Toft, Susan, ed.
    1985   *Domestic Violence in Papua New Guinea*. Law Reform Commission of Papua New Guinea Monograph No. 3. Port Moresby: Papua New Guinea Law Reform Commission.

Tolman, Deborah L., and Lisa M. Diamond
    2001   Desegregating Sexuality Research: Cultural and Biological Perspectives on Gender and Desire. *Annual Review of Sex Research* (12):33–73.

Treichler, Paula A.
    1999   *How to Have Theory in an Epidemic: Cultural Chronicles of AIDS*. Durham, NC: Duke University Press.

Trostle, James A.
    2005   *Epidemiology and Culture*. New York: Cambridge University Press.

Tuzin, Donald
    1980   *The Voices of the Tambaran: Truth and Illusion in Ilahita Arapesh Religion*. Berkeley: University of California Press.
    1991   Sex, Culture and the Anthropologist. *Social Science and Medicine* 33(8):867–74.

UNAIDS
    1999   *Facts about UNAIDS: An Overview*. Geneva: UNAIDS.
    2004   *Report on the Global HIV/AIDS Epidemic 2004*. Geneva: UNAIDS.
    2007   *UNAIDS' Terminology Guidelines*. Geneva: UNAIDS.
    2010   *Global Report: UNAIDS Report on the Global AIDS Epidemic 2010*. Geneva: UNAIDS.

UNAIDS and World Heath Organization
    2009   Global Facts and Figures. Geneva: UNAIDS and World Health Organization.

United Nations
    1996   *Time to Act*. Suva, Fiji: United Nations.

UN/USAID Review Team Mission
    2002   *Review of Papua New Guinea National HIV/AIDS Medium Term Plan, 1998–2002*. Port Moresby, Papua New Guinea: UN/USAID.

Valeri, Valerio
    1994   Buying Women but Not Selling Them: Gift and Commodity Exchange in Huaulu Alliance. *Man,* New Series 29(1):1–26.

Van Dokkum, André
    1997   Belief Systems about Virgin Birth: Structure and Mutual Comparability. *Current Anthropology* 38(1):99–104.

Vance, Carole S.
    1991   Anthropology Rediscovers Sexuality: A Theoretical Comment. *Social Science and Medicine* 33(8):875–84.

Vete, Steven
    1995   Sex and AIDS: Myths that Kill. *Pacific Health Dialog* 2(2):132–39.

Visweswaran, Kamala
    1994   *Fictions of Feminist Ethnography*. Minneapolis: University of Minnesota Press.

Waldby, Catherine
    1996   *AIDS and the Body Politic: Biomedicine and Sexual Difference*. London: Routledge.

Wardlow, Holly
    2002   Giving Birth to *Gonolia:* "Culture" and Sexually Transmitted Disease among the Huli of Papua New Guinea. *Medical Anthropology Quarterly* 16(2):151–75.
    2004   Anger, Economy, and Female Agency: Problematizing "Prostitution" and "Sex Work" among the Huli of Papua New Guinea. *Signs: Journal of Women in Culture and Society* 29(4):1017–40.

2006   *Wayward Women: Sexuality and Agency in a New Guinea Society*. Berkeley: University of California Press.

2008   "You Have to Understand: Some of Us Are Glad AIDS Has Arrived": Christianity and Condoms among the Huli, Papua New Guinea. In *Making Sense of AIDS: Culture, Sexuality, and Power in Melanesia*. Edited by Leslie Butt and Richard Eves, pp. 187–205. Honolulu: University of Hawaii Press.

2009   "Whip Him in the Head with a Stick!" Marriage, Male Infidelity, and Female Confrontation among the Huli. In *The Secret: Love, Marriage, and HIV*. By Jennifer S. Hirsch, Holly Wardlow, Daniel Jordan Smith, Harriet M. Phinney, Shanti Parikh, and Constance A. Nathanson, pp. 136–67. Nashville, TN: Vanderbilt University Press.

Waterston, Alisse
1997   Anthropological Research and the Politics of HIV Prevention: Towards a Critique of Policy and Priorities in the Age of AIDS. *Social Science and Medicine* 44(9):1381–91.

Weiner, Annette B.
1976   *Women of Value, Men of Renown: New Perspectives in Trobriand Exchange*. Austin: University of Texas Press.

1979   Trobriand Kinship from Another View: The Reproductive Power of Women and Men. *Man* 14(2):328–48.

1980a   Reproduction: A Replacement for Reciprocity. *American Ethnologist* 7:71–85.

1980b   Stability in Banana Leaves: Colonialism, Economics and Trobriand Women. In *Women and Colonization: Anthropological Perspectives*. Edited by Mona Etienne and Eleanor Leacock, pp. 270–93. New York: J. F. Bergin.

1983   From Words to Objects to Magic: Hard Words and the Boundaries of Social Interaction. *Man,* New Series 18(4):690–709.

1988   *The Trobrianders of Papua New Guinea*. New York: Holt, Rinehart and Winston.

1992   *Inalienable Possessions: The Paradox of Keeping-While-Giving*. Berkeley: University of California Press.

White, Geoffrey M., and Lamont Lindstrom, eds.
1993   Special Issue, "Custom Today in Oceania." *Anthropological Forum* 6:4.

Whiting, John W. M., Victoria K. Burbank, and Mitchell S. Ratner
1986   The Duration of Maidenhood across Cultures. In *School-Age Pregnancy and Parenthood: Biosocial Dimensions*. Edited by Jane B. Lancaster and Beatrix A. Hamburg, pp. 273–302. New York: Aldine De Gruyter.

Wilde, Charles
2007   "Turning Sex into a Game": Gogodala Men's Responses to the AIDS Epidemic and Condom Promotion in Rural Papua New Guinea. Special Issue, "HIV/AIDS in Rural Papua New Guinea," edited by Alison Dundon and Charles Wilde. *Oceania* 77(1):58–71.

Windybank, Susan, and Mike Manning
2003   Papua New Guinea on the Brink. *Issue Analysis* 30. St. Leonards, New South Wales: Center for Independent Studies.

Wolf, Diane L.
1996   Situating Feminist Dilemmas in Fieldwork. In *Feminist Dilemmas in Fieldwork*. Edited by Diane L. Wolf, pp. 1–55. Boulder, CO: Westview.

World Bank
2004   Control of HIV/AIDS in Papua New Guinea: Situation Assessment and Proposed Strategy. Unpublished report. World Bank Human Development Strategy Mission, June 2004.

World Health Organization

2003   *Guidelines for Implementing Collaborative TB and HIV Programme Activities.* Stop TB Partnership: Working Group on TB/HIV. Geneva: World Health Organization.

2007   *Global Tuberculosis Control: Surveillance, Planning, Financing.* Geneva: World Health Organization. WHO/HTM/TB/2007.376. www.who.int/tb/publications/ global_report/2007/pdf/full.pdf, accessed 10 August 2010.

Worthman, Carol M.

1998   Adolescence in the Pacific: A Biosocial View. In *Adolescence in Pacific Island Societies.* Edited by Gilbert Herdt and Stephen C. Leavitt, pp. 27–52. ASAO Monograph No. 16. Pittsburgh: University of Pittsburgh Press.

Yoder, Stanley P.

1997   Negotiating Relevance: Belief, Knowledge, and Practice in International Health Projects. *Medical Anthropology Quarterly* 11(2):131–46.

Young, Michael W.

1986   "The Worst Disease": The Cultural Definition of Hunger in Kalauna. In *Shared Wealth and Symbol: Food, Culture, and Society in Oceania and Southeast Asia.* Edited by Lenore Manderson, pp. 111–26. Cambridge: Cambridge University Press.

1989   Suffer the Children: Wesleyans in the D'Entrecasteaux. In *Family and Gender in the Pacific: Domestic Contradictions and the Colonial Impact.* Edited by Margaret Jolly and Martha Macintyre, pp. 108–34. Cambridge: Cambridge University Press.

2004   *Malinowski: Odyssey of an Anthropologist, 1884–1920.* New Haven, CT: Yale University Press.

Zatz, Noah D.

1997   Sex Work / Sex Act: Law, Labor, and Desire in Constructions of Prostitution. *Signs: Journal of Women in Culture and Society* 22(2):277–308.

Zimmer-Tamakoshi, Laura

1993   Nationalism and Sexuality in Papua New Guinea. *Pacific Studies* 16(4):61–97.

1997   "Wild Pigs and Dog Men": Rape and Domestic Violence as "Women's Issues" in Papua New Guinea. In *Gender in Cross-Cultural Perspective.* Edited by C. Brettell and C. Sargent, pp. 538–53. Englewood Cliffs, NJ: Prentice-Hall.

FILMOGRAPHY

In a Savage Land

1999   Produced and directed by Bill Bennett. Distributed by PolyGram Filmed Entertainment. 115 min. Color.

Trobriand Cricket: An Ingenious Response to Colonialism

1974   Produced and directed by Jerry W. Leach and Gary Kildea. Distributed by University of California Extension Media Center, Berkeley, CA. 54 min. Color.

Index

Page numbers in bold indicate illustrations.